Ultrasound Biomicroscopy of the Eye

Charles J. Pavlin
F. Stuart Foster

Ultrasound Biomicroscopy of the Eye

With 198 Illustrations and 24 Color Plates

Springer-Verlag
New York Berlin Heidelberg London Paris
Tokyo Hong Kong Barcelona Budapest

Charles J. Pavlin, MD
Department of Ophthalmology
Faculty of Medicine
University of Toronto
Toronto, Ontario M4X 1W3
Canada

F. Stuart Foster, PhD
Department of Medical Biophysics
University of Toronto
Toronto, Ontario M4N 3M5
Canada

Library of Congress Cataloging-in-Publication Data

Pavlin, Charles J.
Ultrasound biomicroscopy of the eye/Charles J. Pavlin, F. Stuart Foster.
p. cm.
Includes bibliographical references and index.
ISBN-13: 978-1-4612-7551-0 e-ISBN-13: 978-1-4612-2470-9
DOI: 10.1007/978-1-4612-2470-9
1. Ultrasonics in ophthalmology. 2. Ocular biomicroscopy.
I. Foster, F. Stuart. II. Title.
[DNLM: 1. Eye Diseases—ultrasonography. 2. Microscopy—methods.
WW 143 P338u 1994]
RE79.U4P38 1994
617.7'1543—dc20
DNLM/DLC
for Library of Congress 93-40948

Printed on acid-free paper.

Production coordinated by Publishing Network and managed by Ellen Seham; manufacturing supervised by Vincent Scelta.
Typeset by ATLIS Graphics, Mechanicsburg, PA.
Color separations and printing by New England Book Components, Inc., Hingham, MA.
Printed and bound by Edwards Brothers, Inc., Ann Arbor, MI.

9 8 7 6 5 4 3 2 1

For	Peggy, Michael, and Jessica Now we can clear the table and shoot some pool. CJP
and for	Diane, Danusha, and Brett With love. FSF

Preface

The history of the use of ultrasound in medicine has been one of evolution of technology and innovative methods of applying this technology to imaging body structures. Many scientists and clinicians have contributed to this evolution. Ophthalmic ultrasound has become an indispensible tool in ophthalmic practice, with its own instrumentation and techniques. Ultrasound frequencies used in ophthalmology have generally been higher than those used in general medicine because of a requirement for higher resolution and a lesser need for deep penetration. Most ophthalmic diagnostic equipment uses frequencies in the 10 MHz range. The use of ultrasound frequencies in the 50–100 MHz range is a relatively new development in ultrasound imaging of the eye. This technique has been developed in our laboratories over the past several years. We have progressed from the theoretical description of the basic science required, past the first in-vitro experiments in eye bank eyes, to the construction of an instrument capable of clinical application. We have gained broad clinical experience with this instrument in normal patients and patients with ocular disease. A commercial instrument based on our original clinical scanner has recently become available, allowing other clinicians to apply this tool to ophthalmic research and clinical practice.

We have applied the term ultrasound biomicroscopy to this new imaging technique because of similarities to optical biomicroscopy, i.e., the observation of living tissue at microscopic resolution. The abbreviation UBM is frequently used in our institution to refer to this process. The ability to observe subsurface ocular structures in their living state at microscopic resolution provides a new way of looking at ocular disease. In some ways it is like looking at living pathological specimens, albeit at low power. This process has provided new insight into many disease processes that we will discuss in this book.

Ultrasound biomicroscopy is a non-specific imaging technique that can be used for any ocular pathology which falls within its penetration limits. This book is meant as a guide for those using this new technology and a summary of the clinical information that has been gained. Because of the new nature of this technology, and the current scarcity of published information on clinical application from sources other than ourselves, this book has, by necessity, a personal tone. It is partially based on our published articles and chapters on the subject, but it also contains much new information not contained in these sources.

The first section of the book covers basic considerations including physics, instrumentation, and examination techniques. Examination techniques are very similiar to those that have evolved for conventional contact B-scan instrumentation, and anyone familiar with these techniques will have little difficulty adapting to ultrasound biomicroscopy. The second section of the book discusses specific ocular conditions in which ocular biomicroscopy has aided understanding of the disease process or been of value in clinical decision making. Glaucoma and anterior segment tumors currently are particularly well-established applications of ultrasound biomicroscopy. New findings related to the cornea, sclera, intraocular lenses, trauma, and adnexal pathology also are presented in this section. We have not attempted to provide a comprehensive bibliography related to every pathological condition that we present clinical information on, because our discussion of these conditions generally is confined to the new information that we have gained using our instrument. We have included a comprehensive bibliography on the physics and engineering aspects of this instrumentation.

We expect the future of this imaging modality to be one of continued technological innovation and development of new methods of applying this technology to research and clinical practice.

Charles J. Pavlin MD
F. Stuart Foster PhD

Acknowledgments

The development of ultrasound biomicroscopy has been a collaborative effort that has included tremendous contributions from many individuals. We are indebted to Michael Sherar, who nurtured the idea from the early beginnings to the first in vitro and in vivo images while persuing his PhD; and Kasia Harasiewicz, whose outstanding engineering and clinical skills moved the project forward rapidly. We also acknowledge the selfless efforts of Brian Starkoski, who designed all of the signal processing hardware; Shigong Ye, who made basic measurements of ocular tissue properties; and Karen Hahn, who managed the day-to-day clinical activities.

Without the generous contributions of the National Cancer Institute of Canada it is very unlikely that this new ophthalmic imaging technique would have been possible. Finally, and perhaps most importantly, we thank our wives and families for their patience, encouragement, and support during the course of this work.

Charles J. Pavlin, MD
F. Stuart Foster, PhD

Contents

Preface vii
Acknowledgments ix
Color plates following front matter

Part 1 Basic Considerations

1 Basic Physics of High-Frequency Ultrasound Imaging 3
The Acoustic Spectrum 3
Fundamental Properties of Acoustic Waves 5
Acoustical Properties of Ocular Tissues at High Frequencies 6
Principles of Pulse Echo (Backscatter) Imaging 11
Resolution and Penetration 13
Summary 14
References 15

2 Instrumentation for Ultrasound Biomicroscopy 17
Scanner Design 17
Transducers 17
Image Quality 23
Measurement Accuracy 23
Safety of High-Frequency Ultrasound 25
Future Development 27
References 28

3 Examination Techniques 30
Patient Preparation 30
Examination of the Eye 35
Use of the Commercial Scanner 41
Image Storage and Retrieval 44
Measurement Techniques 44
References 46

4 Ultrasound Biomicroscopic Anatomy of the Normal Eye and Adnexa 47

The Cornea 47
The Sclera 49
Anterior Chamber 50
The Angle 51
The Iris 52
The Ciliary Body and Posterior Chamber 55
The Peripheral Retina 60
Ocular Adnexa 60
References 60

Part 2 Ultrasound Biomicroscopy of Ocular Disease

5 Glaucoma 63
Angle Closure Glaucoma 63
Open Angle Glaucoma 88
Glaucoma Surgery 93
Summary 97
References 97

6 Anterior Segment Tumors 98
Iris Tumors 98
Ciliary Body Tumors 119
Cysts 123
Peripheral Choroidal Tumors 127
Lymphoma and Leukemia 136
Summary 139

7 Trauma 140
Angle Recession 140
Iridodialysis 140
Cyclodialysis 140
Hyphema 148
Vitreous Hemorrhage 148
Corneal Blood Staining 150
Foreign Bodies 152
Epithelial Downgrowth 153
Summary 154
References 154

8 Corneal Disease 155
Corneal Edema 155
Corneal Opacification and Underlying Changes 155
Conjunctival Flaps 160
Corneal Grafts 161
Corneal Dystrophies 163
Refractive Surgery 166
Summary 169
References 169

9 Scleral Disease 170
Localized Scleral Staphyloma 170
Episcleritis 170
Diffuse Scleritis 175
Nodular Scleritis 176
Necrotizing Scleritis 178
Summary 181
References 181

10 Intraocular Lenses 182
Anterior Chamber Lenses 182
Posterior Chamber Lenses 182
Intraocular Lens Complications 186
Summary 195
References 195

11 Conjunctival and Adnexal Disease 196
Conjunctival and Limbal Disease 196
Tumors in the Superotemporal Quadrant 202
Eyelid Disease 206
Summary 208
References 208

Index 209

Color Plates

A short history of ultrasound biomicroscopy

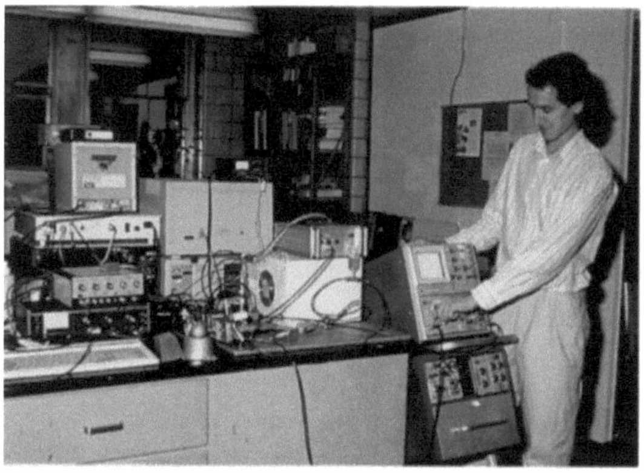

C1-1. Early instrumentation with Michael Sherar at the controls.

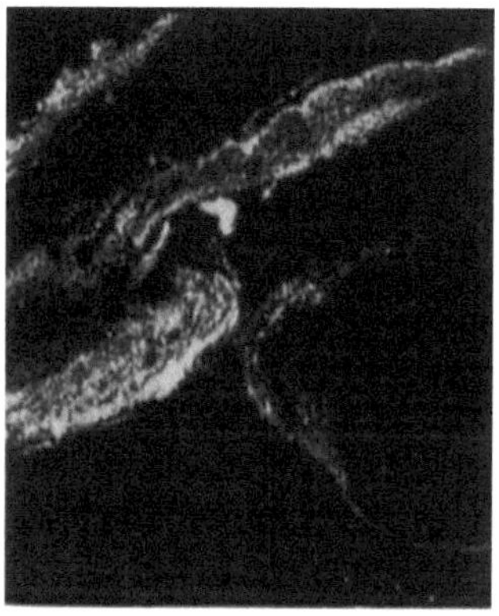

C1-2. The first ocular image produced in our laboratories. This image is a C-scan of a section of the angle and lens in an eye bank eye.

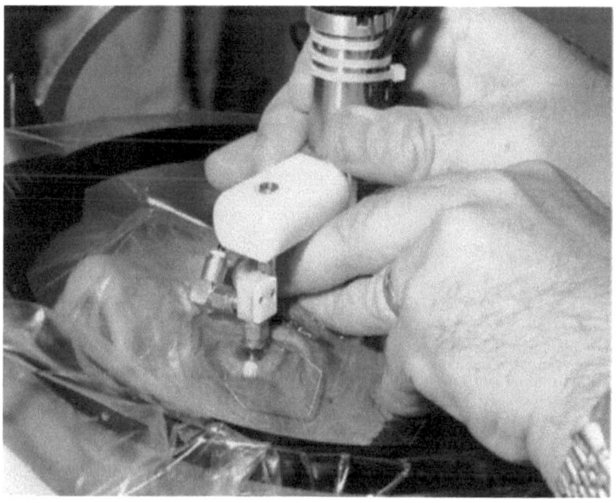

C1-3. The first B-scan probe being used to produce clinical images in a water bath.

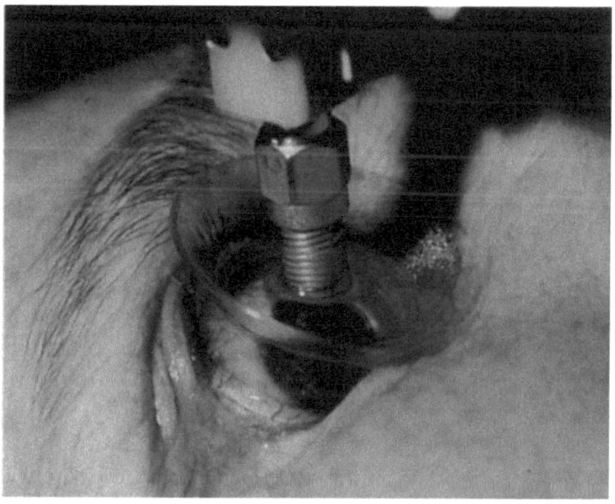

C1-4. The use of specially designed eye cups made patient setup easier.

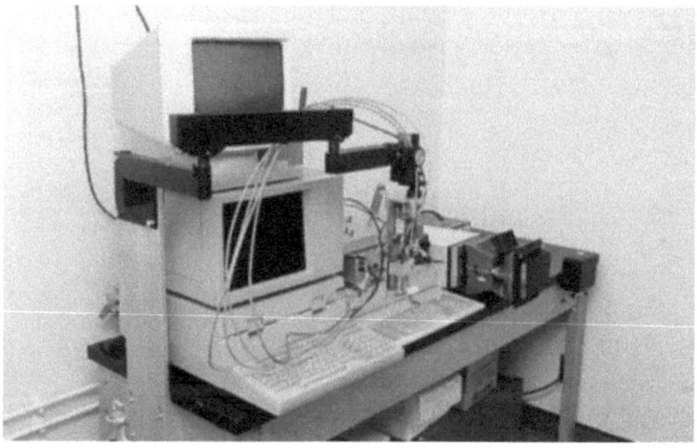

C1-5. The clinical instrument constructed in our laboratories that was used to make the majority of images in this book. An articulated arm supports the scanning head.

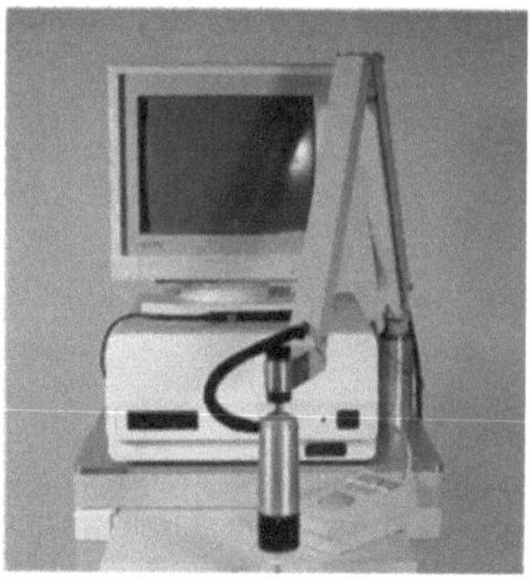

C1-6. The commercial version of our instrumentation.

Ultrasound biomicroscopy in glaucoma (see Chapter 5)

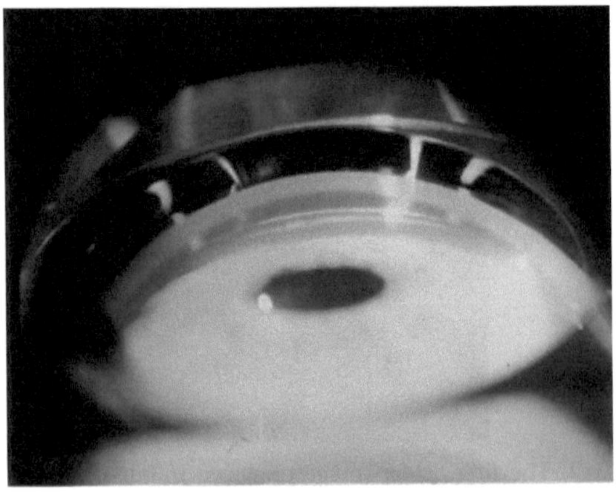

C2-1a. Gonioscopic view of a narrow angle.

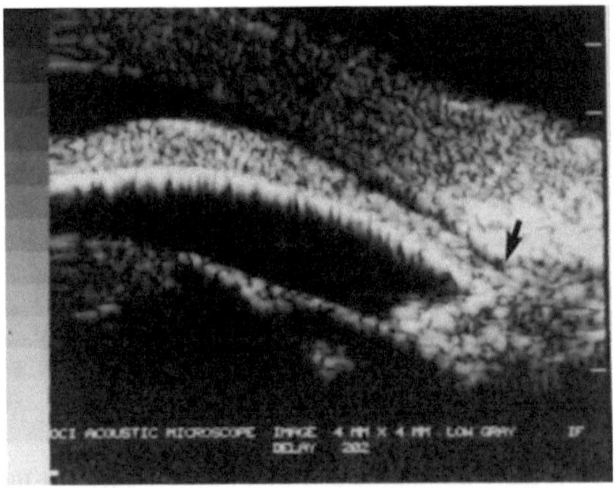

C2-1b. Ultrasound biomicroscopic image shows pupil block with anterior iris bowing. The entire angle can be visualized to the scleral spur (arrow). Image size is 4mm × 4mm.

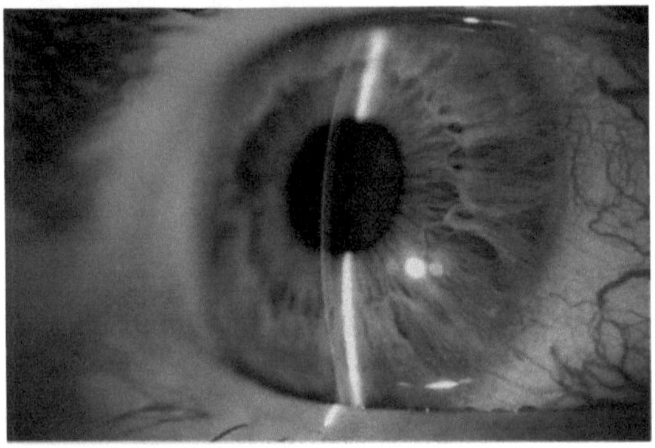

C2-2a. A patient presenting with a shallow anterior chamber.

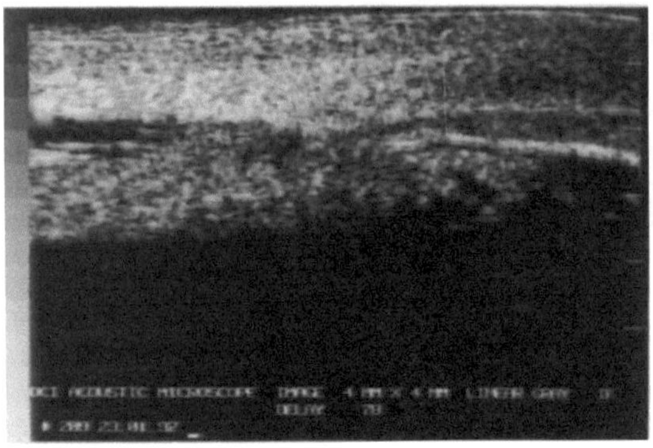

C2-2b. Ultrasound biomicroscopic image shows fluid present over the ciliary body and anterior rotation of ciliary processes closing the angle.

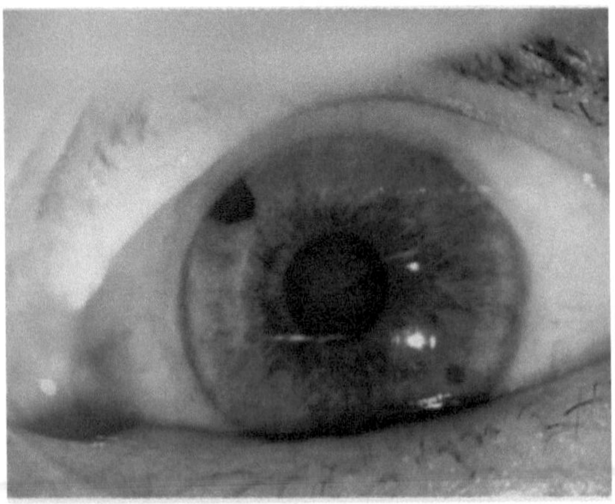

C2-3a. The first case of plateau iris syndrome described by Chandler in 1955. The angles are narrow in spite of patent iridectomies.

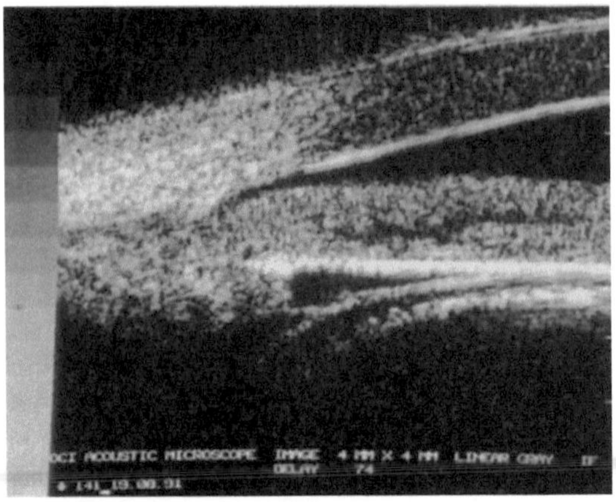

C2-3b. Ultrasound biomicroscopic image shows the anterior location of the ciliary processes supporting the peripheral iris.

Ultrasound biomicroscopy of anterior segment tumors (see Chapter 6)

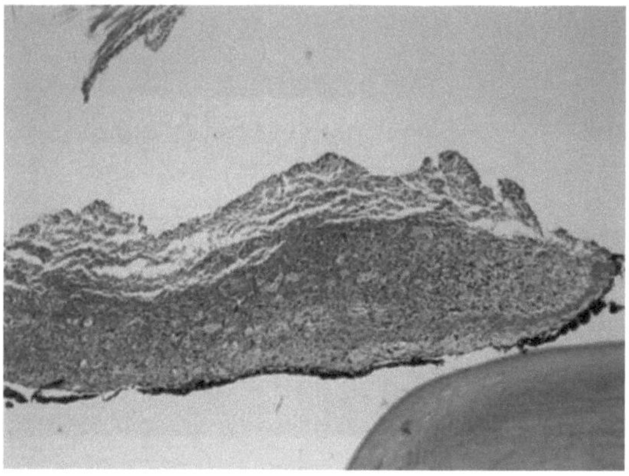

C3-1a. Histological section of an iris melanoma.

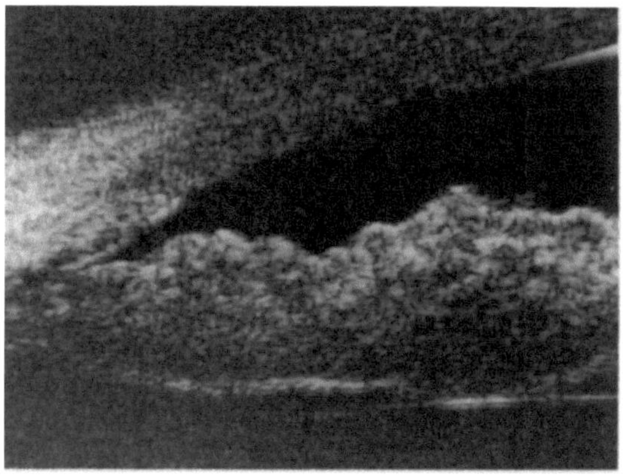

C3-1b. Ultrasound biomicroscopic image of iris melanoma in cross section. Note close correlation to histological section.

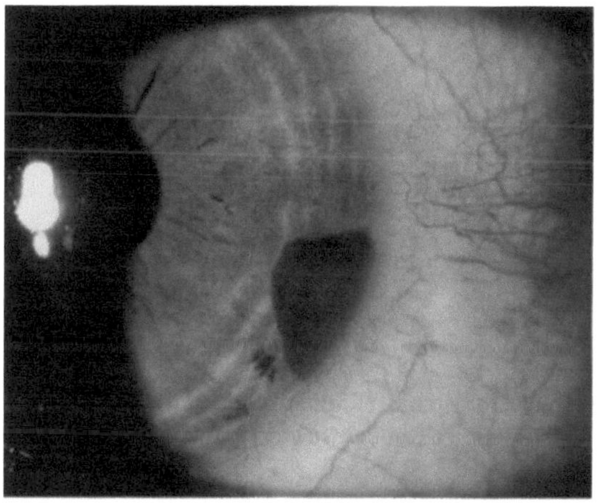

C3-2a. Peripheral iris nevus.

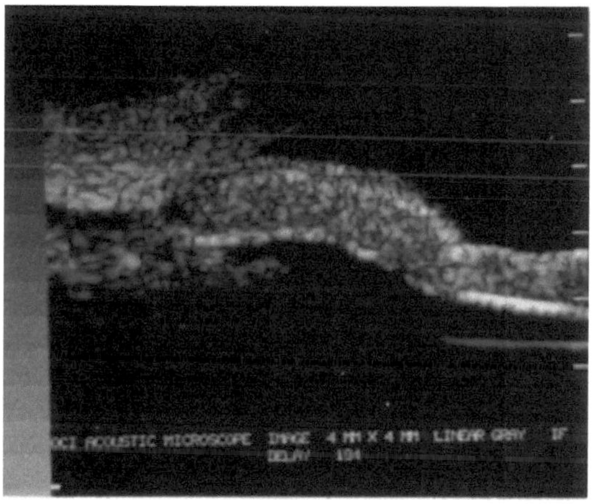

C3-2b. Ultrasound biomicroscopic image shows the bowed appearance typical of peripheral iris nevi. The ciliary body is not involved.

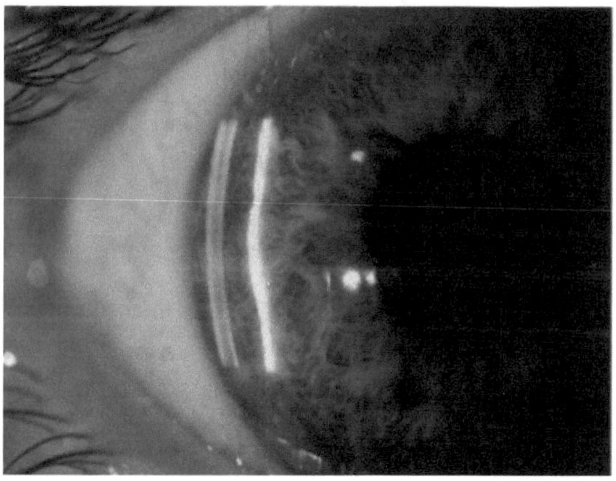

C3-3a. Irido-ciliary cysts appear clinically as localized iris elevations.

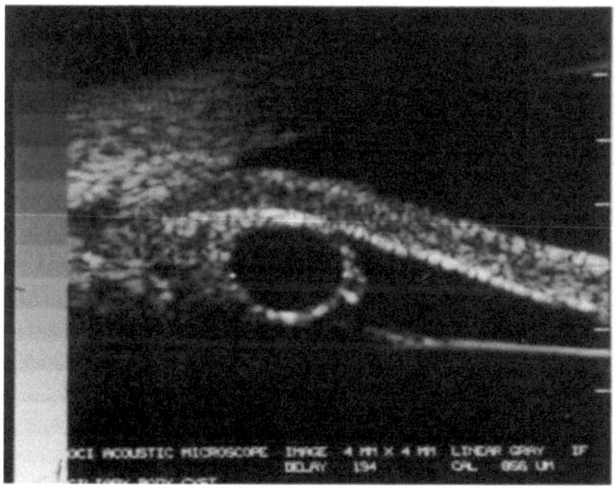

C3-3b. Ultrasound biomicroscopic appearance of an irido-ciliary cyst.

Ultrasound biomicroscopy in scleral disease (see Chapter 9)

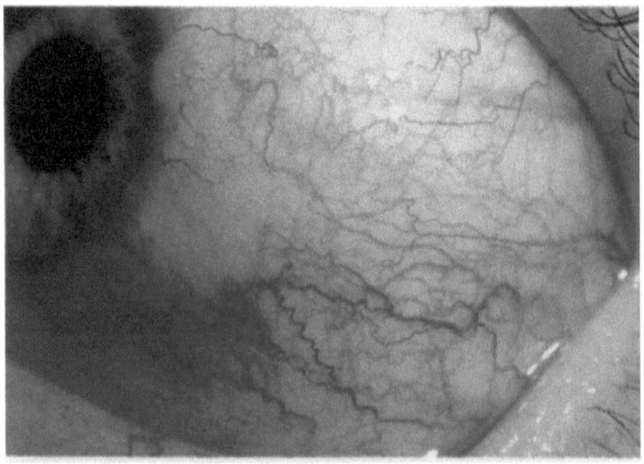

C4-1a. A patient with episcleritis.

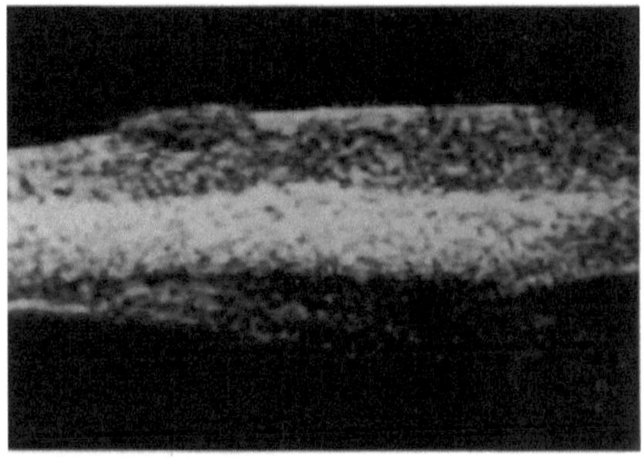

C4-1b. Ultrasound biomicroscopy shows episcleral thickening without scleral involvement.

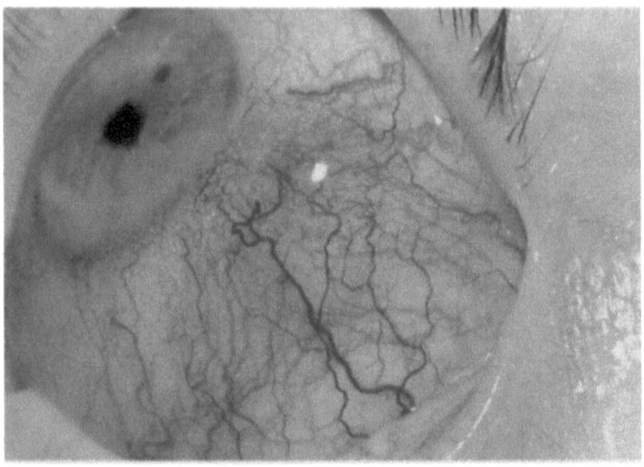

C4-2a. A patient with nodular scleritis.

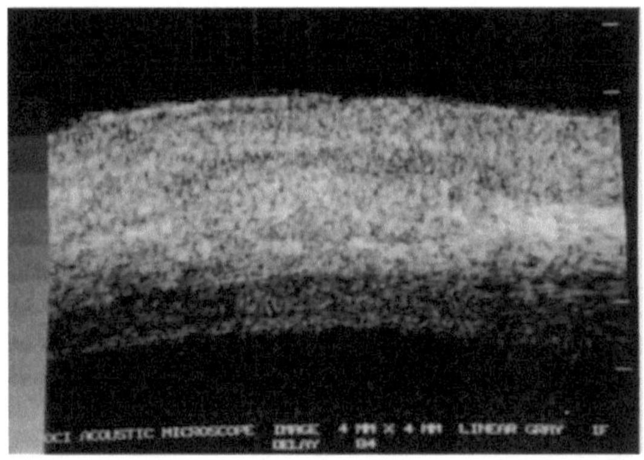

C4-2b. Ultrasound biomicroscopy shows a relatively weakly reflective nodule involving scleral tissue.

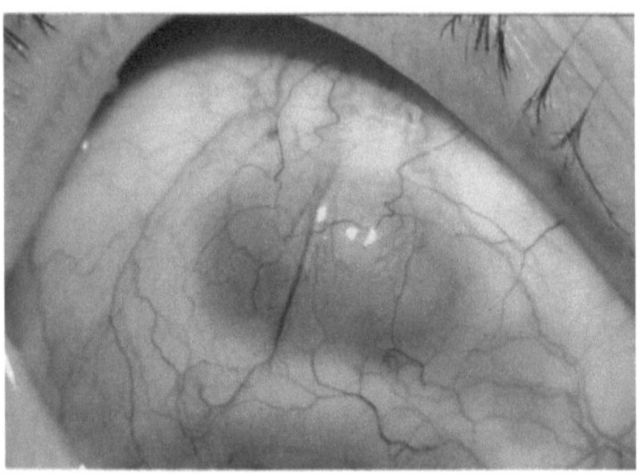

C4-3a. A patient with necrotizing scleritis.

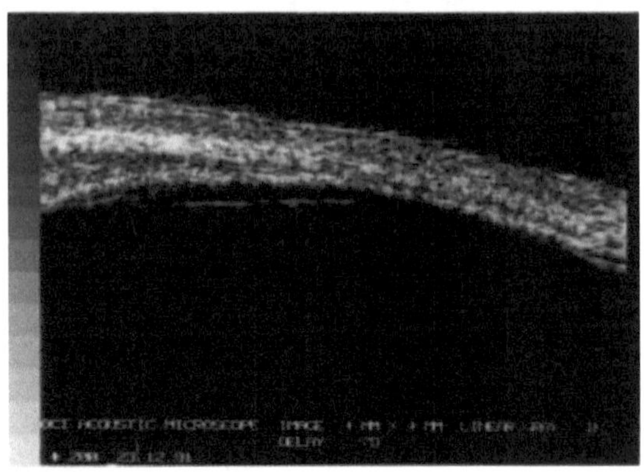

C4-3b. Ultrasound biomicroscopy shows thinned sclera in the affected region.

Part 1
Basic Considerations

1
Basic Physics of High-Frequency Ultrasound Imaging

The sensation of hearing represents a fundamental connection between ourselves and the world around us. As Lord Rayleigh stated in the introduction of his famous treatise, *The Theory of Sound* [1], "the sensation of sound is a thing *sui generis*, not comparable with any other of our senses." At the basic level sound and hearing, however, represent only a small window on the broad science of vibration. Our ability to appreciate and understand vibration is in turn tied to the physical and mathematical concepts of mechanics. In a sound wave, periodic variations in pressure cause the individual molecules of the medium in which the wave is propagating to oscillate about their equilibrium positions. The energy of the wave is transferred to neighboring molecules by means of the elastic properties of the medium, resulting in a wave that propagates at a characteristic speed called the speed of sound. In ideal liquids, gases, and to a large extent in tissues, these waves are compressional in nature; that is, the displacement of the molecules is along the longitudinal axis of propagation. Unlike other forms of propagating wave energy such as light and heat, sound is unique in that it requires a medium in which to propagate.

The Acoustic Spectrum

Mechanical waves and vibrations occur over a wide range of frequencies called the acoustic spectrum. This spectrum extends from the audible range (10 to 20,000 Hz), with which we are all familiar, to the range of phonons ($> 10^{12}$ Hz), which comprise the vibrational states of matter. A graphical interpretation of the acoustic spectrum is given in Figure 1.1, in which frequency is shown in powers of 10 on the horizontal axis from 10^0 to 10^{13} Hz. Sound occupies the range from 10 Hz to 20 KHz. We are all familiar with the fabulous wealth of information that we extract from verbal communication, music, and other sources of sound. It is not surprising, therefore, that frequencies greater than 20 KHz, the ultrasonic frequencies, have similar potential. In the frequency range from 20 to 100 KHz many animals use ultrasound to communicate and navigate and to track their prey. Bats, for instance, perform unbelievably sophisticated processing in a fraction of a second to locate insects equal to or less than the wavelengths of ultrasound used to detect them. This frequency range is also used in a number of commercial applications such as sonicators, ultrasonic cleaners, and range finders for instruments such as cameras.

From 100 KHz (10^5 Hz) to 1 MHz (10^6 Hz), ultrasound has numerous applications. Perhaps the most important of these is SONAR (sound navigation and ranging), which is the human imitation of the echolocation methods of many animals. A patent for this idea was granted to Paul Langevin in 1917 [2]. It is unlikely that he could even have dreamed of how successful this approach would be in its intended application, or that it would become the basis of a powerful diagnostic imaging method that would be used to study over 100 million patients per year in 1992. The medical applications occupy only a tiny sliver of the spectrum between 1 and 10 MHz. Even in this range the choice of frequency is closely tied to the intended application. For example, frequencies between 3.5 and 5

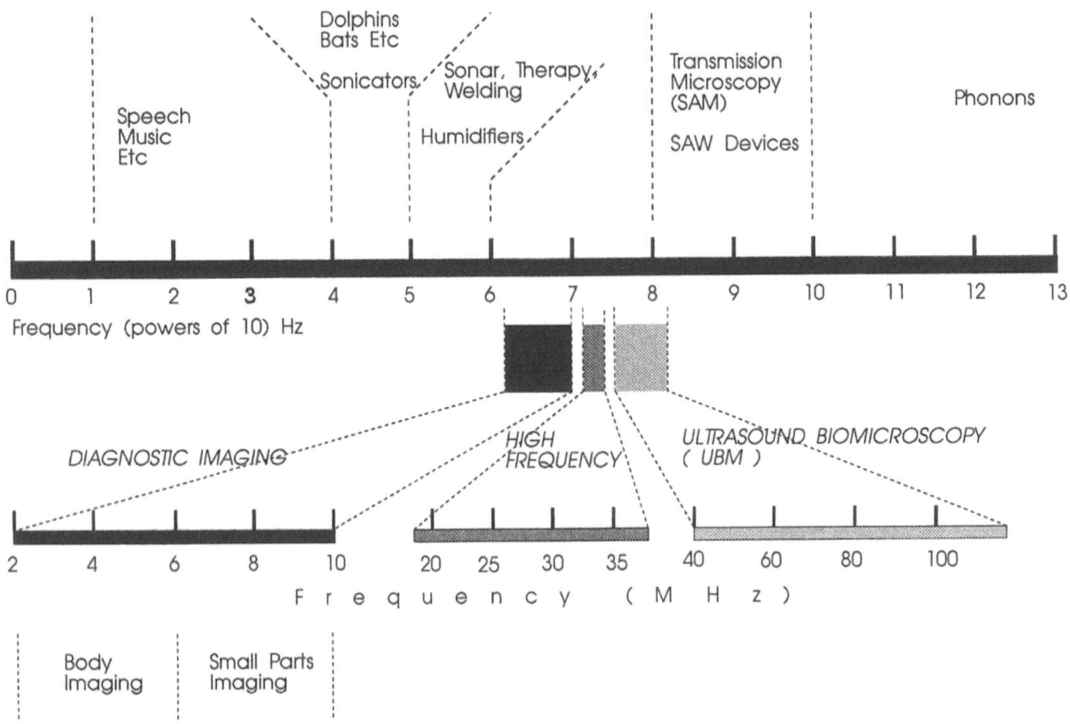

FIGURE 1.1. The acoustic spectrum. Diagnostic applications are clustered in the 1–10 MHz range, whereas ultrasound biomicroscopy applications occur in the range from approximately 40 to 100 MHz.

MHz are used in body imaging applications where significant penetration of the tissues is needed. These frequencies have the ability to penetrate the tissues to a depth of 15 to 20 cm and still return signals of sufficient strength to form an image. As the frequency increases, the ultrasound is more strongly attenuated, reducing penetration. Higher frequencies (7 to 10 MHz) can be used in small parts imaging such as visualization of the eye, where penetration of 4 to 5 cm is sufficient. The exact relationship between resolution and wavelength will be considered in more detail later in this chapter.

Although the vast majority of clinical ultrasound imaging is performed between 1 and 10 MHz, new applications are beginning to emerge in the high-frequency range between 10 and 40 MHz. These include systems designed to image the skin [3–5], the gastrointestinal tract [6–8], and intravascular imaging of blood vessels [9–12]. The commercial systems for skin and intravascular applications in the 20 to 30 MHz range have transverse resolution ranging from approximately 200 to 500 μm and are still considered experimental.

The development of transducers for very-high-frequency ultrasound imaging began in our laboratory in 1979 with the development of transducers based on the polymer polyvinylidene difluoride [13]. These transducers had the advantage of being well matched to the body and were sensitive over a very broad range of frequencies. By 1984 13 MHz polymer devices were being used to map the acoustical properties of human tissues [14], and experimental devices with center frequencies as high as 100 MHz were tested. The continued development of these probes culminated in the publication of a paper in *Nature* by Sherar et al. [15] in 1987, which showed the enormous potential of ultrasound imaging of tissue in the frequency range from 40 to 100 MHz. This system demonstrated microscopic (15 μm) subsurface resolution in living tissue and showed information that was unobtainable using any other noninvasive approach. The success of this technique rapidly led to the development of the first real time B-scan imaging systems for microscopic imaging by Sherar, Starkoski, Taylor, and Foster in Toronto [16]. This system was refined for ocular imaging in collaboration with Dr. Pavlin, resulting in the technology that is the subject of this book. We have used the term *ultrasound biomicroscopy* (UBM) to distinguish these imaging systems from conventional ultrasound B-scan imaging approaches and scanning acoustic microscopy (SAM), which is basically a transmission imaging method. Given the reduced penetration of high-frequency ultrasound, the eye was an ideal clinical application for ultrasound biomicroscopy. Before we present some of these early results it is useful for the reader to gain an understanding of the basic physics of ultrasound in general and high-frequency ultrasound in particular. In the following sections the interactions of acoustic waves with ocular tissue including attenuation, speed of sound, and reflectivity are examined. These studies lead to an appreciation of the critical factors affecting the design of high-frequency transducers and imaging equipment. The effects of these factors on imaging performance such as resolution and penetration are discussed.

The acoustic spectrum above 100 MHz also has diverse and interesting applications. For example, surface acoustic wave (SAW) devices operating up to hundreds of MHz are essential components in a wide variety of signal processing and communications instruments. By using frequencies up to several gigahertz (GHz or 10^9 Hz), transmission scanning acoustic microscopes have been developed that provide submicron resolution on thin sections of tissue in vitro; however, this approach is not suitable for in vivo applications. It is also important to note that all of the frequencies between 1 MHz and 1 GHz are used extensively in nondestructive evaluation applications for nonbiological materials.

Fundamental Properties of Acoustic Waves

If we take a snapshot of a propagating compressional sound wave it might look like the drawings of Figure 1.2. Here the propagation direction is along the horizontal axis and the relative positions of the molecules are indicated by the small circles in Figure 1.2a. In the regions of high pressure the molecules are tightly packed, whereas in the regions of low pressure (rarefaction) the molecules are widely separated. By encoding the wave as shades of gray it is easy to appreciate the fact that the crests or peaks of the pressure wave are separated by a characteristic distance called the wavelength, λ. Mathematically the pressure wave of Figure 1.2 can be represented as:

$$p(z) = \sin\left(\frac{2\pi}{\lambda} z\right) = \sin(kz) \tag{1.1}$$

where $k = 2\pi/\lambda$ is called the wave number and z is the direction of propagation. A plot of Eq. (1.1) reveals that it is a simple sine wave with wavelength

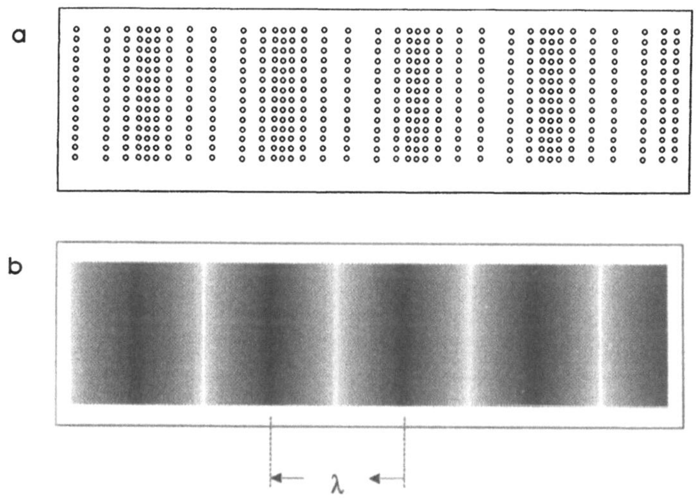

FIGURE 1.2. **(a)** Molecules of the propagation medium, and **(b)** pressure distribution for a planar continuous compressional wave with wavelength λ.

λ, as shown in Figure 1.3a. However, because we have taken a "snapshot" of the wave we have essentially frozen time and have not considered its role. To examine the time dependence of the pressure wave it is convenient to fix our position in space, for example at the dashed line in Figure 1.3a, and ask how the pressure varies at that point with time. Again a sinusoidal variation is observed, as shown in Figure 1.3b and described by the equation:

$$p(t) = \sin\left(\frac{2\pi}{T}t\right) = \sin(2\pi ft) \quad (1.2)$$

where T is the period of the wave (time between pressure peaks), f is the frequency (the inverse of the period), and t is time. By combining Eqs. (1.1) and (1.2) an expression for the time and spatial dependence of the pressure wave is derived:

$$p(z,t) = \sin(2\pi ft - kz) \quad (1.3)$$

where the negative sign reflects the fact that the wave is propagating in the positive z direction. Further consideration of the physics of the wave allows us to determine the important relationships between the speed of sound, the frequency, and the wavelength. These are:

$$\lambda = cf \qquad f = \frac{\lambda}{c} \qquad c = \frac{\lambda}{f} \quad (1.4)$$

Thus, the wavelength of ultrasound is linearly proportional to both frequency and speed of sound. For example, assuming a speed of sound of 1500 m/s, the wavelength of ultrasound at 5 MHz is 300 μm, whereas at 100 MHz the wavelength is 15 μm. As we will see later, wavelength is the critical factor in determining image resolution.

Acoustical Properties of Ocular Tissues at High Frequencies

Tissues possess three important properties that are of fundamental importance in ultrasound imaging: attenuation, reflectivity, and speed of sound. Attenuation processes consist of any interaction that removes energy from the beam. In general, attenuation processes can be divided into two forms, absorption and reflectivity, as illustrated schematically in Figure 1.4. Energy that is absorbed is converted to heat, whereas reflectivity, perhaps the most important acoustical property of tissue from the imaging point of view, can be further subdivided into specular and scatter components. At the larger tissue interfaces, specular reflections take place. The strength of these signals depends on the characteristic acoustic properties of the tissues forming the interface and the angle of the interfaces with respect to the transducer. At small tissue structures, ultrasound is scattered over a wide range of angles. The strength of the scattered ultrasound depends on the size, acoustical impedance, and number density of the scattering structures. Of

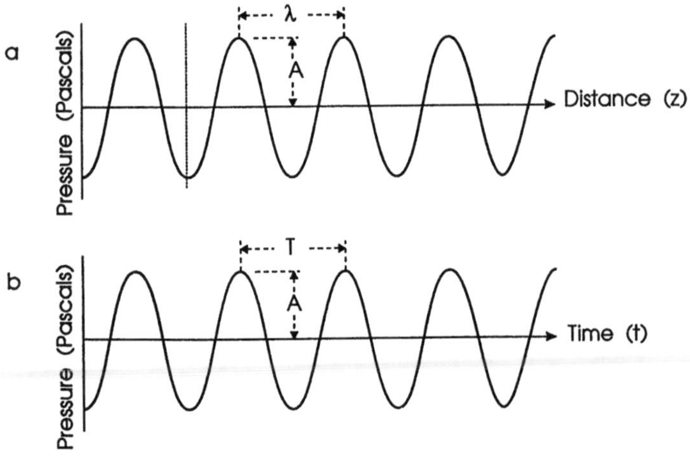

FIGURE 1.3. **(a)** Spatial distribution of pressure at constant time [Eq (1.1)] and **(b)** temporal distribution of pressure at constant position.

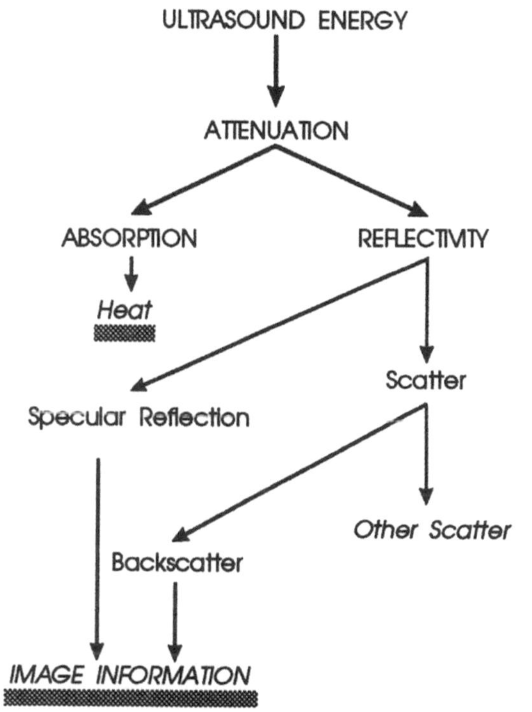

FIGURE 1.4. Schematic diagram showing the interactions of ultrasound with tissue. Loss of energy in the ultrasound beam is due to absorption and reflectivity processes. Of the reflectivity processes only backscatter and near normal incidence specular reflection are eventually converted into image information.

the reflected ultrasound, only a small fraction will be ultimately detected and converted into image information.

The accuracy of distance measurements in ultrasound images is determined by our knowledge of the speed of sound in tissues. Fortunately, this parameter only varies by a few percent for most soft tissues. Studies of the ultrasonic properties of eye tissues have usually emphasized estimation of the sound velocity, which is very important in various biometry techniques. Early in the 1950s, the speeds of sound of some liquidlike ocular tissues were measured with an ultrasound interferometer [17]. Since 1960 many investigators have measured the speed of sound in vivo and in vitro with different methods [18–21]. In spite of this effort, there is still debate over the correct speeds of sound for ocular tissues. This is particularly true for the cornea, where values range from 1550 m/s [22] to 1650 m/s [20]. Efforts to extract tissue parameters such as scatter number density and scatter size have been undertaken by Fellepa, Lizzi, and coworkers [23,24], who have analyzed calibrated backscattered radiofrequency spectra from ocular tissue. Encouraging success in differentiating ocular masses using this approach has been reported [23,24]. At present there is little literature concerning the quantitative measurement of either attenuation coefficients or backscatter. It is also important to note that all of the above measurements have been made at frequencies below 20 MHz. We have recently reported on the ultrasonic properties of ocular tissues (Ye et al. [25]) including sclera, ciliary body, iris, and cornea in the frequency range from 50 to 100 MHz at 37°C. The following sections will introduce the concepts of attenuation, speed of sound, and tissue reflectivity and will summarize the results of the Ye study, which are directly relevant to ultrasound biomicroscopy.

Attenuation

Attenuation describes the loss of energy in the ultrasound beam as it propagates through tissue. As noted above, there are two general processes that result in attenuation: absorption and reflectivity. Absorption refers to the conversion of acoustic energy to heat. Ultimately all acoustic energy is degraded into thermal energy via this process. The mechanisms by which absorption takes place are: (1) frictional (viscous) losses, (2) heat conduction losses (conduction from regions of high pressure to regions of low pressure), and (3) molecular exchange of energy (transient changes in molecular structure, changes in internal rotational, and vibrational states). Scattering contributes to attenuation by redirecting ultrasonic energy off the axis of the ultrasound beam. Thus, we must consider both components in deriving an expression for the pressure distribution in an ultrasound field. Fortunately homogeneous tissues exhibit a simple exponential loss of pressure amplitude due to attenuation as the ultrasound wave propagates. A simple modification of Eq. (1.3) results in:

$$p(z) = p_0 e^{-\alpha' z} \tag{1.5}$$

where p_0 is the initial pressure amplitude and the attenuation coefficient α' consists of the sum of contributions from absorption and scattering. That is,

$$\alpha' = \alpha_a + \alpha_s \tag{1.6}$$

The units of the attenuation coefficient are nepers/mm. Although these units are perfectly adequate for the comparison of attenuation coefficients, the logarithmic units of decibels/mm (dB/mm) are more commonly used because of their ready association with commonly applied electrical engineering formulae. For pressure amplitude, A, the decibel is defined as

$$A_{(\text{dB})} = 20 \text{ Log}_{10}\left(\frac{A}{A_{\text{ref}}}\right) \tag{1.7}$$

where A is the measured amplitude and A_{ref} is the reference amplitude. It is useful to note that 6 dB represents a factor of 2 and 20 dB represents a factor of 10, and similarly that −6 dB represents a factor of 0.5 and −20 dB represents a factor of 0.1. The attenuation coefficient expressed in units of dB/mm can be written:

$$\alpha\left(\frac{\text{dB}}{\text{mm}}\right) = 8.686\ \alpha'(\text{mm}^{-1}) \tag{1.8}$$

Figure 1.5 shows plots of the attenuation coefficients for sclera, cornea, ciliary body, and iris at a temperature of 37°C over the frequency range from 50 to 100 MHz. These in vitro measurements by Ye et al. [25] demonstrate that scleral tissue has the highest attenuation among the four eye tissues, and that the cornea has the lowest. It has been shown that there is an empirical relationship between ultrasonic propagation properties and the structural components of tissue. Collagen plays an important role in attenuating ultrasound energy [26]. The sclera consists of bundles of flat plates of collagen. The dense imbrication of these bundles gives the sclera its strength. Although the cornea also contains collagen fibers, the extracellular matrix is less dense and contains a high proportion of sulfated compounds. This structural difference between sclera and cornea results in the large difference in attenuation. The ciliary body, which is a form of smooth muscle, and the iris, which is a sheetlike diaphragm with loose fibrous support, are viscoelastic tissues. Their attenuation characteristics, therefore, fall in between those of the cornea and the sclera. At 50 MHz the attenuation in ocular tissues ranges from 1.3 dB/mm (cornea) to 4.3 dB/mm for sclera. This is a factor of 2.6 to 8.6 times the attenuation coefficient of fresh water at this frequency.

Speed of Sound

In ultrasound imaging our knowledge of the speed of sound allows us to convert times of flight into distance in the image. The speed of sound is proportional to the inverse of the compressibility and density of a material. Because the soft tissues of the body are largely composed of water, it is not surprising that the speed of sound in soft tissue is very

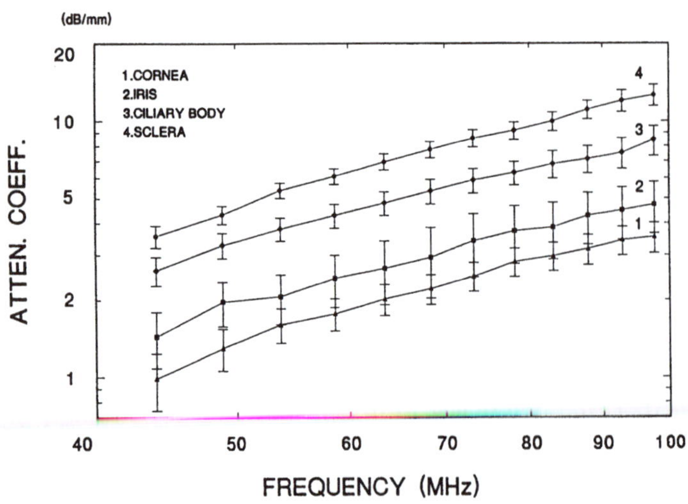

FIGURE 1.5. Measured attenuation coefficients for cornea, sclera, ciliary body, and iris at 37°C. Reprinted from Ye et al. [25] with permission.

similar to that of water. At 37°C the speed of sound in water is 1524 m/s, whereas the accepted average speed of sound for soft tissues is 1540 m/s. The measured speeds of sound for ocular tissues are somewhat higher, as shown in Figure 1.6. The highest speed of sound is observed in scleral tissue (1622 m/s), whereas comparatively low speeds of sound are observed in the ciliary muscle (1554 m/s) and iris (1542 m/s). These results are somewhat lower than those reported by Tschewnenko [20] and Thijssen et al. [21] for the diagnostic frequency range. However, the measured value of ultrasound velocity for the ciliary body is consistent with results for other muscle tissues obtained at lower frequency [27]. Literature values for cornea range from 1550 m/s [22] to 1620 m/s [20]. The measured value at 60 MHz falls between these extremes at 1575 m/s. The reason for this wide variation may be due to the state of the tissue. Corneal tissue changes rapidly under nonphysiological conditions, even in saline becoming edematous. Such changes could easily affect the measurements. Measurements on fresh and previously frozen cornea in this study did not show any significant difference in ultrasound velocity.

Tissue Reflectivity

In an ideal material with uniform elastic properties, an ultrasound wave will propagate in an undisturbed fashion. However, the presence of any material with differing elastic properties will cause the ultrasound wave to be partially reflected and partially transmitted. This reflected energy is the basis of the ultrasound image. Clearly, in tissues there exist a vast number of structures that would reflect ultrasound, ranging from organ boundaries to small vessels to cellular and even intracellular structures. These structures can be grouped into two major classes depending on the size of the target. In situations in which there is an interface between organs or tissue types where the interface is large compared to the wavelength of ultrasound, the reflection is specular in nature. That is, it behaves like a partially reflecting mirror. In situations in which there is an interface that is similar to or smaller than the wavelength the reflected wave is referred to as scatter. The information in ultrasound images is primarily due to scatter.

Geometrical (Specular) Reflection and Transmission

Ultrasonic waves obey many of the laws of geometrical optics. For example, if we consider an ultrasound pulse with amplitude A_i impinging on an interface between two media at an angle of θ_i to the normal, the reflected pulse has an angle equal to that of the incident pulse. That is:

$$\theta_i = \theta_r \tag{1.9}$$

and Snell's law, which describes the bending of the ultrasound beam, holds

$$\frac{\sin \theta_j}{c_1} = \frac{\sin \theta_r}{c_2} \tag{1.10}$$

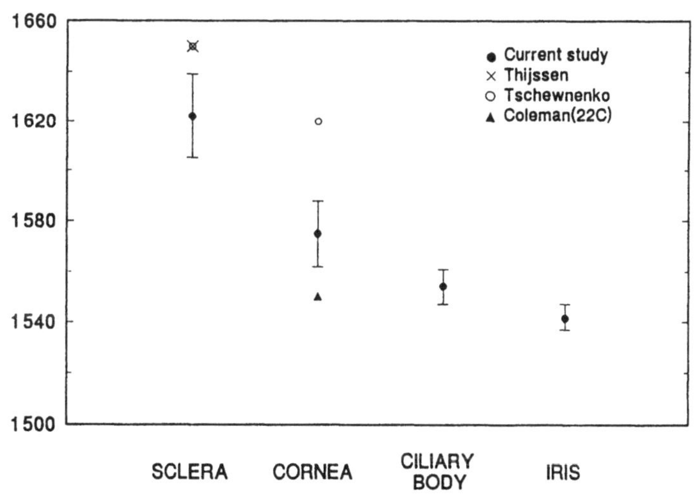

FIGURE 1.6. Speeds of sound in ocular tissues at 60 MHz, 37°C. Reprinted from Ye et al. [25] with permission.

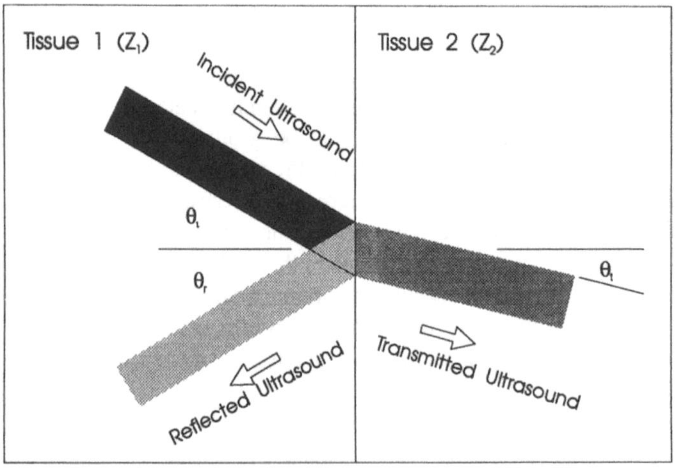

FIGURE 1.7. Reflection and refraction of an ultrasound pulse.

This is shown schematically in Figure 1.7 for two tissues with differing acoustic properties. If we define the pressure reflection coefficient R as the ratio of the reflected pressure amplitude to the incident amplitude, then a simple expression can be derived to determine its magnitude. Assuming normal incidence ($\theta_i = \theta_r = 90°$), this expression is:

$$R = \frac{Z_2 - Z_1}{Z_2 + Z_1} \quad (1.11)$$

where the symbol Z refers to a parameter called "acoustial impedance," which describes the elastic properties of the tissue. For a plane wave propagating in tissue the acoustical impedance is given by:

$$Z = \rho c \quad (1.12)$$

where ρ is the density of the tissue and c is the speed of sound in the tissue. Table 1.1 gives the acoustical impedances of several eye tissues as tabulated by Thijssen [21] and the strength of the reflection coefficient relative to a perfect reflector using Eq. (1.11). Note that the the reflected pressure is comparatively small for each of these tissues, ranging from approximately −20 dB (a factor of one-tenth) for the lens to approximately −40 dB (a factor of one one-hundredth) for the cornea, vitreous, and retina.

TABLE 1.1.

Tissue	Relative acoustical impedance	Reflection coefficient in water at 37°C (dB)
Cornea	1.55	−41.8
Sclera	1.61	−31.3
Vitreous humour	1.54	−46.2
Lens	1.73	−24.0
Retina	1.55	−41.8

Scattering from Tissue

Scattering of ultrasound from targets whose sizes are comparable to or smaller than the wavelength of ultrasound makes an important contribution to ultrasound images of soft tissue. It can be argued that this form of reflected ultrasound constitutes the critical information in an ultrasound image. Because these scatterers are, by their nature, pointlike, and because there are many of them in a given volume of tissue, we must consider the statistical sum of their contributions to the image. This concept is illustrated schematically in Figure 1.8, in which the scatter from a single resolution volume is observed to have a random nature. Most of the scattered ultrasound is absorbed by the tissue but some of these randomly scattered waves (the backscattered portion) arrive back at the transducer where their contributions are summed. This summing process occurs in such a way that both constructive interference and destructive interference take place, resulting in an image that has a distinct speckled texture for each tissue being imaged. The quantitative parameter that characterizes the amount of backscattered ultrasound is called the backscatter coefficient μ_b and is defined as:

$$\mu_b = \frac{\text{backscattered energy from tissue}}{\text{(reference energy)(solid angle)(distance)}} \quad (1.13)$$

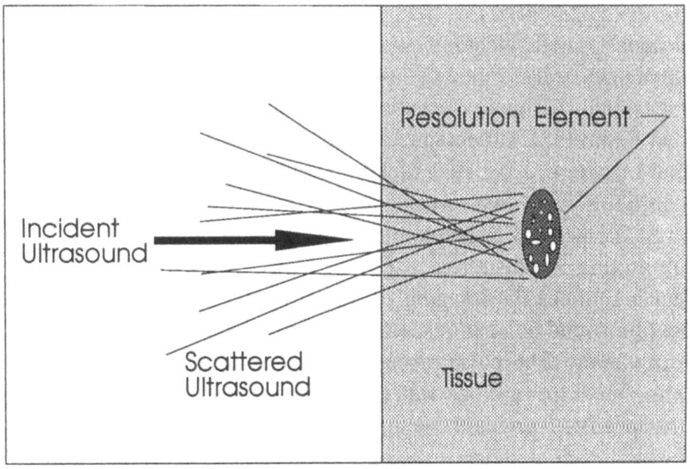

FIGURE 1.8. Schematic diagram showing the random nature of scattering from the small targets (cells, small blood vessels, extracellular matrix, etc.) that exist within the smallest resolvable volume of an ultrasound source (resolution volume). The fraction of these randomly scattered waves arriving back at the transducer (called backscatter) cause interferences that give ultrasound images a speckled texture.

where the reference energy is equal to the total energy in the pulse. The brightness of a given tissue on the scanner monitor is directly proportional to the backscatter coefficient. Backscatter coefficients vary in a characteristic fashion with frequency. This information can sometimes be used to differentiate tissues on the basis of their ultrasonic properties. Figure 1.9 shows plots of backscatter coefficients for various ocular tissues over the frequency range relevant to ultrasound biomicroscopy imaging. This figure, again from the work of Ye et al. [25], shows that the amount of backscatter increases with frequency for all of the tissues. The sclera has a backscattering coefficient that is a factor of 2 to 5 times higher than the other ocular tissues. The large variability in these data indicate that it would be difficult to distinguish iris, cornea, and ciliary body tissue on the basis of backscatter alone. The backscatter properties of tumor tissues at high frequencies have not yet been investigated.

Principles of Pulse Echo (Backscatter) Imaging

Although the pioneering work in medical imaging applications of reflected ultrasound energy was originally reported by Wild and Reid [28] and Howry and Bliss [29] in the early 1950s, it was not long before Mundt and Hughes [30] demonstrated the first applications to ocular imaging in 1956. A number of groups made important contributions to

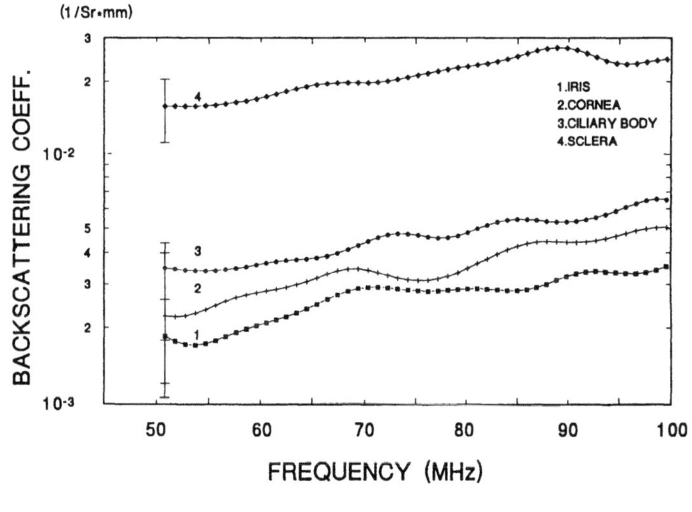

FIGURE 1.9. Measured backscattering coefficients for several ocular tissues over the frequency range from 50 to 100 MHz. Note the general increase with frequency and the clear separation of sclera from the other tissues. Reproduced from Ye et al. [25] with permission.

the development of this field during the succeeding decades. These include Ossoinig [31] who developed standardized methods of interpreting one-dimensional (A-mode) ultrasound images of the eye, and Baum [32], Coleman et al. [33], Purnell [34], and Lizzi et al. [35], each of whom made important contributions to two-dimensional (B-mode) imaging. The general principle of ocular imaging with ultrasound is illustrated in Figure 1.10. A transducer initiates the imaging process by generating an ultrasound pulse in response to a brief electrical stimulation. The pulse propagates through a coupling medium (such as water or artificial tears) at the speed of sound and encounters the tissues of the eye. At each impedance discontinuity, such as that between the couplant and the cornea, ultrasound is partially reflected back toward the transducer. Some of these reflections or echoes return to the transducer and are reconverted back into radiofrequency electrical signals, as shown in Figure 1.10b. The radiofrequency signal can be used to determine the distances to the various interfaces by virtue of the fact that we know the speed of sound in the medium. For example, the distance, z, to the first interface is given by substituting the value of t_{cornea} for t in the expression:

$$z = \frac{ct}{2} \tag{1.14}$$

The factor of 2 in this equation results from the fact that ultrasound must travel to and return from the interface. Once the radiofrequency signal has been received by the transducer it is "detected" by an electronic circuit that calculates its envelope, as shown in Figure 1.10c. This information is often referred to as an amplitude scan or A-scan and it represents the reflectivity along one line of sight in the eye. By coding the A-scan line as a brightness along one line of a video monitor a single line image is formed. A two-dimensional image or B-scan is then formed by rotating the transducer

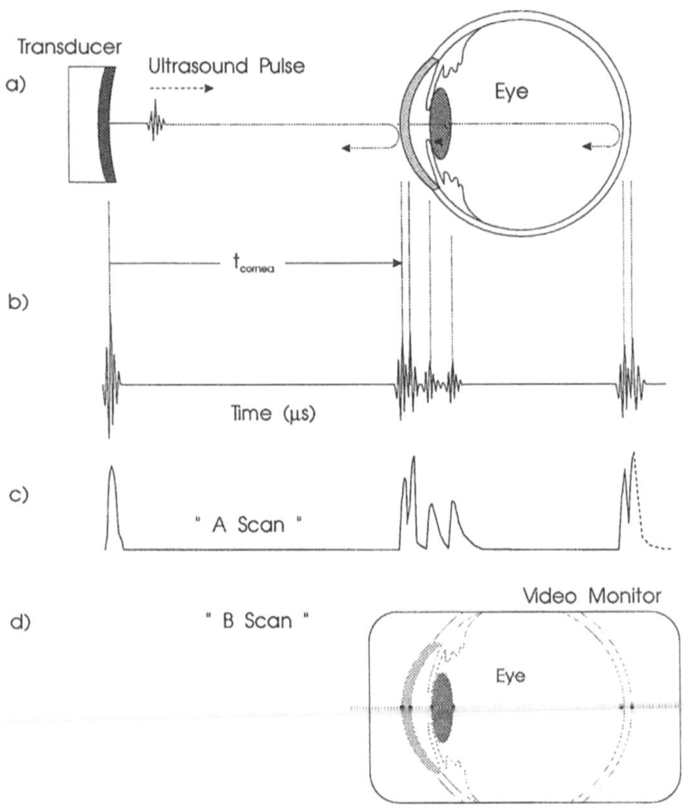

FIGURE 1.10. Basic principle of pulse echo (backscatter) imaging. A transducer initiates the imaging process by generating an ultrasound pulse in response to a brief electrical stimulation **(a)**. The pulse propagates through a coupling medium (such as water or artificial tears) at the speed of sound and encounters the tissues of the eye. The backscattered ultrasound returned from the tissue is converted by the transducer into a radiofrequency signal **(b)**. The radiofrequency signal is envelope detected, resulting in the A-scan signal **(c)**, which is encoded as brightness in the final image **(d)**.

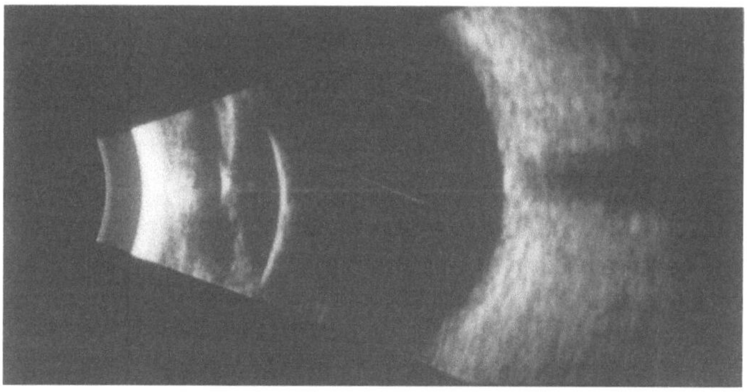

FIGURE 1.11. Conventional B-scan image of the eye at 10 MHz. Shown are the lens, vitreous cavity, and optic nerve. Resolution is approximately 0.5 mm laterally and 0.25 mm axially.

about a fixed axis and writing new lines of sight in correct registration such that the final video image presents a two-dimensional cross section through the eye. This imaging process can be performed as fast as 10 to 20 times a second, resulting in "real time" image frame rates. An example of a state-of-the-art ultrasound image of the eye is shown in Figure 1.11. Here, the lens, vitreous cavity, and the optic nerve are well imaged and, from a qualitative examination of the image, it appears that detail on the order of 0.5 mm can be resolved. This is consistent with the wavelength at 10 MHz, which is 0.15 mm according to Eq. (1.4), assuming a speed of sound of 1500 m/s in the tissue. An excellent guide to the principles and physics of ultrasound image formation can be found in the work of Hill [36].

Resolution and Penetration

The limits in current clinical imaging have been set as a result of the need to provide the maximum resolution consistent with the need for the ultrasound beam to penetrate the globe of the eye and to a certain extent penetrate the orbit. Thus, there is a constant need to make a compromise between resolution and penetration. In an ultrasound imaging system, the lateral resolution can be related via diffraction theory to the full width of the ultrasound beam at half maximum amplitude (FWHM), as illustrated in Figure 1.12 and is given by the equation:

$$\text{FWHM} = \frac{cR}{fd} = \lambda(f - \text{number}) \quad (1.15)$$

where c is the speed of sound, R is the focal length of the transducer, f is the frequency of ultrasound, d is the diameter of the focused transducer, λ is the wavelength, and f-number is the ratio of the focal length to the diameter of the transducer. This fixed focus situation is analogous to the focusing of light by an optical lens. It is not surprising that the best focus is achieved at the focal length of the transducer and that the width of the beam expands as we move away from the focal plane, as shown in Figure 1.12. The region over which the beam remains reasonably well focused is called the depth of field (DOF). The focusing characteristics of the imaging transducer are usually chosen such that the tissue of interest lies within the depth of field.

The foundation for the compromise between resolution and penetration is illustrated in Figures 1.13 and 1.14, in which plots of resolution and penetration versus frequency are shown. Figure 1.13 represents a plot of resolution as defined by Eq. (1.15) for transducers with f-numbers of 1.0,

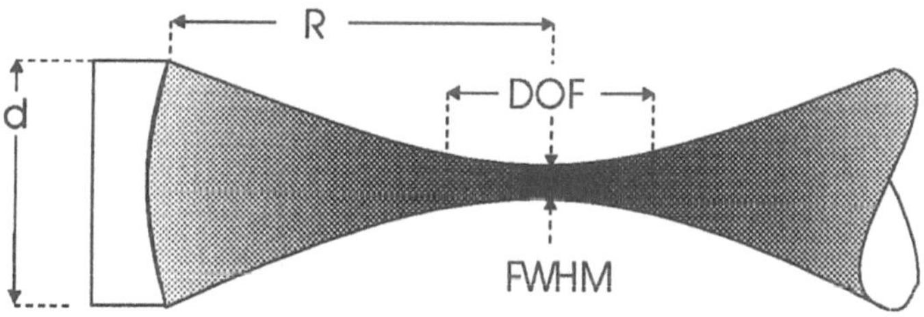

FIGURE 1.12. A focused ultrasound beam reaches its narrowest point at the focal length, R, and maintains adequate resolution over a distance called the depth of field (DOF). The width of the beam at R is a measure of lateral resolution and is given by Eq. (1.15).

2.0, and 4.0. A typical ophthalmic transducer with a frequency of 10 MHz and an f-number of 4.0 would have lateral resolution of 600 μm at the focus (Figure 1.13a). It has been appreciated for some time that Eq. (1.1,) allows almost unlimited freedom in achieving arbitrarily high resolution by simply selecting the appropriate frequency. For example, if we want 60 μm resolution, an operating frequency of 60 MHz would be chosen, as shown in Figure 1.13b. This is approximately 10 times the resolution obtained using conventional clinical instrumentation.

The penalty to be paid for this increase in resolution is loss of penetration. All human tissues exhibit ultrasound attenuation coefficients that increase with frequency. If we assume an attenuation coefficient of 0.5 dB/mm $MHz^{1.2}$, which is consistent with typical soft tissues [36], the maximum penetration that could be achieved for the 10 MHz system is approximately 50 mm for an 80 dB dynamic range, as shown in Figure 1.14a. For the 60 MHz system, penetration is only 5 mm (Figure 1.14b). This reinforces the need to optimize transducer sensitivity and performance in ultrasound biomicroscopy systems development.

Thus far we have concerned ourselves only with lateral resolution. In the direction along the axis of the beam (axial direction) resolution is proportional to the length of the pulse. The smallest distance between two planar surfaces that can be resolved, Δz, is defined by modifying Eq. (1.14)

$$\Delta z = \frac{ct_{-6\text{ dB}}}{2} \tag{1.16}$$

where $t_{-6\text{ dB}}$ is the temporal width of the pulse at one-half maximum. The axial resolution of a typical 10 MHz system is 187 μm, whereas a 50 MHz system has axial resolution of 37 μm, as illustrated in Figure 1.15.

Summary

In this chapter we have presented a basic introduction to ultrasound and its propagation in tissue. The wave nature of ultrasound is similar, in many re-

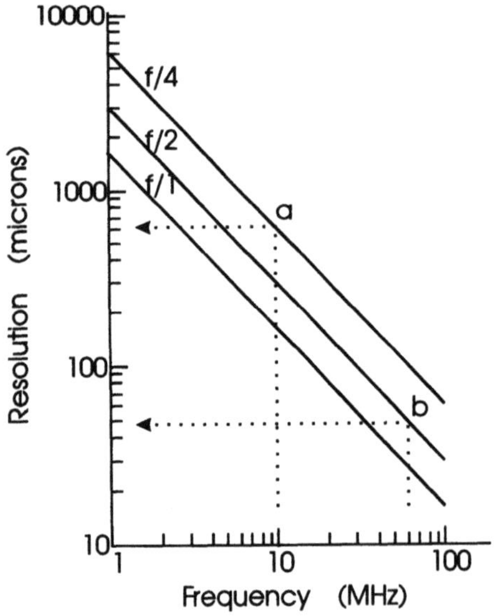

FIGURE 1.13. Plot of lateral resolution versus frequency for transducers with *f*-numbers (*R*/*d*) ranging from f/1 to f/4. At conventional imaging frequencies of 10 MHz **(a)**, lateral resolution of approximately 600 μm can be achieved using an *f*/4 transducer. However, at 60 MHz **(b)** lateral resolution of 60 μm is possible with an *f*/2 transducer.

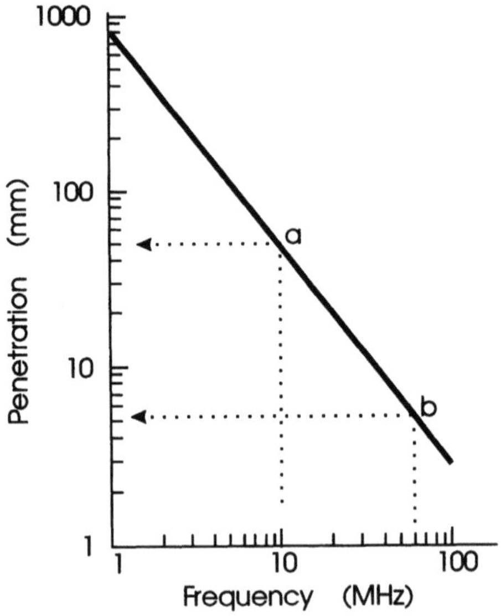

FIGURE 1.14. Plot of penetration versus frequency under realistic imaging conditions. Increased resolution at elevated frequencies is accompanied by reduced penetration due to increased losses in the tissues. Although it is possible to achieve penetration of nearly 50 mm at 10 MHz **(a)**, only 5 mm can be penetrated at 60 MHz **(b)**.

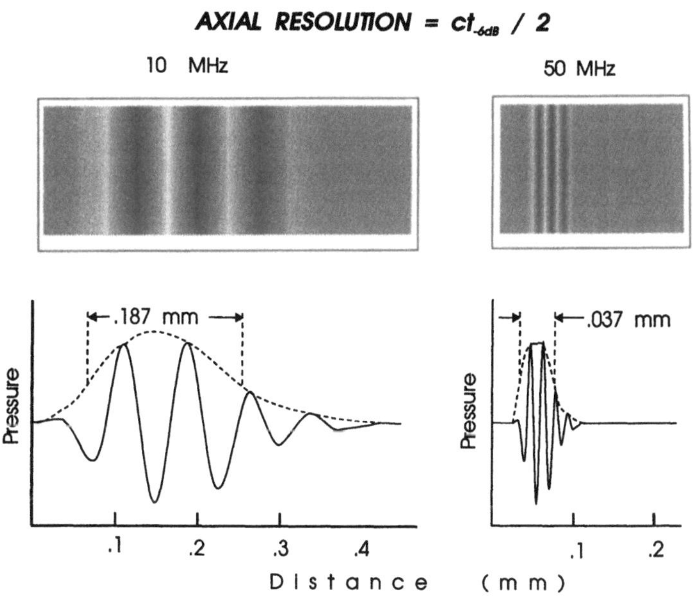

FIGURE 1.15. Axial resolution is defined as the pulse echo length (at half maximum) of the ultrasound echo from a planar interface. The axial resolution of a typical 10 MHz system is 187 μm, whereas a 50 MHz system has axial resolution of 37 μm.

spects, to optical radiation, in that it obeys the fundamental laws of reflection and refraction. This means that it is possible to focus ultrasound, according to classical diffraction theory, to achieve beamwidths on the order of 20 to 80 μm in the frequency range from 40 to 80 MHz. This is approximately 10 times the resolution achieved at conventional ophthalmic ultrasound imaging frequencies. Because losses due to attenuation increase almost linearly with frequency, the total imaging depth is significantly reduced, leading to fields of view of 4–5 mm. We have used the term ultrasound biomicroscopy to describe the concept of realtime microscopic visualization of living tissue over a limited range.

References

1. Rayleigh JWS. *The Theory of Sound*, 2nd Ed., 1984. Macmillan Co., London.
2. Langevin P, Chilowski MC. Procedes et appareils pour la production de signaux sous-marins direges et pour la localisation a distance d'obstacles sous-marins. French Patent 1916, No. 502913.
3. Forster FK, Olerud JE, Pomajevich GR, Holmes AW, Sharar SR. High frequency ultrasonic imaging and backscatter attenuation techniques for determination of thermal injury to the skin. *IEEE Ultrasonics Symposium Proceedings 1986*; IEEE Cat. No. 86CH2791–2, pp. 845–848. IEEE, New York.
4. Yano T, Fukukita H, Uneo S, Fukomoto A. 40 MHz ultrasound diagnostic system for: Dermatologic examination, *IEEE Ultrasonics Symposium Proceedings 1987*; IEEE Cat. No. 87CH2791–2, pp. 875–878. IEEE, New York.
5. Altmeyer P, el Gammal S, Hoffman K, Eds. *Ultrasound in Dermatology*, 1992. Springer-Verlag, Berlin.
6. Wiersema MJ, Reilly CR, Sanghvi NT, Hawes R, Wiersema L, Aust C. Twenty-five MHz gastrointestinal ultrasonography. *IEEE Ultrasonics Symposium Proceedings 1989*; IEEE Cat. No. 89CH2791–2, pp. 845–848. IEEE, New York.
7. Silverstein FE, Martin RW, Kimmeym MV, Jiranek GC, Franklin DW, Proctor A. Experimental evaluation of an endoscopic ultrasound probe: In vitro and in vivo canine studies. *Gastroenterology* 1989; 88:1058–1062.
8. Sanghvi NT, Wiersema M, Reilly CR, Smith PE, Franklin TD. PC based high resolution, high frequency US system for gastroenterology. *IEEE Ultrasonics Symposium Proceedings 1990*, pp. 1477–1479. IEEE, New York.
9. Pandian NG. Intravascular and intracardiac ultrasound imaging: An old concept, now on the road to reality. *Circulation* 1989;88:1091–1094.
10. Yock PG, Linker DT, Angelsen BA. Two dimensional intravascular ultrasound: Technical development and initial clinical experience. *J Am Soc Echo* 1989;2:296–304.
11. Hodgson JM, Graham SP, Savakus AD, Dame SG, Stephens DN, Brand D, Sheehan H, Eberle MJ.

Clinical percutaneous imaging of coronary anatomy using an over-the-wire ultrasound catheter system. *Int J Card Imaging* 1989;4:186–193.
12. Lockwood GR, Ryan LK, Gotlieb AI, Lonn E, Hunt JW, Lui P, Foster FS. In vitro high resolution intravascular imaging in muscular and elastic arteries. *J Am Coll Cardiol* 1992;20:153–160.
13. Brown LF. Ferroelectric polymers: Current and future applications. *IEEE Ultrasonics Symposium Proceedings 1992*, pp. 539–545, IEEE, New York.
14. Foster FS, Strban M, Austin G. The ultrasound macroscope. *Ultrasonic Imaging* 1984;6:243–261.
15. Sherar MD, Noss MB, Foster FS. Ultrasound backscatter microscopy images the internal structure of living tumor spheroids multicellular tumour spheroids. *Nature* 1987;330:493–495.
16. Sherar MD, Starkoski BG, Taylor WB, Foster FS. A 100 MHz B-scan ultrasound backscatter microscope. *Ultrasonic Imaging* 1989;11:95–105.
17. Begui ZE. Acoustic properties of refractive media of the eye. *J Acoust Soc Am* 1954;26:365–372.
18. Jansson F, Sundmark E. Determination of the velocity of ultrasound in ocular tissues at different temperatures. *Acta Ophthalmol* 1961;39:899–911.
19. Rivara A, Sanna G. Determination of the velocity of ultrasound in the ocular tissues of human and swine (in Italian). *Ann Ottalmol Clin Ocul* 1962;88:675–680.
20. Tschewnenko AA. Über die Ausbreitungsgeschwindigkeit des Ultraschalls in den augengeweben (in German). *Z Humbolt Univ Berlin Math Naturwiss Reihe* 1965;14:67–69.
21. Thijssen MJ, Mol MJ, Timer MR. Acoustic parameters of ocular tissues. *Ultrasound Med Biol* 1983;11:157–161.
22. Coleman DJ, Lizzi FL, Jack R. Ultrasonography of the Eye and Orbit. 1977. Lea & Febiger, Philadelphia.
23. Feleppa EJ, Lizzi FL, Coleman DJ, Yaremko MM. Diagnostic spectrum analysis in ophthalmology: A physical perspective. *Ultrasound Med Biol* 1986; 12:623–631.
24. Lizzi FL, Ostromogilsky M, Feleppa FJ, Rorke MC, Yaremko MM. Relationship of ultrasonic spectral parameters to features of tissue microstructure. *IEEE Trans UFFC* 1987;33:319–329.
25. Ye SG, Harasiewicz KA, Pavlin CJ, Foster FS. Ultrasound characterization of ocular tissue in the frequency range from 50MHz to 100 MHz. *IEEE Trans UFFC* 1993. In press.
26. Bamber JC. Attenuation and absorption. In: Hill CR, Ed. Physical Principles of Medical Ultrasonics. 1986, Chapter 4. Ellis Horwood Limited, London.
27. Goss SA, Johonston RL, Dunn F. Comprehensive compilation of empirical ultrasonic properties of mammalian tissues. *J Acoust Soc Am* 1978;64:423–457.
28. Wild JJ, Reid JM. Application of echo-ranging techniques to the determination of the structure of biological tissues. *Science* 1952;115:226–230.
29. Howry DH, Bliss WR. Ultrasonic visualization of soft tissue structures of the body. *J Lab Clin Med* 1952;40:579–592.
30. Mundt GH, Hughes WF. Ultrasonics in ocular diagnosis. *Am J Ophthalmol* 1956;42:488–498.
31. Ossoinig KC. Standardized echography: Basic principles, clinical applications, and results. *Int Ophthalmol Clin* 1979;19:127–210.
32. Baum G. The effect of ultrasonic radiation upon the eye and ocular adnexa. *Am J Ophthalmol* 1956; 42:696–706.
33. Coleman DJ, Lizzi FL, Jack R. *Ultrasonography of the Eye and Orbit*. 1977. Lea & Febiger, Philadelphia.
34. Purnell EW. Ultrasonic biometry of the posterior ocular coats. *Trans Am Ophthalmol Soc* 1980; 78:1027–1078.
35. Lizzi FL, Feleppa EJ, Coleman DJ. Ultrasonic ocular tissue characterization. In: Greenleaf JF, Ed. *Tissue Characterization with Ultrasound: Volume 11, Results and Applications*. 1986, pp. 41–60. CRC Press, Boca Raton.
36. Hill CR, Ed. *Physical Principles of Medical Ultrasonics*. 1986. Ellis Horwood Limited, London.

2
Instrumentation for Ultrasound Biomicroscopy

Scanner Design

The essential component blocks of an ultrasound biomicroscope are identical to those of a conventional B-mode imaging system except that the operating frequency is approximately an order of magnitude higher. Achieving the goal of real time B-mode imaging at these frequencies required development of new technology in three important areas: (1) transducers, (2) high-frequency signal processing, and (3) precise motion control. Figure 2.1 shows a block diagram of the principal components of an ultrasound biomicroscope. A 40 to 100 MHz transducer is moved linearly over the imaging field (typically 4 mm), collecting radiofrequency ultrasound data at each of 512 equally spaced lines (8 μm between lines). A monocycle high voltage (200 V peak to peak) 40 to 100 MHz pulse is used to excite the transducer. The resulting 40 to 100 MHz ultrasound pulse is transmitted into the tissue and the backscattered ultrasound is detected by the same transducer. The radiofrequency signal (see Figure 1.10b) is received and amplified in proportion to the depth from which it originated using time-gain compensation (TGC), as shown in Figure 2.1. By amplifying signals from deeper structures more than superficial structures it is possible to compensate for the attenuation of the ultrasound beam in the tissue. After the radiofrequency signal is nonlinearly processed to enhance the low-level signals, its envelope is "detected" to produce the A-scan signal corresponding to Figure 1.10c. This signal is then converted from analog to digital format and transferred to a special high-speed scan converter, stored, and displayed as brightness on a video monitor. Only signals returning from a 4 mm region centered at the focal depth are stored. The servo motion system and signal processing are controlled and synchronized by a computer. B-mode imaging is currently performed at 5 to 10 frames/second. Additional details on the scanner design are given in References [1] to [4].

Transducers

The critical job of transforming electrical energy into acoustical energy and vice versa is performed by an ultrasound transducer. It can be argued that the transducer is the single most important component in an ultrasound imaging system. As such, it is directly responsible for image resolution, contrast, and sensitivity. The main components of an ultrasound transducer are illustrated in Figure 2.2. The active piezoelectric material has a thickness that causes it to vibrate at the resonant frequency of the scanner. By appropriately choosing the acoustic properties of the backing and matching layers (Figure 2.2) it is possible to generate ultrasound pulses that are well suited for high-frequency imaging applications. The development of high-frequency transducers has been central to the progress achieved in ultrasound biomicroscopy. We have used the piezoelectric polymer, polyvinylidene difluoride (PVDF) [2] and copolymer, polyvinylidene difluoride/trifluoroethylene, as the active piezoelectric materials for imaging applications such as the eye. The construction of this type of transducer is illustrated in Figure 2.3. The polymer transducers are built into a connector and have an

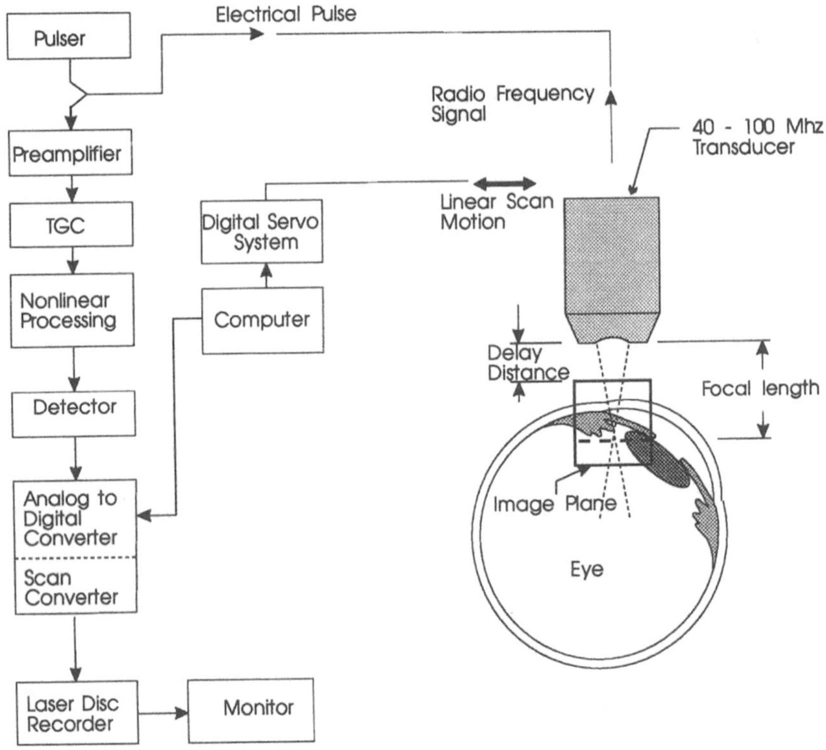

FIGURE 2.1. Schematic diagram of an ultrasound biomicroscope. The transducer executes a linear scan over a 4 mm field of view. At each position in the linear motion an ultrasound pulse is transmitted. Backscatter returned to the transducer is converted to a radiofrequency signal. The radiofrequency signal is amplified, processed to detect the envelope, and displayed on a video monitor at a rate of 5 to 10 frames per second.

active surface approximately 3 mm in diameter and a conductive epoxy backing. For a 10 μm thick polymer film, this configuration results in a device that produces short, wide bandwidth pulses with good sensitivity in the frequency range from 50 to 100 MHz. The device illustrated in Figure 2.3 has a resonant frequency of 60 MHz (wavelength = 25 μm) and an f-number (ratio of focal length to diameter) of 2.0. Thus, by substitution into Eq. (1.15) the lateral resolution is approximately 50 μm. An example of the pulse produced by this transducer is given in Figure 2.4. The temporal width of the pulse is approximately 30 ns at half maximum amplitude. Substituting this time into Eq. (1.14) we see that this corresponds to a distance of 25 μm. In effect, this is the resolution in the direction of pulse

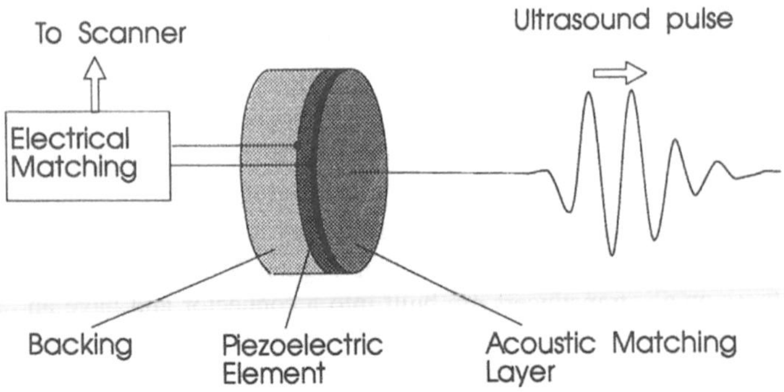

FIGURE 2.2. An ultrasound transducer consists of four major components: an active piezoelectric element, a backing on which the piezoelectric element is mounted, acoustic matching layers (if neccessary), and an electrical matching circuit. The acoustic and electrical properties are chosen to optimize pulse characteristics for a given imaging application.

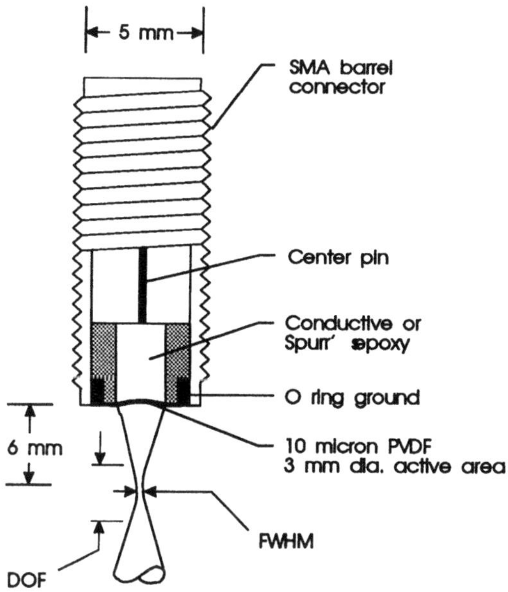

FIGURE 2.3. Schematic diagram of a high-frequency polymer transducer. The width of the beam at the focus, given by Eq. (1.15), is 50 μm.

propagation (axial resolution). More discussion on axial resolution will be given later in this chapter. From the above discussion it is clear that the choice of transducer parameters will have a significant impact on image quality. It is therefore necessary to optimize the transducer characteristics for each application to obtain the best compromise for resolution, contrast, and depth of field. More detail on the development of high-frequency polymer transducers is given in References 5 and 6.

Early Images

A photograph of the first ultrasound biomicroscope is shown in Figure 2.5. This system, which became operational in mid-1988, was originally designed to have a field of view of 2 mm × 2 mm and a frequency of 100 MHz. With it, we obtained our first views of enucleated eyes unsuitable for corneal transplantation. The results revealed fascinating detail of the angle of the eye and other structures that were partially dissected from these eyes. Examples of some of the early images are given in Figures 2.6 and 2.7 and in Reference 7. Figure 2.6 shows an image plane through the corneoscleral junction, demonstrating the appearance of the cornea (C), sclera (S), iris (I), and ciliary body (CB). The visualization of Schlemm's canal (arrow) at these frequencies was quite variable.

At 100 MHz, with resolution of approximately 30 μm, it was possible to visualize the layers of the choroid and retina (Fig. 2.6) through the scleral tissue. An example of a 100 MHz image of a dissected portion of retinal tissue is given in Figure 2.7a. The ultrasound biomicroscope image shows three distinct layers plus a fourth less well resolved layer. Histologically (Figure 2.7b, magnification ×40) the three major layers corresponded to the surface ganglion cell layer (top layer in B-scan), the inner nuclear layer (middle), and outer nuclear layer / outer limiting membrane (bottom). Less ev-

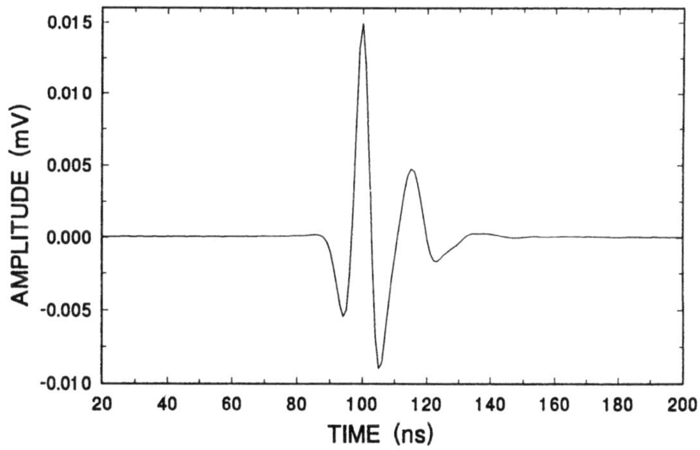

FIGURE 2.4. Pulse shape from a transducer similar to that illustrated in Figure 2.3. The center frequency is 62 MHz and the pulse length is 30 ns corresponding to an axial resolution of 25 μm. This device would be suitable for corneal imaging or tissue characterization studies.

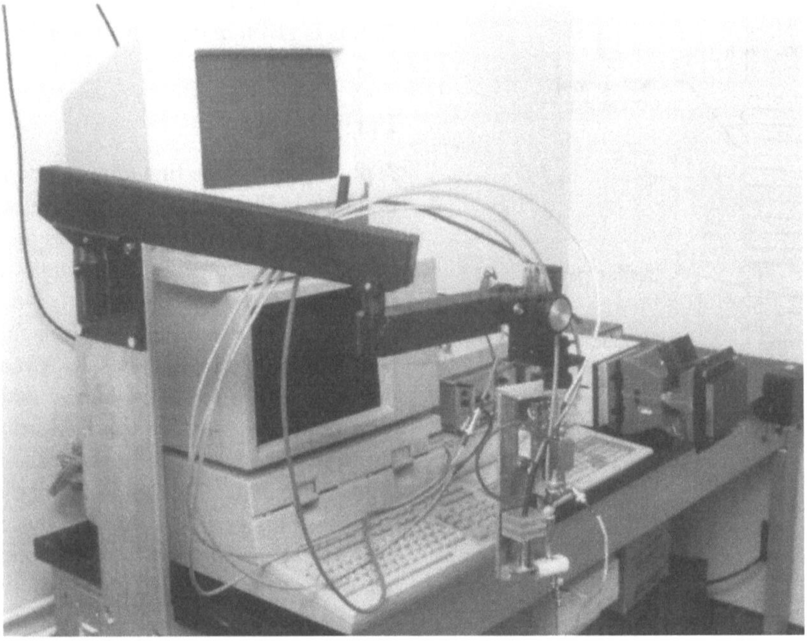

FIGURE 2.5. The first ultrasound biomicroscope became operational in mid-1988. This system was used to image over 400 patients and is still used for special high-frequency studies of the cornea.

ident are the visual processes that can be seen as a fourth peak in the A-scan along the dashed line of the biomicroscope image (Figure 2.7c). Only remnants of the visual processes are seen in the histological image due to the hematoxylin and eosin fixation process.

Imaging at 100 MHz with a 2 mm × 2 mm field of view provided outstanding resolution but did not

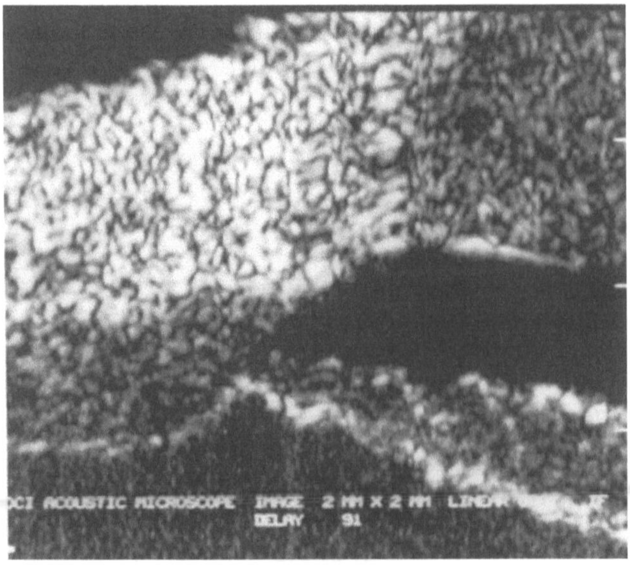

FIGURE 2.6. An early ultrasound biomicroscopic image of the angle of the eye in vitro. This image was made at an operating frequency of 100 MHz and has a 2 mm × 2 mm field of view. The sclera (S), cornea (C), iris (I), and ciliary body (CB) are clearly visualized. Resolution on the order of 30 μm is displayed. Published courtesy of *Ophthalmology* (1990;97:244–250).

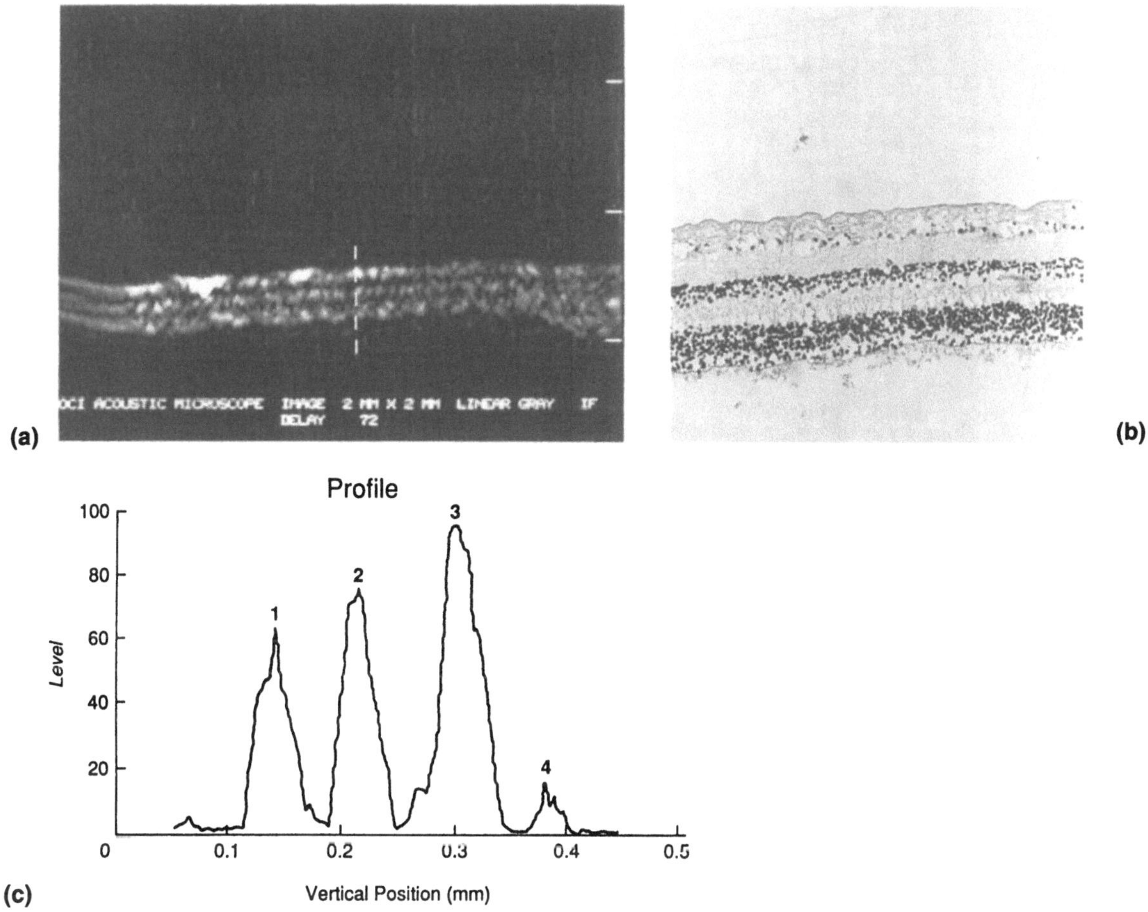

FIGURE 2.7. 100 MHz image of a dissected portion of retinal tissue. The ultrasound biomicroscope image **(a)** shows three distinct layers plus a fourth less well resolved layer. Histologically **(b)** (magnification ×40) the three major layers corresponded to the surface ganglion cell layer (top layer in B-scan), the inner nuclear layer (middle), and outer nuclear layer / outer limiting membrane (bottom). Less evident are the visual processes that can be seen as a fourth peak in the A- scan along the dashed line of the biomicroscope image **(c)**. Only remnants of the visual processes are seen in the histological image due to the hematoxylin and eosin fixation process. Published courtesy of *Ophthalmology* (1990;97:244–250).

permit appreciation of larger deeper structures. Accordingly, the next design incorporated transducers ranging from 50 to 80 MHz with a field of view of 4 mm × 4 mm. This proved to be a useful compromise that allowed all of the important structures of the anterior globe to be well visualized. The images from the new system were so clear that they almost appeared to have come from an anatomy textbook. We were ready for our first patient!

The first clinical images were made in March of 1990 using a water bath approach similar to that described by Coleman et al. [8]. The opening in a standard surgical drape was attached to the periocular region with the aid of colloidon and the edges of the drape suspended from a metal hoop. Scanning was then performed by placing the probe close to the area of interest and observing the resulting image on the screen. Fine movement of the probe was done by hand with reference to the screen image. Surprisingly, this was no more difficult than in conventional ultrasound imaging. Figure 2.8 shows an early clinical examination using the water bath method. Notice that the probe and preamplifier are supported by a mechanical arm assembly to

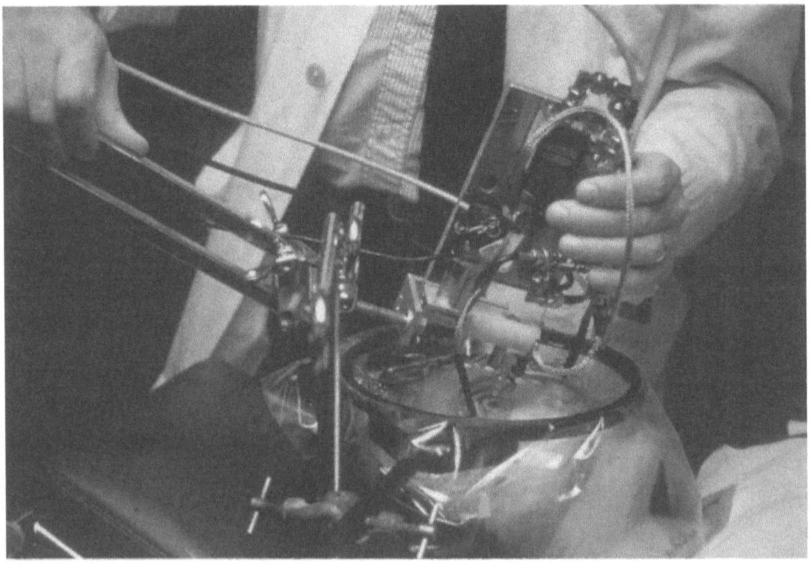

FIGURE 2.8. Early clinical examinations like the one shown here were performed using a water bath method. Published courtesy of *Ophthalmology* (1991;98:287–295).

help reduce motion artifacts. An example of an early clinical image made using this approach showing an 860 μm diameter cyst in the posterior chamber is given in Figure 2.9. This 60 MHz image demonstrates the expected resolution of approximately 50 μm. Early clinical results are reported in Reference 9.

Recently a commercial version of the biomicroscope has become available through Ziess-Humphrey Inc. (San Leandro, CA). This system has a more compact probe and signal processing box than our previous prototype and operates at a frame rate of 8 Hz. It will be described in more detail in the next chapter.

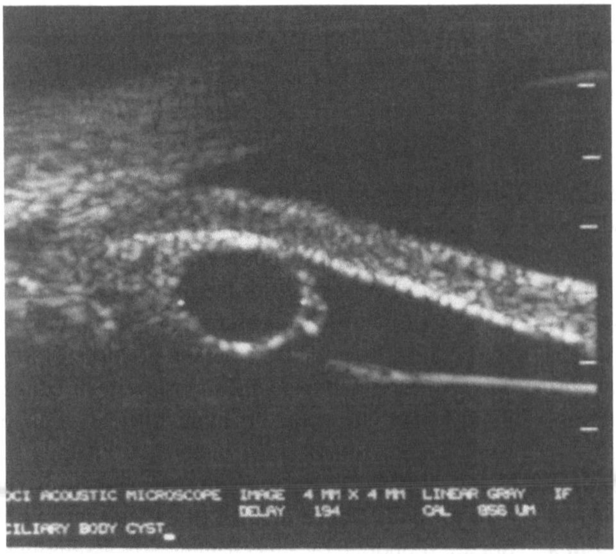

FIGURE 2.9. Clinical imaging at 60 MHz proved to be a useful compromise between resolution and depth of penetration. Images such as the one shown here showed excellent definition of the posterior chamber and in this case the 860 μm diameter cyst with its 100 μm diameter satellite.

Image Quality

As indicated in the previous discussion, image quality is primarily governed by the frequency (wavelength) of the ultrasound, the ratio of the focal length to the transducer diameter (f-number), and the length of the pulse. A number of transducers have been fabricated to examine the trade-offs in the choice of these parameters. These devices range from 50 to 80 MHz center frequency and have f-numbers ranging from 1.2 to 2.2, as illustrated in Figure 2.10. Examples of images of the cornea made with these transducers are given in Figure 2.11. The 50 MHz f/2.2 transducer gives an image (Figure 2.11, top) with fairly coarse speckle and is unable to resolve the corneal epithelium. In contrast, the 80 MHz f/1.2 device (Figure 2.11, bottom) provides an image with extraordinary sharpness showing the 50 μm thick epithelial layer (arrow) clearly. However, a bright band corresponding to the narrow focal zone of the transducer is evident in the image. A good compromise is achieved by the 80 MHz f/2.2 transducer (Figure 2.11, middle) for this particular application. This choice permits both the epithelium and the depth of the cornea to be well visualized. We typically employ transducers with center frequencies of 60 to 80 MHz with an f-number of 2.2 for most of our ophthalmic studies.

Measurement Accuracy

Measurement accuracy in ultrasound biomicroscopy is limited by the lateral and axial resolution of the system, the stability of the mechanical motion, the pixel size in the image, and by our knowledge of the speed of sound in ocular tissues. In the lateral direction (transverse to the direction of pulse propagation) the fundamental limit in accuracy will be dictated by the distribution of ultrasound in the field of the transducer. As discussed in the previous section, this distribution has a width at half maximum given by the product of the wavelength and the f-number [Eq. (1.15)]. A test of lateral measurement accuracy at the focus can be made by scanning a phantom consisting of a number of small fibers spaced a known distance apart and comparing the screen measurements with the known measurements between fibers. Examples of images of a phantom consisting of parallel 20 μm diameter glass fibers spaced 500, 400, 300, 200, 100, and 50 μm apart are given in Figures 2.12a, b, and c. These images were made with the transducers illustrated in Figure 2.10c, b, and a, respectively. For the 50 MHz f/2.2 probe the fibers separated by 50 μm are not resolved but the 100 μm spacing is easily resolved and is measured by the cursors as 104 μm. The 80 MHz f/2.2 transducer is just capable of resolving the 50 μm fibers and the

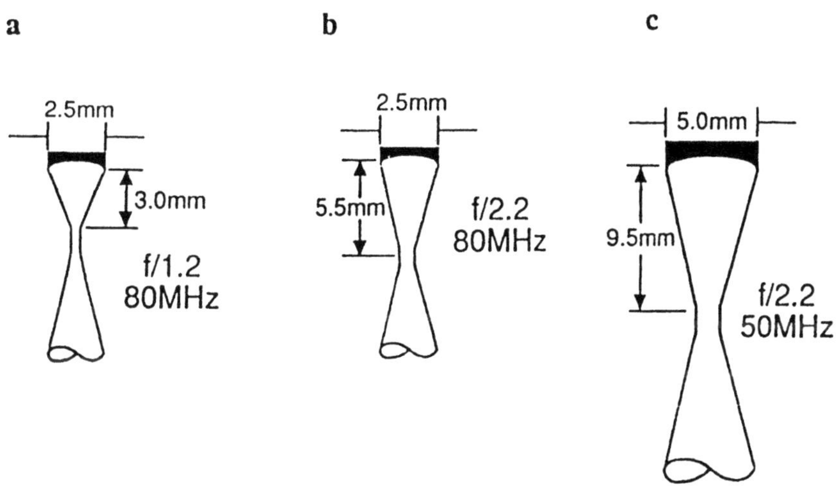

FIGURE 2.10. Several transducer geometries used in image evaluation.

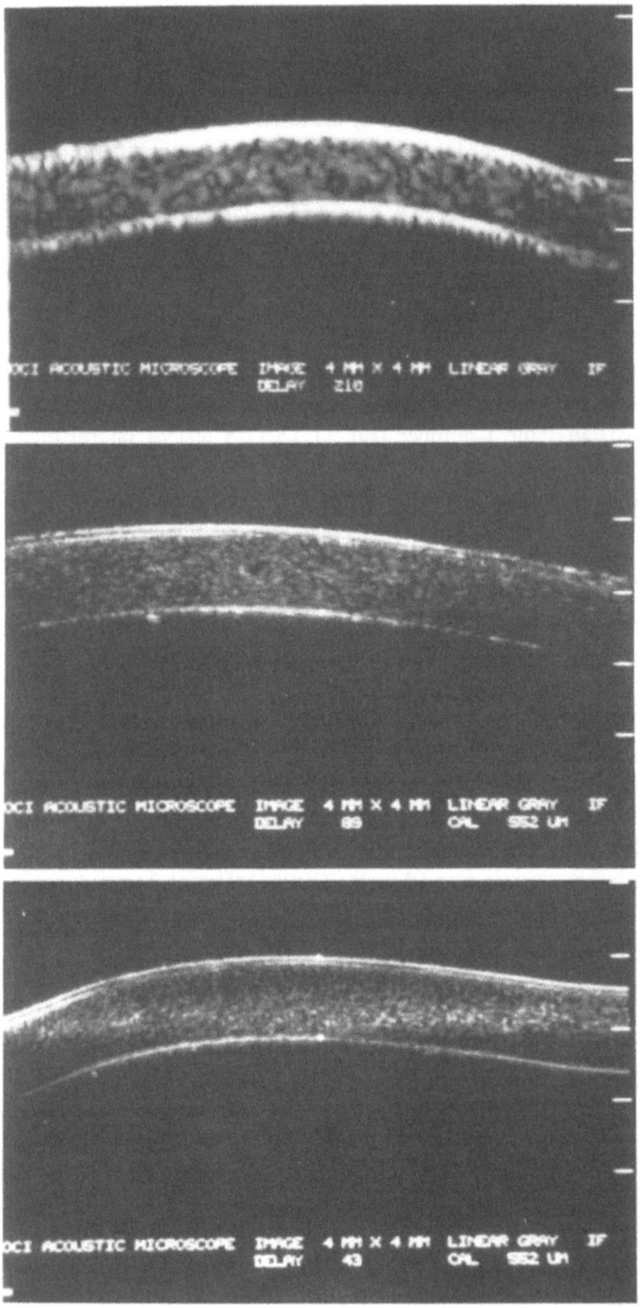

FIGURE 2.11. Imaging of the cornea using the devices shown in Figure 2.10. At 50 MHz, f/2.2 the image has fairly coarse speckle and is unable to resolve the corneal epithelium (top). By contrast the 80 MHz f/1.2 device (bottom) provides an image with extraordinary sharpness showing the 50 μm thick epithelial layer (arrow) clearly. However, a bright band corresponding to the narrow focal zone of the transducer is evident in the image. A good compromise is achieved by the 80 MHz f/2.2 transducer (center) for this particular application.

80 MHz f /1.2 device easily resolves the 50 μm fibers with the cursors measuring 52 μm.

In the axial direction measurement accuracy will be governed by the axial resolution and our knowledge of the speeds of sound in the various tissue layers. As discussed in Chapter 1 the speeds of sound range from 1542 m/s in the iris to 1620 m/s in the sclera. Accurate distance measurements in the axial direction (vertical direction on the screen) therefore require correction by a factor equal to the speed of sound for the particular tissue being measured divided by the speed of sound constant used in the scanner (usually 1540 m/s). The correction factor is usually only a few percent. It is important

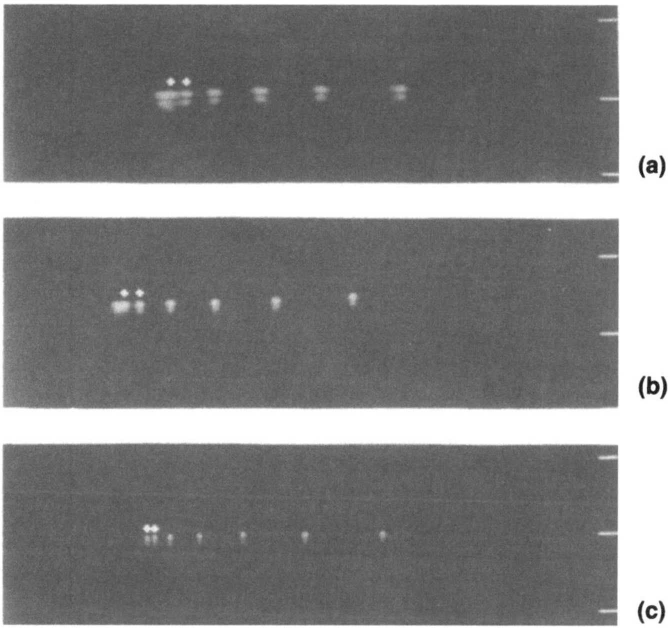

FIGURE 2.12. Phantom images of 20 μm diameter glass fibers spaced 500, 400, 300, 200, 100, and 50 μm apart for the three transducers shown in Figure 2.10. The influence of frequency and f-number on image sharpness are clearly evident.

to recognize the difference between instrument axial resolution and measurement precision. In this context axial resolution refers to the instruments capability to distinguish between two surfaces as they are brought closer and closer together. If the interfaces are truly planar and parallel, it is possible to use frequency domain techniques such as those developed by Lizzi and Elbaum [10] to increase the axial resolution significantly depending on the bandwidth of the transducer. Measurement precision can be significantly better than the axial resolution under the special condition that the two planar interfaces are well resolved and parallel (e.g., anterior and posterior surfaces of the cornea). In this situation a cursor can be positioned at half the maximum envelope amplitude of the leading or trailing edge of each signal with a precision of approximately one-half wave period for each cursor with the result that the thickness of the cornea is precise to within 10 μm at 75 MHz. If the radiofrequency signal is available, the use of cross correlation analysis should permit extraordinary precision on the order of a few microns to be achieved.

Safety of High-Frequency Ultrasound

In recent years, diagnostic ultrasound has come under considerable scrutiny for any potentially harmful effects. Current studies indicate two mechanisms that can, at sufficiently high power levels, cause irreversible cell damage: thermal mechanisms and mechanical mechanisms. Thermal damage occurs as a result of temperature increases due to absorption of ultrasound, whereas mechanical damage is the result of various cavitational and acoustic streaming phenomena. The net result of investigations of these processes has been the development of "onscreen labeling" showing estimated in vivo thermal and mechanical indices for clinical ultrasound instrumentation. Temperature rises of less than 1°C (thermal index = 1.0) are considered safe. In spite of these measures the Food and Drug Administration still adheres to an archaic standard based on "preamendment" power levels. That is, if an instrument does not exceed the

TABLE 2.1. Colony-forming ability for EMT6 cells.

	Monolayers plating efficiency (%)	Spheroids plating efficiency (%)
Unexposed	71 ± 6	49 ± 8
Exposed	70 ± 7	53 ± 3
Exposed × 10	74 ± 4	———

power levels of instruments manufactured before 1978 it is considered safe. For ophthalmic imaging this number is 17 mW/cm^2 spatial peak intensity averaged over time (SPTA). At the present time it is not possible to measure SPTA for the ultrasound biomicroscope accurately because it would require the development of a calibrated measurement probe on the order of 25 μm in size! However, calculations based on the measured efficiency of the transducer and the measured beam distribution indicate that the SPTA for our transducers is similar to the recommended preenactment levels and thermal modeling indicates that temperature rises will be much less than 1°C.

In addition to the above estimates of power levels, experiments were carried out in biological systems to confirm the expected lack of toxicity. Initially, the survival of EMT6 cell monolayers was evaluated at up to 10 times the power levels used in imaging. In these tests, the plating efficiency (number of colonies per unit area / number of cells plated per unit area × 100%) was evaluated for untreated cells, cells treated at normal imaging in-

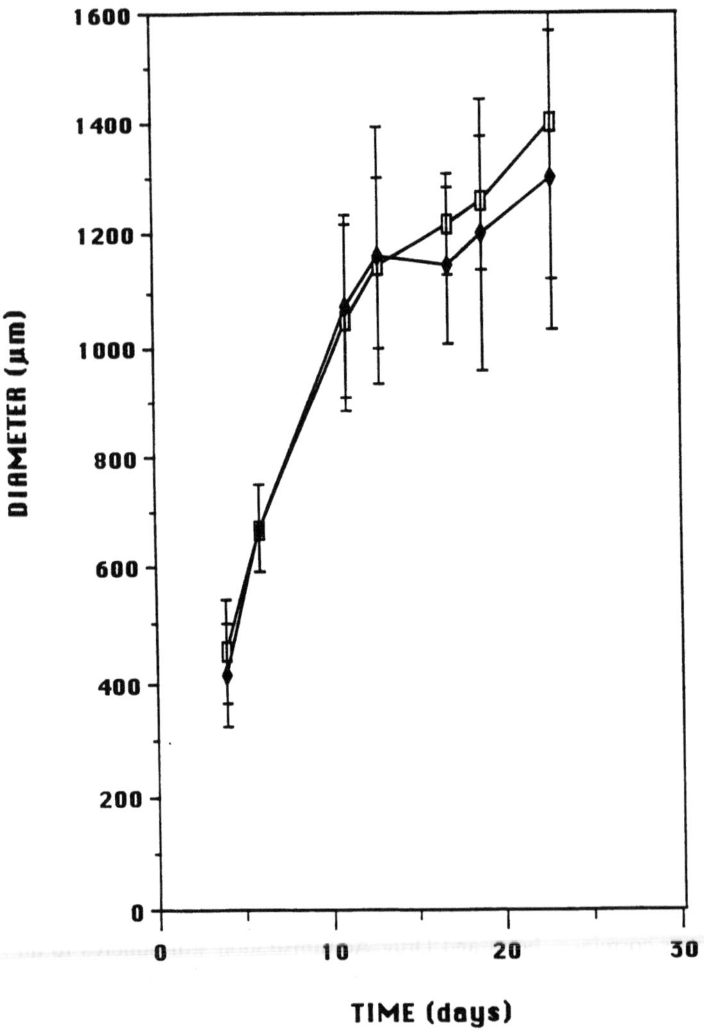

FIGURE 2.13. Growth curves for spheroids unexposed to ultrasound (□) and spheroids exposed under typical imaging conditions (♦).

tensities, and cells treated at 10 times normal imaging intensity. Similar experiments were performed for cellular aggregates called spheroids, which more closely represent tissue. Spheroids with diameters of 300 to 500 μm were exposed as outlined above, disaggregated, and tested for plating efficiency. The results shown in Table 2.1 indicated no difference in colony-forming ability in three independent experiments for cells in monolayer or in spheroids.

The effect of high-frequency ultrasound on the growth of spheroids was also evaluated. Figure 2.13 shows a comparison of sham-exposed spheroids and ultrasound-exposed spheroids (at a diameter of approximately 400 μm) under typical imaging conditions. The results for both sets of conditions are not significantly different. The above data were reported by Berube et al. [11]. Overall there is no indication that high-frequency ultrasound has any significant biological effects when used at the intensity levels for normal imaging.

Future Development

The current implementation of ultrasound biomicroscopy is at a very early stage of development in which simple single element transducers with fixed foci are mechanically scanned to generate the image. Future developments in transducer technology may permit the development of linear array devices that would vastly increase the flexibility of the

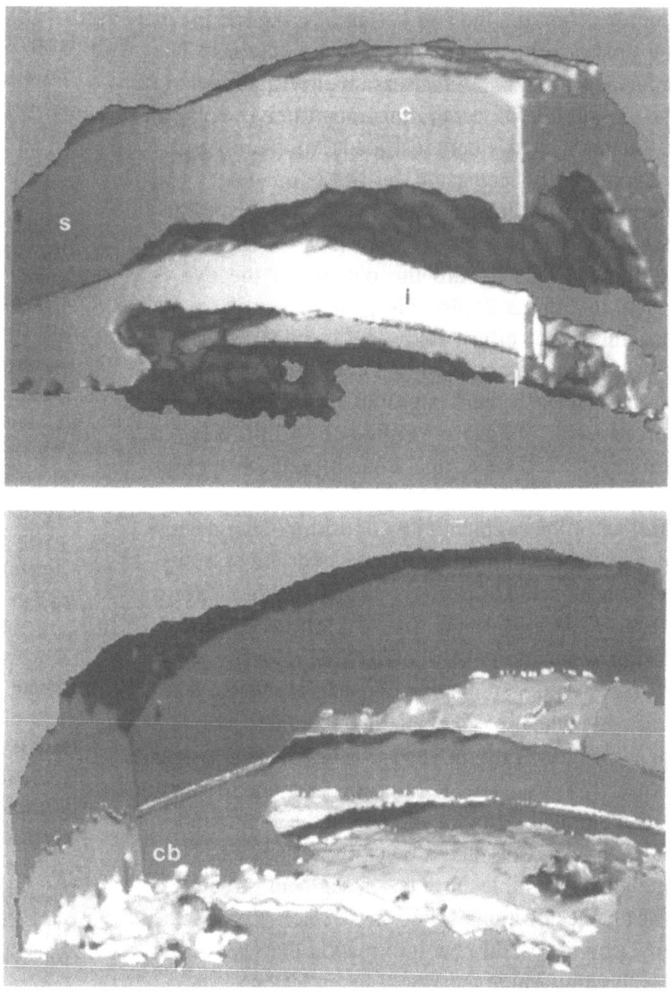

(a)

(b)

FIGURE 2.14. Two examples of early three-dimensional reconstructions of high-frequency ultrasound biomicroscopic images of the anterior segment. (**a**) view showing cornea (c), iris (i), sclera (s), and lens surface (l), with the pupilary space evident. (**b**) Rotated view showing additional detail of the ciliary body (cb).

scanner by increasing frame rates, widening the field of view, and eliminating the hazard of corneal abrasion caused by the moving probe. The addition of a second mechanical axis at right angles to the image plane of an ultrasound biomicroscopy system would permit the acquisition of serial sections over a region of tissue. Image sets acquired in this manner could be reconstructed into volumetric images [12]. Such visualization might provide a more accurate means of assessing changes in lesion volume and would clarify the relationship of abnormal tissues to adjacent healthy tissue. An example of an early three-dimensional study is shown in Figure 2.14. These views have been reconstructed from a set of 25 image planes spaced 200 μm apart using an experimental volume imaging ultrasound biomicroscope operating at 50 MHz. A time of approximately 5 seconds was needed to acquire the images. Figure 2.14a is a view of the anterior chamber showing the lens surface (l), the iris in (i), the cornea (c), and sclera (s) in tan shades. The anterior segment structures are well visualized and the possibility of generating quantitative volume estimates is clearly demonstrated. Another interesting possibility suggested by these images is the mapping of corneal topography following refractive surgery [13]. A second view looking from behind the lens toward the outside of the eye is given in Figure 2.14b. Here more detail in the structure of the ciliary body (cb) is evident.

Although the potential of three-dimensional imaging is clear, there are many problems to be solved. The images of Figure 2.14 still have a limited field of view, and smooth surfaces such as the cornea and lens display roughness that is an artefact of the segmentation algorithm. The design of new segmentation approaches that are less susceptible to speckle noise is clearly needed. Methods to suppress effects due to motion of the eye during acquisition also should be developed.

At conventional imaging frequencies interest is increasing in the use of Doppler ultrasound to map and quantify blood flow in normal and abnormal ocular tissues [14–16]. The addition of Doppler to ultrasound biomicroscopy should permit the identification of smaller vessels and slower flow than has been previously possible in anterior segment structures. The characterization of flow on the microscopic scale may provide useful new information that will aid in the classification of anterior segment lesions.

The possibility of combining ultrasound biomicroscopy with a therapeutic intervention offers some interesting opportunities. For example, if the focal region of a laser probe intersected the image plane of the ultrasound biomicroscope we should be able to observe the progress of a treatment in realtime permitting effective optimization and verification of the results.

References

1. Sherar MD, Foster FS. A 100 MHz PVDF ultrasound microscope with biological applications. *Acoustical Imaging* 1987;16:511–520.
2. Sherar MD, Starkoski BG, Taylor WB, Foster FS. A 100 MHz B-scan ultrasound backscatter microscope. *Ultrasonic Imaging* 1989;11:95–105.
3. Lockwood GR, Hunt JW, Foster FS. Design of protection circuitry for high frequency ultrasound systems. *IEEE Trans UFFC* 1991;38:48–55.
4. Foster FS, Pavlin CJ, Lockwood GR, Ryan LK, Harasiewicz KA, Berube LR, Rauth AM. Principles and applications of ultrasound backscatter microscopy. *IEEE Trans UFFC* 1993;40:608–617.
5. Sherar MD, Foster FS. The design and fabrication of high frequency poly(vinylidene fluoride) transducers. *Ultrasonic Imaging* 1989;11:75–94.
6. Brown LF. Ferroelectric Polymers: Current and future applications. *IEEE Ultrasonics Symposium Proceedings* 1992, pp. 539–545. IEEE, New York.
7. Pavlin CJ, Sherar MD, Foster FS. Subsurface ultrasound microscopic imaging of the intact eye. *Ophthalmology* 1990;97:244–250.
8. Coleman DJ, Dallow RL, Smith ME. Immersion ultrasonography: Simultaneous A and B scan. *Int Ophthalmol Clin* 1979;19:67–103.
9. Pavlin CJ, Harasiewicz KA, Sherar MD, Foster FS. Clinical use of ultrasound biomicroscopy. *Ophthalmology* 1991;98:287–295.
10. Lizzi FL, Elbaum ME. Clinical spectrum analysis techniques for tissue characterization II. National Bureau of Standards Special Publication #525 1980:111–119.
11. Berube LR, Harasiewicz KA, Foster FS, Dobrowski E, Sherar MD, Rauth AM. Use of a high frequency ultrasound microscope to image the action of 2-nitroimidazoles in multi cellular spheroids. *Brit J Cancer* 1992;65:633–640.
12. Coleman DJ, Woods S, Rondeau MJ, Silverman RH. Ophthalmic ultrasonography. *Radiol Clin North Am* 1992;30:1105–1114.
13. Reinstein DZ, Silverman RH, Trokel SL, Coleman

DJ. Corneal pachymetric topography. *Ophthalmology* (in press).
14. Canning CR, Restori M. Doppler ultrasound studies of the ophthalmic artery. *Eye* 1988;2:92–95.
15. Guthoff RF, Berger RW, Winkler P, Helmke K, Chumbley LC. Doppler ultrasonography of the ophthalmic and central retinal vessels. *Arch Ophthalmol* 1991;109:532–536.
16. Lieb WE, Cohen SM, Merton DA, Shields JA, Michell DG, Goldberg BB. Color doppler imaging of the eye and orbit. Technique and normal vascular anatomy. *Arch Ophthalmol* 1991;109:527–531.

3
Examination Techniques

The ultrasound biomicroscopic examination has many similarities to other types of B-scan ultrasound examinations. The technique of placing the transducer opposite the area of interest and using fine manipulations of the probe with reference to the screen image to produce optimal ultrasonic sections is similar to that used with conventional ultrasound. The main differences are the presence of a moving transducer without a covering membrane, the necessity for a water bath technique, the finer movements required, and a relatively short working distance.

Patient Preparation

It is important to explain the elements of the procedure to the patient. The examination generally produces minimal discomfort and does not take long. The possibility of some residual transient irritation from the eye cup, solution, or inadvertent corneal contact should be discussed.

Positioning the Patient

The patient is usually examined in a supine position looking up at the ceiling. The patient can be lying on any type of bed or stretcher that allows the operator to sit at the head of the bed and approach the eye at a comfortable level. We use a stretcher that changes from the sitting position to the lying position, which makes patient access simple, including those with limited mobility.

Fixation Device

Some form of fixation device that the patient can look at with the eye not being examined is helpful because this produces stability in the eye being examined. It is difficult for patients to hold their eye in one position for long without fixation, especially in extremes of gaze. A ceiling target or a fixation device on a flexible arm may be used.

Positioning Machine Controls and the Monitor

The monitor should be placed at a comfortable height that can be observed by the operator without undue contortion. The monitor can be on the machine itself located to the side of the patient, or moved from the machine to a shelf suitable for good visibility. The hand controller should be in an easily accessible position. Figure 3.1 shows a patient being examined with good visibility of the monitor and easy access to the controls. Adjustments to scanning parameters can be made with the left hand while controlling the probe with the right hand. Generally one would lift the scanning head from the eye cup for safety reasons if any major adjustments were to be made. It is useful to have the controls preset to optimal positions so that intra-examination adjustments can be kept to a minimum. The foot pedal should be in a comfortable position.

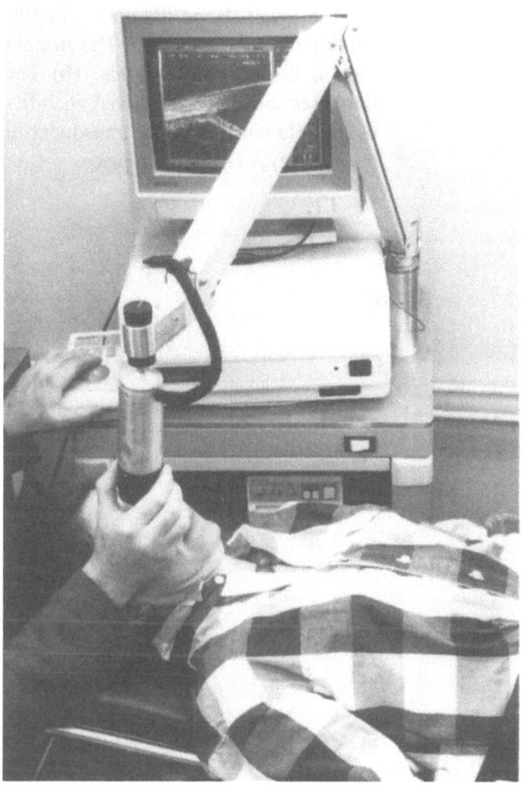

FIGURE 3.1. Patient being examined by ultrasound biomicroscopy. The patient is lying down with the examiner seated behind the patient's head. The monitor is in an easily observed position, and the hand controller is accessible to the left of the instrument.

Creating a Fluid Standoff

Eye Cups

The authors, in conjunction with K. Harasiewicz, P.Eng, have designed a series of eye cups that make setup simple and allow for a more rapid completion to the examination [1]. A series of these eye cups are illustrated in Figure 3.2. They are similar to eye cups used for A-scan biometry [2] with a smooth flanged inferior margin that fits between the lids and holds them open. They differ from conventional biometry eye cups by the presence of a flared superior opening and somewhat shallower height. Figures 3.3a and b show a closer view of the details of cup construction. The cups do not have to be as high as conventional biometry cups because of the relatively short working distance. The flared opening allows the operator a better view of the position of the transducer in relation to the eye and allows improved mobility. These cups come in different diameters. We find that cups with diameters of 24 and 22 mm are suitable for virtually all adult eyes. Smaller diameters may be necessary for pediatric use. Figure 3.3c shows an eye cup in place on the patient's eye.

Figure 3.4 shows the technique for placing one of these eye cups in the eye. Topical anesthetic is instilled (Figure 3.4a). The superior lip of the eye cup is placed under the upper lid with the patient looking down (Figure 3.4b). Maintaining upward pressure on the eye cup to hold it in place under the upper lid, the lower lid is drawn down with a finger and placed over the inferior lip. Occasionally the use of a tissue is helpful to grip the lower lid and place it in position. The eye cup is then filled with fluid (Figure 3.4c), and the examination is begun (Figure 3.4d).

Eye cups can be used for most intraocular structures, and the conjunctiva. They can also be used for adnexal structures by placing the cup around the structure to be examined. If the base of the region to be examined is too irregular to hold fluid, a water bath made with a surgical drape can be used.

Fluid Coupling Medium

Fluid is required to produce a coupling medium between the transducer and the eye. Ultrasound traverses air very poorly. The fluid used should

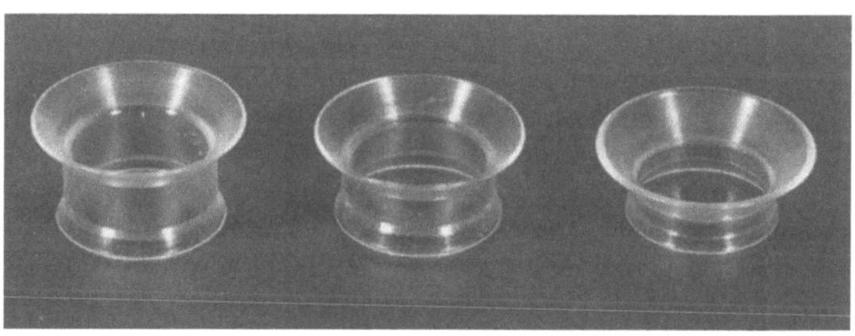

FIGURE 3.2. Eye cups for ultrasound biomicroscopy designed by the authors in conjunction with K. Harasiewicz, P.Eng.

FIGURE 3.3. Details of eye cup design. **(a)** The lower flange fits under the lids holding the cup on the eye. The straight section fits between the lids. **(b)** The flared section allows improved visibility of the relationship of the transducer to the eye. **(c)** An eye cup in place.

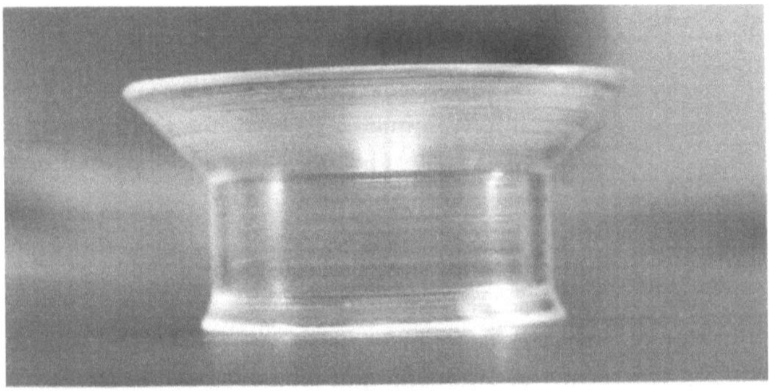

(a)

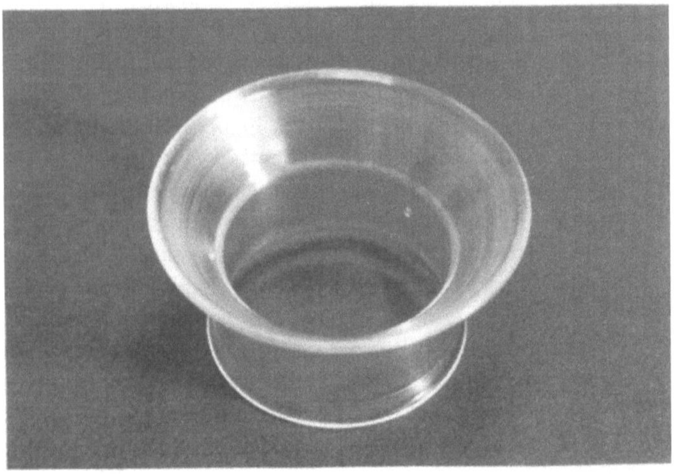

(b)

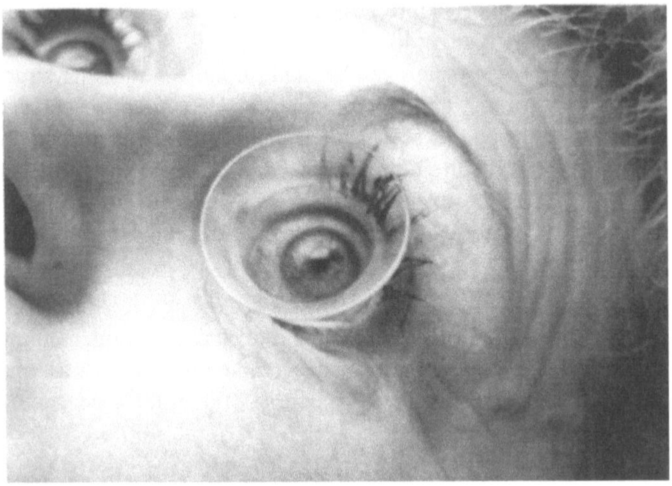

(c)

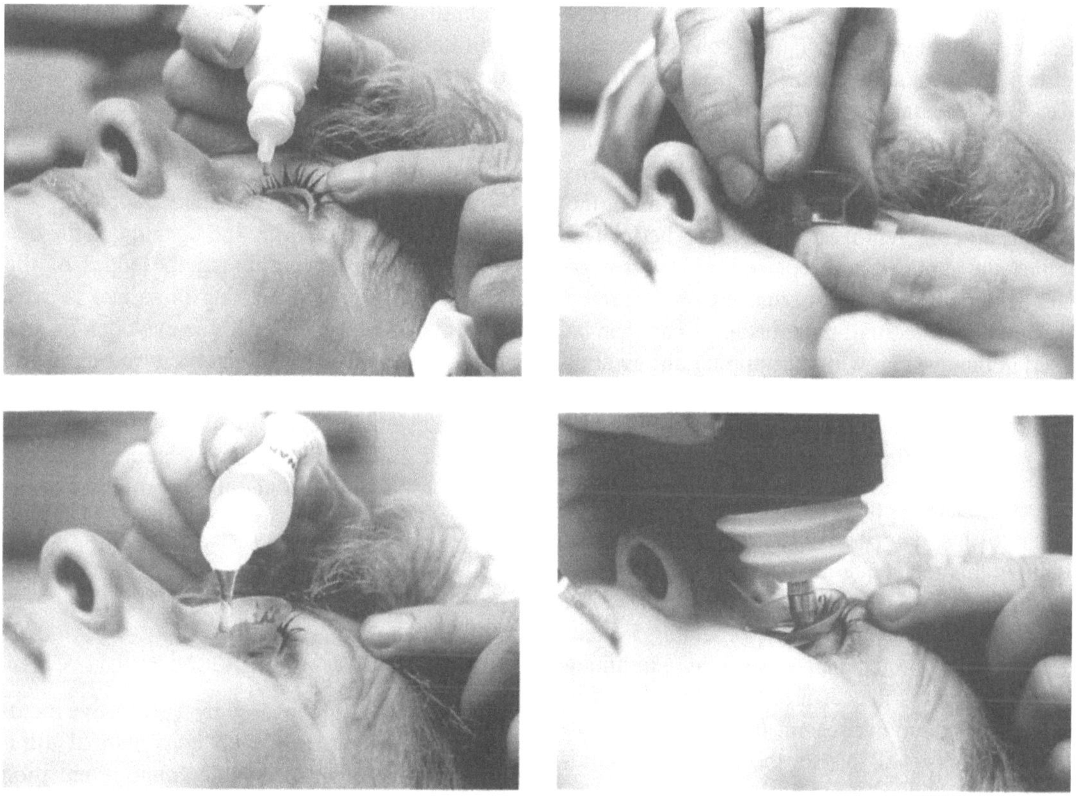

(a) (b) (c) (d)

FIGURE 3.4. Preparing the fluid standoff. **(a)** Local anesthetic is instilled in the eye. **(b)** The eye cup is placed in position following instillation of local anesthetic. The lip of the cup is placed under the superior lid, and the lower eyelid drawn down and placed over the lip interiorly. **(c)** Methyl cellulose is poured into the cup from a dropper bottle with the tip removed. **(d)** The transducer tip is placed in the fluid opposite the pathology of interest after being cleared of bubbles.

have low sound attenuation, be safe for use on the eye for short periods of time, and have a certain degree of viscosity to prevent rapid fluid loss as the cup is moved around to examine different parts of the globe. We use 1 to 2.5% methyl cellulose for the majority of examinations. Methyl cellulose has minimal sound attenuation, and has sufficient viscosity to prevent fluid loss during examination. Lower viscosity methyl cellulose is less irritating, but escapes more easily. Both viscosities are available as commercial preparations. Saline can be used to fill the cup after using a small amount of 2.5% methyl cellulose to seal the base as suggested by C. Tello and colleagues. Leakage is more common using this technique.

Removing Air Bubbles

Sound travels very poorly through air. Air bubbles in the fluid or on the tip of the transducer can produce attenuation of sound. If a commercial preparation of methyl cellulose in a squeeze bottle is being used, it is helpful to remove the small bore top before pouring, as shown in Figure 3.4c. The subsequent lack of turbulence decreases air bubble formation. Larger air bubbles that find their way into the solution can be removed with a cotton swab.

Air bubbles on the tip of the transducer will produce unacceptable sound attenuation. Because the transducer surface is concave (required for proper ultrasound focusing), dipping the tip into the fluid without prior preparation will frequently produce a bubble caught in this concave space. Figure 3.5 shows a bubble on the tip of the transducer. It is necessary to remove these bubbles prior to examination by immersing the tip in water and massaging the tip very gently with a bent swab. Figures 3.6a and b show a bubble on the tip of the transducer being removed in a water bath. The bubbles are removed and replaced with a drop of water held in place by surface tension, as illustrated in Figure 3.7. The tip of the transducer can then be placed in the eye cup without trapping air. Examination can then proceed.

Using a Water Bath

Our early cases were performed in a water bath similar to that described by Coleman et al. [3]. Although this technique requires a greater amount of equipment and takes somewhat longer to set up, it is an effective method and is something we still use in special circumstances such as examining adnexal structures that do not lend themselves to placing an eye cup over them. It is helpful to have the components available for these special circumstances. Material required includes topical anesthetic, colloidon to place around the eye to produce a watertight seal, sterile normal saline, a small wire speculum, an operating room drape with a small central hole, a ringlike structure to hold the edges of the drape up, and clips to clip the edges of the drape to the ring. The ring can be a specific design for this purpose or a retort holder of adequate size obtained from the chemistry lab. The technique consists of instilling local anesthetic, applying colloidon to the skin, sticking the opening of the eye drape around the eye, clipping the edges of the drape to the ring, and pouring in saline. A wire speculum can be used to hold the eye open if indicated, or relevant adnexal pathology brought into the field by pressure from a cotton swab. Figure 3.8 shows an eye being examined in a water bath with one of our early probes. This technique produces optimal probe mobility, and the opportunity to examine adnexal structures with an irregular base such as the lid margin.

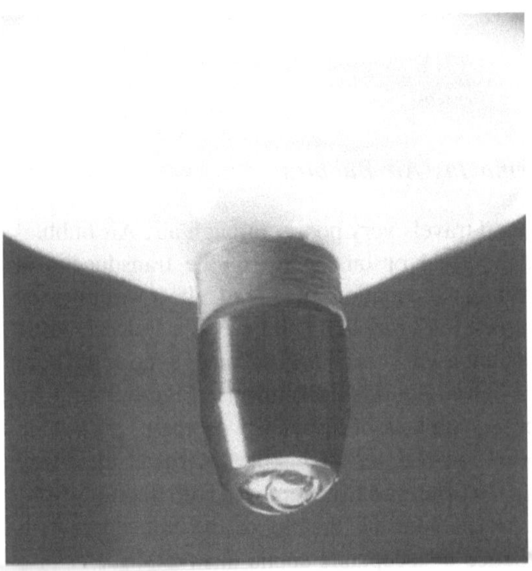

FIGURE 3.5. Tip of the concave transducer with an air bubble present.

Using a Protective Contact Lens

The transducer is not covered by a protective membrane such as that used with conventional ultrasound because of unacceptable sound attenuation from the membrane. The transducer is moving at a rate of 8 passes per second. Although the edges of the transducer are smooth, contact with the cornea could produce a corneal abrasion. An extra margin of safety is provided by the use of a soft contact lens on the cornea prior to examination to provide a barrier between the transducer and the cornea. A high water content disposable soft contact lens (Figure 3.9) produces the least attenuation. Figure 3.10 shows an image with a contact lens in place. Attenuation of sound by the lens is modest, but still present. We have estimated a sound attenuation of between 20% and 30% in our laboratory studies. An interesting caveat is that examination of deep structures requires the transducer to be placed very close to the cornea and deeper structures are most likely to suffer minor quality degradation from this attenuation. Tello and colleagues have described a modification of our eye cup that incorporates a contact lens attached to the base. This could be useful in special circumstances, but presents a difficult sterilization problem. We currently do not use a contact lens for the majority of our examinations, but rely on precise control of the scanning head with reference to the screen image. We do,

FIGURE 3.6. Removing air bubbles from the transducer. **(a)** The tip of the transducer is immersed in water and gently wiped with the tip of a swab. **(b)** An air bubble being pushed off the edge of the transducer by the tip of the swab.

(a)
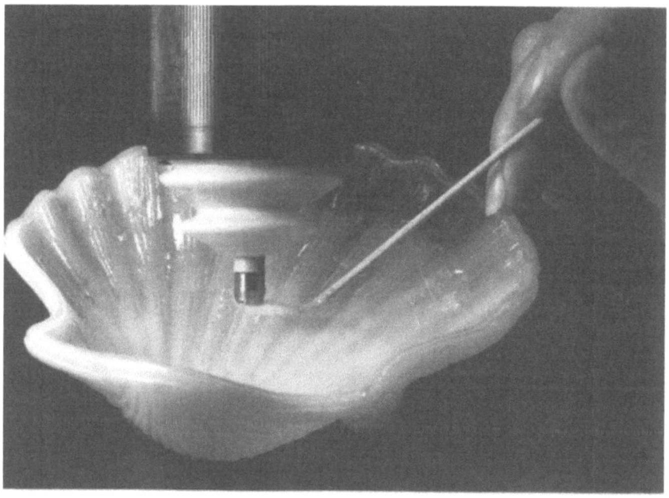

(b)
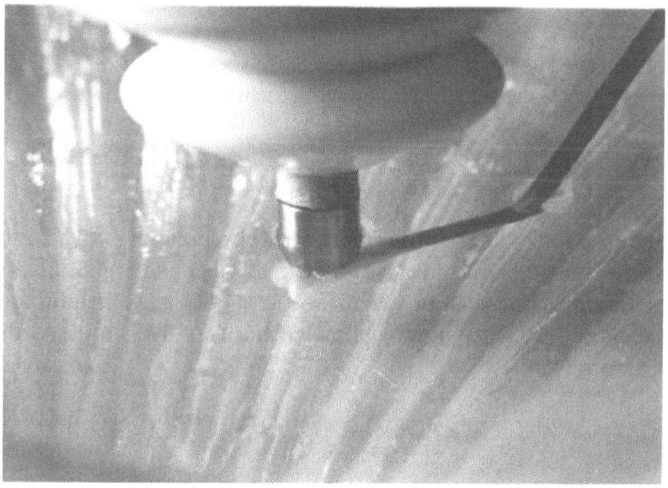

however, recommend a contact lens for those operators who are learning the technique, and for special circumstances. In practice we have found corneal contact to be extremely rare when examination is performed by an experienced operator.

Examination of the Eye

Examination Procedure

After the patient has been set up with the proper fluid bath and the transducer cleared of bubbles, the examination is begun. It is important that the patient and the operator are comfortable. The patient must be lying down facing the ceiling with the head supported by a headrest.

The articulated arm that supports the probe should be checked to make sure it is stable. It should be easily movable, but when released it should remain stable or rise slightly. We originally added the articulated arm to aid the operator in controlling the weight of the scanning head, and have found that it is absolutely critical in preventing inadvertent corneal touch. If attention is diverted from the examination for any reason, the probe should be removed from the water bath. It is helpful to have scanning parameters preset as much as possible to minimize the need to set them during the examination.

The operator is usually seated behind the patient's head with one hand resting on the patient's forehead for stability. The small indentation in the scanning head allows one to place a finger or

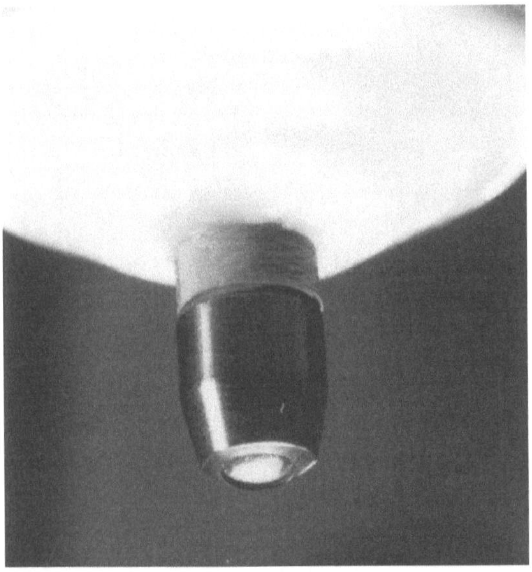

FIGURE 3.7. The tip of the transducer contains a bubble-free drop of water held in place by surface tension.

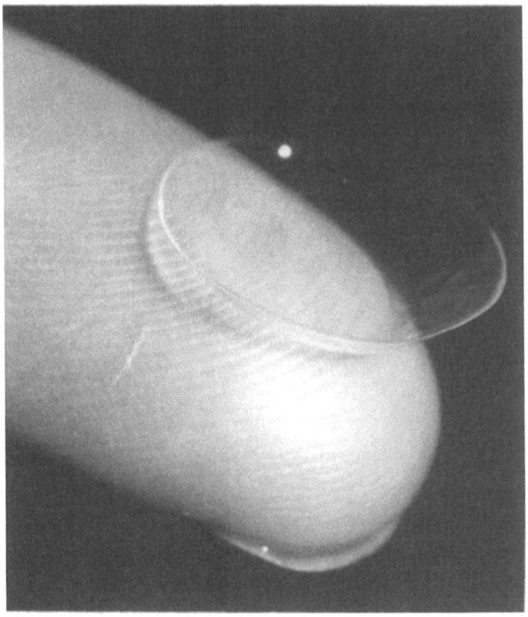

FIGURE 3.9. A high water content disposable contact lens can be placed on the eye prior to examination.

thumb in it to hold the probe more securely (Figure 3.11). The probe is held close to the transducer end to improve fine control. Figure 3.12 shows the hand position that allows optimal control of the scanning head.

The transducer is placed in the water bath opposite the area of interest and close to the eye. It is helpful to have the patient look away from the site of the pathology to bring the pathological area into an easily examined position (Figure 3.13). The op-

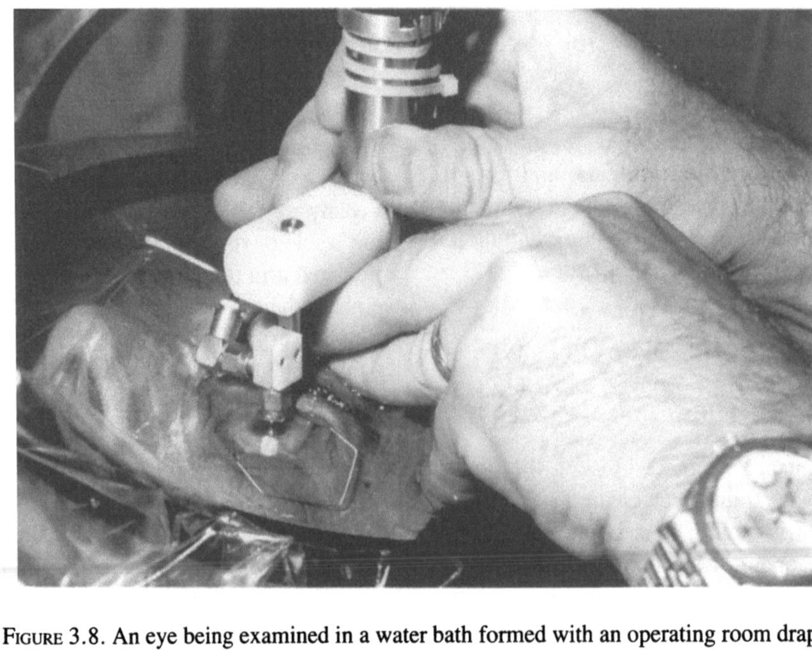

FIGURE 3.8. An eye being examined in a water bath formed with an operating room drape.

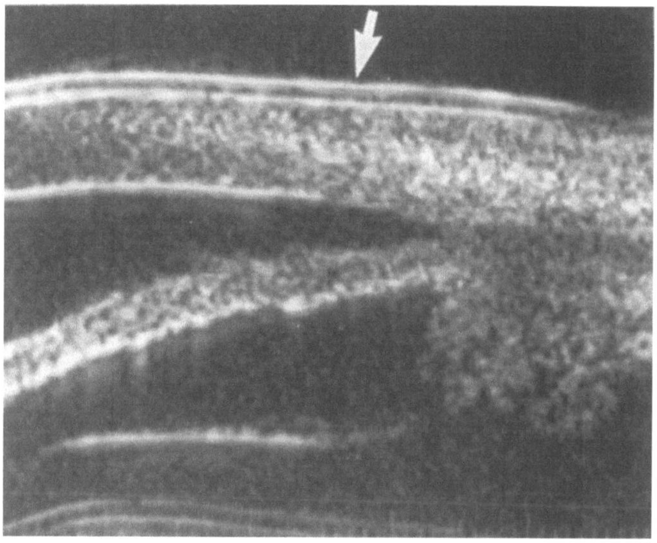

FIGURE 3.10. Ultrasound biomicroscopic image shows the contact lens on the surface of the eye (arrow). The underlying image is reasonably good with slight sound attenuation.

erator's attention is then turned to the screen and further fine adjustments are made in reference to the screen image. The cornea can generally be visualized on the top of the screen when examining the globe. It is important to be aware of the corneal position to avoid inadvertent abrasion. We tend to set the focal zone of the transducer near the bottom third of the screen so that deeper pathology can be in optimal focus while the corneal image is still on the screen. Further information on these adjustments can be found in the section on machine controls.

Producing Optimal Images

The best images are obtained in any ultrasound examination when the ultrasound beam is perpendicular to the structures being examined. This orientation produces the greatest return of reflected sound to the transducer. This is especially critical in the measurement of intraocular structures, because obliquity will make measurement more difficult both from the standpoint of defining clear endpoints and from the distortion of true distance that occurs with an oblique section. Perpendicularity can be accomplished by first lining the probe up as perpendicularly as possible to the area being examined by observing the probe and eye from the side. Subsequently, perpendicularity is produced by performing subtle probe movements until the screen

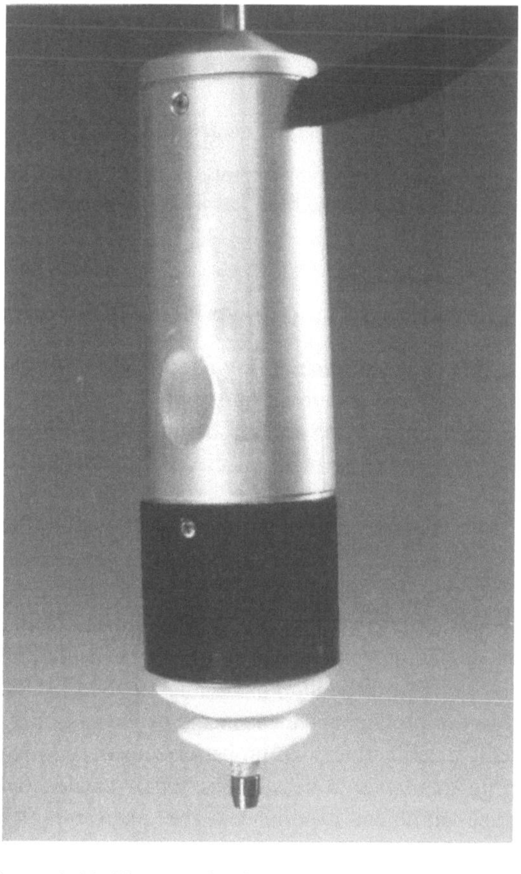

FIGURE 3.11. The scanning head of the commercial scanner. The small indentation on the side allows one to hold the probe more securely.

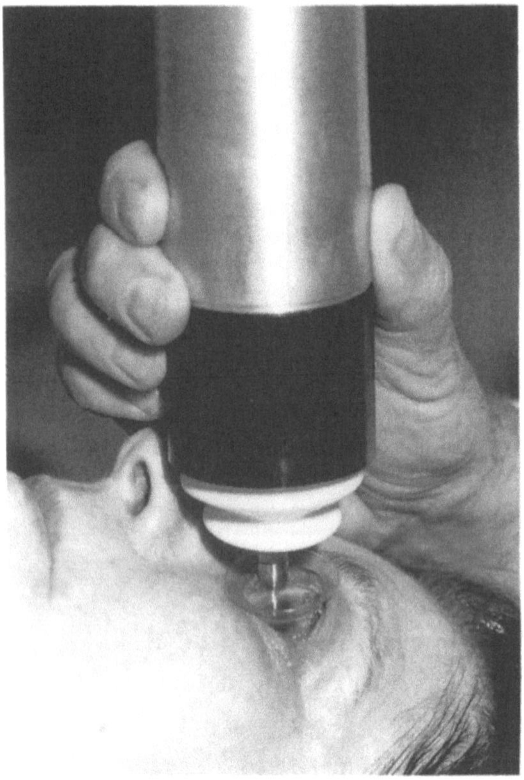

FIGURE 3.12. The transducer probe is held close to the transducer end with the hand resting on the forehead to improve control.

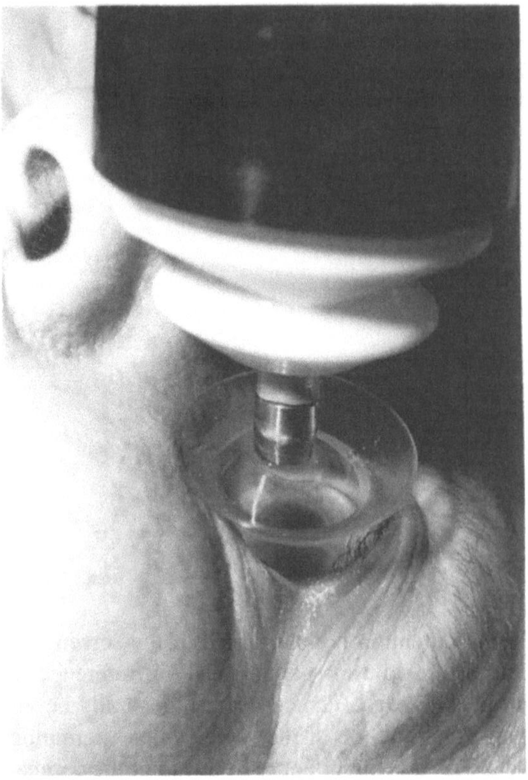

FIGURE 3.13. The transducer is placed in the water bath opposite the region to be examined under direct visualization. It is often helpful to have the patient look away from the site of the pathology to bring the desired region into an easily approached position.

images of the surfaces being examined are bright and clear. Images are brightest when the probe is perpendicular to the surface being examined and reflected sound is returned directly to the transducer.

The number of possibilities in orienting the probe is large. The probe can be moved in a vertical direction, translated in a horizontal direction, tilted, or rotated. These adjustments depend on exactly what information one is seeking. In actual use it is not that difficult. Positioning is ruled by the object of producing a clear image of the pathology being examined and the probe movement required to do this tends to be subconsciously carried out given sufficient experience. The main rule for making fine probe movements is, "if the image is getting better, keep going; if it is getting worse, go the opposite way." This rule also applies to accomodation and life.

Probe Orientation Versus Screen Appearance

It is helpful when examining the anterior segment to use a set technique that allows designation of the examination site for future reproducibility, and easier comparison of serial examinations of ocular disease.

Conventional ophthalmic B-scan ultrasound machines have a different screen orientation than the ultrasound biomicroscope. In conventional B-scan devices the front of the probe corresponds to the left side of the screen (i.e., pathology on the left side of the screen is closer to the probe). The probe has a mark that designates the plane of transducer movement. The two-dimensional section of the eye produced is displayed on the screen with the top of the screen coinciding with the mark on the probe. Thus if the probe is held with the mark toward the top of the globe, the top of the screen image shows pathology in the superior aspect of the globe. Any oblique section of the globe is done with the mark in a superior position. By convention if the probe is held directly horizontally, the mark is placed to the nasal side, making the top of the screen nasal and the bottom of the screen temporal. Other conventions exist including those for longitudinal sections, which orient the probe mark (top of screen) toward a certain clock hour where the pathology is located [5].

In ultrasound biomicroscopy, the relationship of the screen image to the probe position is different from conventional ophthalmic B-scan. In ultrasound biomicroscopy the front of the transducer corresponds to the top of the screen. Pathology displayed at the top of the screen is thus closer to the probe. As the probe is lowered into the water bath to produce an image of the globe, one can see an image of the cornea on the screen and use this corneal image to control the proximity of the probe to the eye. There is a mark on the probe that indicates the plane of the scanning motion. This mark coincides with the left side of the screen. Thus if the probe is held with the mark oriented toward the temporal aspect of the eye, the left side of the screen would display pathology located in the temporal side of the globe. Figure 3.14 shows these relationships in a diagrammatic form.

Examination Conventions

Because ultrasound biomicroscopy is a relatively new field and uses different image orientation as outlined above, a direct transfer of examination conventions from conventional B-scan ultrasound is not possible. It is not absolutely essential to have a set routine for orientation of the probe. Some gen-

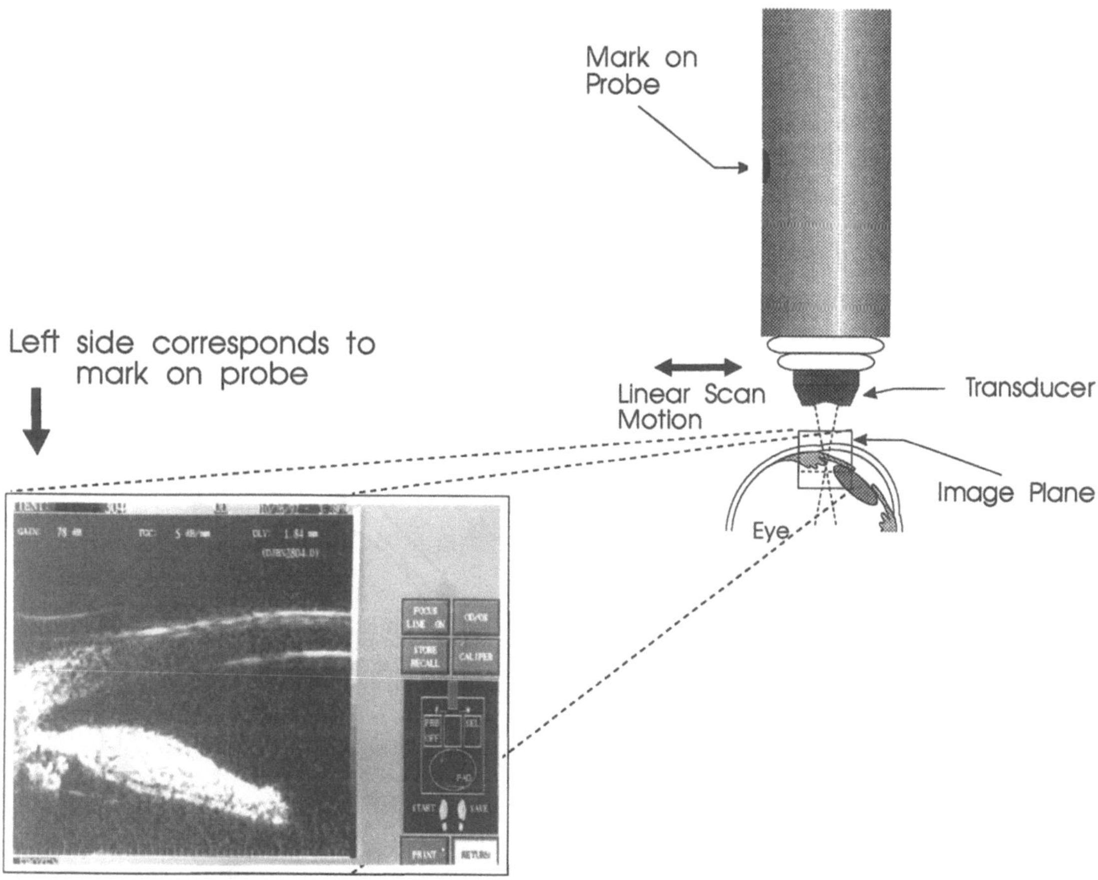

FIGURE 3.14. Probe orientation in relation to screen orientation. The superior aspect of the image correlates to the face of the transducer. The left side of the screen image correlates to the marker on the probe.

eral rules are helpful, however, from the standpoint of reproducibility on serial examinations. For example, if one is imaging an iris tumor, and the first set of images has the iris root on the left, it is helpful when comparing subsequent images to have them in the same orientation. For this reason we present here a method of accomplishing this goal.

Radial Sections of the Globe

The transducer in an ultrasound biomicroscope moves in a linear fashion, creating a two-dimensional cross section of the eye on the screen. The side of the probe contains a marker that designates the left side of the image. If the probe is placed over the limbus in a radial fashion, with the marker on the scleral side, the left side of the picture on the screen would correspond to the scleral side and the right side of the screen would correspond to the corneal side. This orientation is one of the most common sections taken with the ultrasound biomicroscope.

The technique we use for designating probe position with this type of section is as follows. We always place the marker on the probe toward the outer (scleral) side when doing a radial section of the globe (Figure 3.15). The probe position is designated in clock hours.

Transverse Sections of the Globe

If the probe is not radially oriented other methods of designating probe position must be used. These sections would most commonly be transverse, at 90° to the radial section. As stated above, for transverse sections using conventional B-scan, the convention is to have the probe marker superior for all transverse sections with the exception of the totally horizontal plane. Because of the different orientation of the screen image in ultrasound biomicroscopy this technique is not quite as inherently logical. We prefer to place the probe marker on the counterclockwise side, which would allow reproducible orientation in this type of section. Again the clock hour can be used to designate the center of the transducer position. This technique is illustrated in Figure 3.16. The convention for transverse sections is not as important as that for radial sections, but can be useful when one is defining the lateral extent of lesions.

These conventions apply to examination of the globe only and may not apply in every situation. Many variations can exist in which the probe position that produces the best image and provides the most easily performed examination is probably the best one.

The Art of Ultrasound Examination

Eye ultrasound differs from other imaging methods such as X-ray, computed tomographic (CT) scanning, and magnetic resonance imaging (MRI) by virtue of the intimate involvement of the operator in producing and interpreting images simulta-

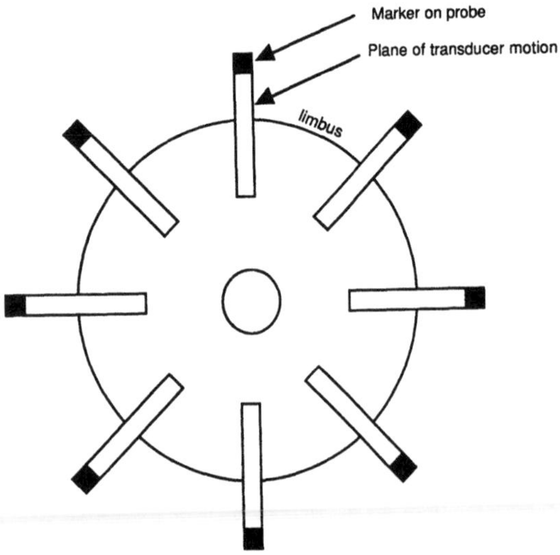

FIGURE 3.15. Radial sections of the globe are performed with the probe marker on the scleral side.

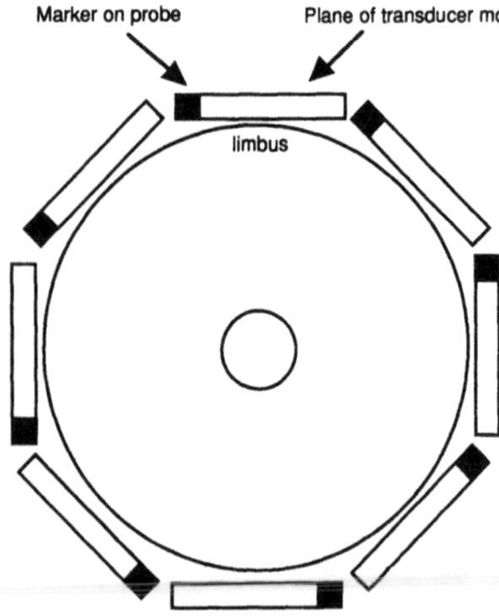

FIGURE 3.16. Transverse sections of the globe are performed with the probe marker on the counterclockwise side.

neously. The ultrasound operator is constantly making fine adjustments to aim the beam accurately and produce sections that show pathological changes clearly. This requires a knowledgeable observer, experience, and a certain amount of coordination. A simple twist of the wrist can produce a very different appearance of an image. The art lies in producing the best image that tells the story of the pathological process in the clearest fashion. The skill with which the examination is carried out is also important from the standpoint of reproducibility. It is impossible to rely on the accuracy of serial quantitative measurements unless the operator is capable of accurately reproducing sections. Ultrasound examination is an art, but an art that everyone is capable of learning.

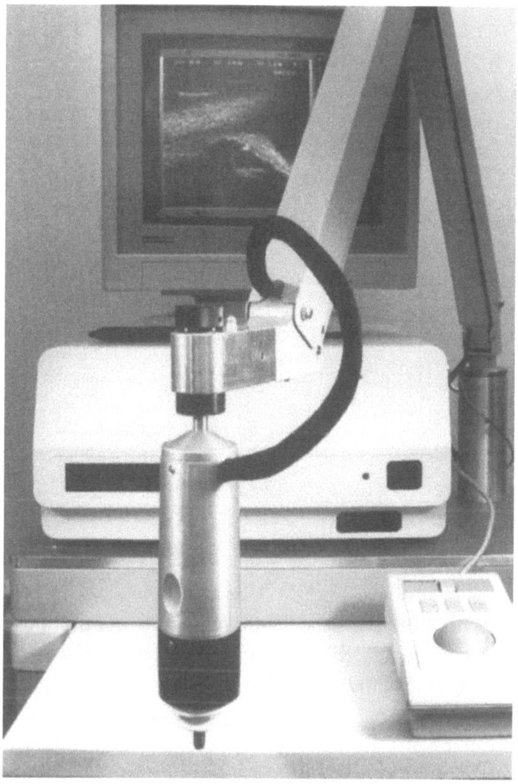

FIGURE 3.17. The commercial scanner designed by Zeiss-Humphrey in cooperation with the authors.

Use of the Commercial Scanner

Because the only commercial instrument available at the time of writing is that designed by Zeiss-Humphrey Inc. (San Leandro, CA) in conjunction with the authors (Figure 3.17), it seems appropriate to relate some of our experience in working with this scanner. This instrument is currently somewhat limited as to available frequencies, and runs at approximately 50 MHz. Other frequencies will most likely be available in the future. The 50 MHz frequency offers a reasonable compromise between resolution and penetration that works very well for general diagnostic use.

We will not attempt to recreate a user manual, but rather give our advice regarding control settings that we find effective, and give our rationale for choosing them. Advice regarding examination techniques has been given above, and measurement techniques will be dealt with in the following section.

Controlling Devices

The first requirement is to become familiar with the control system. Unlike most ultrasound instruments that present us with a panel of knobs and switches, this machine is entirely software controlled using a graphical user interface. This has advantages and disadvantages. On the positive side, it allows the controls to be moved to a comfortable position within easy reach, and allows a wide range of parameters to be controlled from one location. On the negative side, the mixed nature of the controlling devices (i.e., a trackball, thumbwheel, foot pedal, and light pen) can be a bit confusing at first. Do not be surprised if you try to do something with the light pen, and find you need the trackball instead. Onscreen guidance is present, but some experience is required to develop proficiency. The golden rule of ultrasound equipment is in effect, i.e., find the settings that produce the best results and do not move them unless you have to. It is hoped that this section will aid in this process.

The Hand Controller

The hand controller is shown in Figure 3.18a. The presence of a trackball, thumbwheel, and three buttons makes for a large number of possibilities. The first key is that the trackball is used to choose most options and the right button is used to select them. It is necessary to become familiar with the other

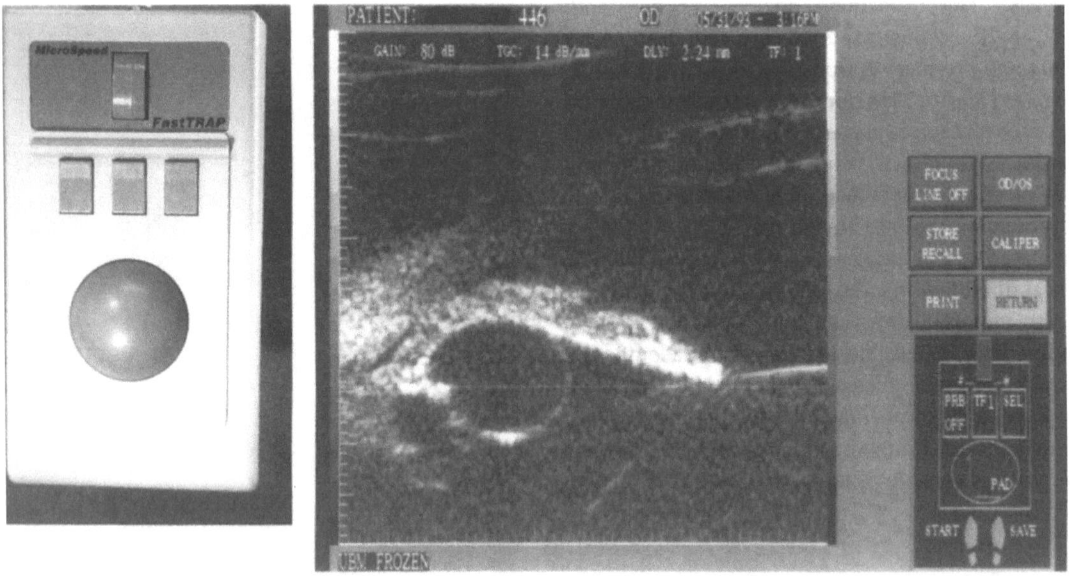

(a) (b)

FIGURE 3.18. (a) The hand controller used to control most scanner functions. (b) A view of the operating screen. The right side of the screen displays choices and supplies prompts that delineate which element of the hand controller performs a specific function at any given time.

controls by experience and reference to the screen prompts. The right side of the screen contains a graphic representation of the hand and foot controller (Figure 3.18b), which prompts the user as to the various options that can be chosen using these devices.

The Light Pen

A light pen is used to enter patient information on the displayed keyboard. This is all it does and touching other controls with the light pen will not produce a response.

Foot Switch

The foot switch (Figure 3.19) is easily operated. The left button toggles between running mode and a frozen image, and the right side saves the image.

The Operating Screen

When in the imaging mode the image display section of the screen is on the left and consists of a square area with rules on the side (Figure 3.20). The rules are set as a millimeter scale using a speed of sound in tissue of 1530 m/s to convert time to distance measurement. The area encompassed by the image display section represents 5 mm × 5 mm. Current settings are displayed on the top of this area.

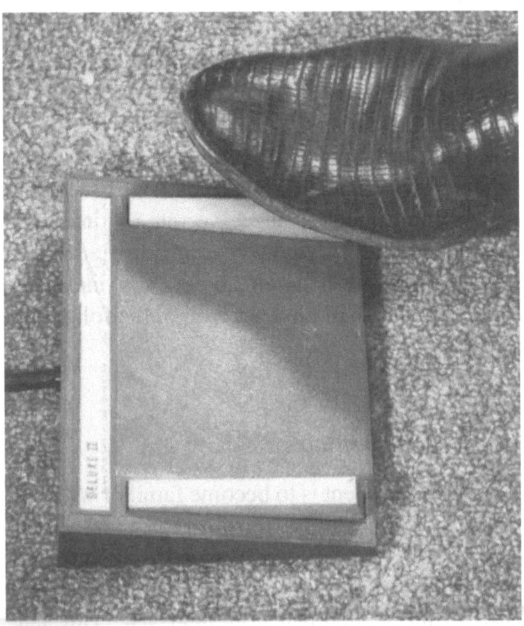

FIGURE 3.19. The foot switch controls image freezing and storage.

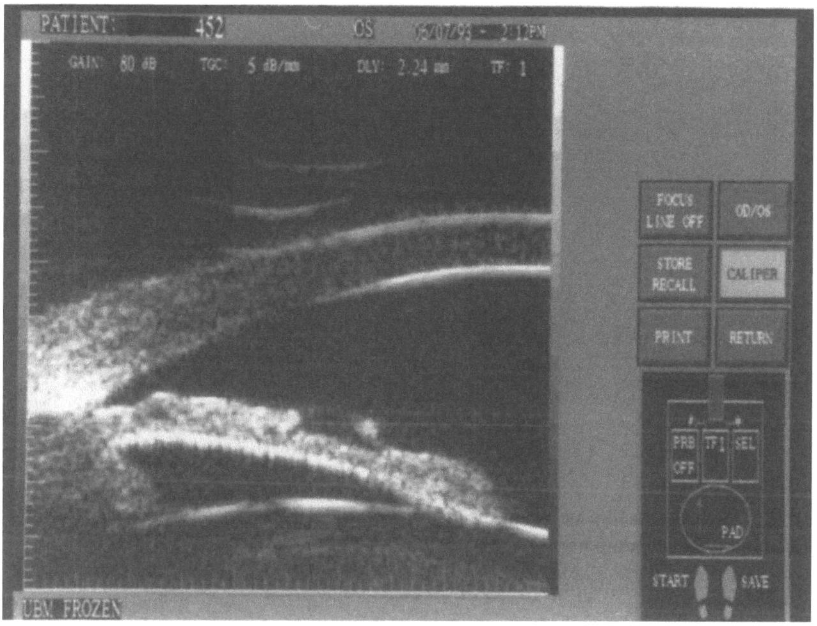

FIGURE 3.20. The imaging part of the operating screen on the left is square and represents an area 5 mm × 5 mm. Rules in millimeters are present on the margins. Current control settings are displayed at the top of the screen.

Preferred Settings

System Configuration

The basic system configuration settings can be accessed from the opening screen. Make sure settings conform to those recommended in the manual. After these are set, no further adjustment should be required.

Focal Zone and Delay

The instrument displays a line representing the focal point of the transducer that can be toggled on and off . Objects displayed near this line will have the best resolution. The position of this line can only be set with the instrument running and is controlled by the delay setting. The term *delay* refers to the time between the pulsing of the transducer and the acquisition of image information. Physically this represents the distance between the transducer and the top of the displayed image. This is not to be confused with the focal line displayed on the screen. Figure 3.21 graphically represents these relationships. We like to set the focal line to the "on" position and place it about 2 mm from the bottom of the screen. When examining a deeper structure this generally allows the corneal image to be displayed simultaneously, allowing the operator to be aware of its position at all times. The focal line is 5.5 mm from the tip of the transducer usually used. Thus, if an observed structure is located 3 mm from the top of the screen at the focal line, and the cornea is visible just at the top of the screen, the transducer would be 2.5 mm from the corneal surface.

Transfer Functions (TF)

These alter the relative brightness of echoes displayed on the screen. We generally use the default setting (TF1)

Time Gain Control

The time gain control allows us to compensate for attenuation of ultrasound in the tissue by increasing the amplification of the signal with time. Signals originating from deep structures that otherwise would be of low magnitude will receive increased amplification. We usually place this setting at 5 dB/mm.

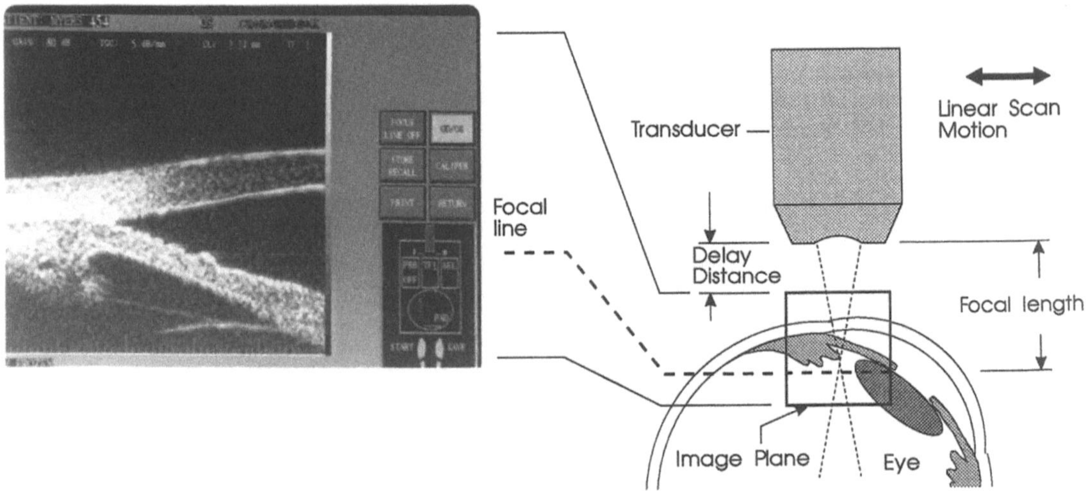

FIGURE 3.21. The relationship between the delay, the focal zone of the transducer, and the screen representation of these parameters.

Gain

Gain refers to the base level of amplification. We generally use 80 dB as our starting point. This can be increased to bring out particularly low level echoes, or decreased to make particularly reflective objects such as foreign bodies stand out from surrounding tissue.

Image Storage and Retrieval

The storage requirements for ultrasound biomicroscopy are governed by a similar rule to that which applies to computers: it is impossible to have too much. Ordinary hard drives can be filled extremely quickly, and even though images can be downloaded to floppy diskettes, this will create a painful archiving and retrieval problem. The images can be printed to an optical printer allowing hard copy but these images will not have the quality one might desire for publication or other uses. High-capacity optical drives with removable media are a reasonable solution. We use a very-high-capacity optical drive to store images. We also use a video capture board in a Macintosh computer (Apple Computer, Cupertino, CA) to capture images, allowing a typical image to become a permanent part of the patient's record. We have written a hypercard (Claris Corporation, Santa Clara, CA) based database that allows an image to pop up on the patient's record at the touch of a button. Figure 3.22 shows a typical screen with a representative image displayed. Copies of this database are available to anyone who wishes to send us a diskette.

Measurement Techniques

Optimizing Measurement Accuracy

Ultrasound biomicroscopy provides increased axial and lateral resolution by a factor of 5 to 10 compared to conventional ultrasound. The basis of this improvement is related to both the frequency and the degree of focusing of the transducers, as outlined in Chapters 1 and 2. Ultrasound biomicroscopy is capable of measuring a large number of structures that could not previously be measured in the living eye. Some of these structures cannot be imaged at all with conventional ultrasound, such as the zonule, and some structures cannot be resolved with sufficient accuracy to produce meaningful measurements, such as the iris and ciliary body. To measure a structure one must be capable of distinguishing it from adjacent tissue. For example, the sclera cannot be distinguished from overlying and underlying tissue using conventional ultrasound. The increased resolution of ultrasound biomicroscopy allows the borders of structures such as the sclera to be defined. In structures that can be measured with conventional ultrasound such as anterior

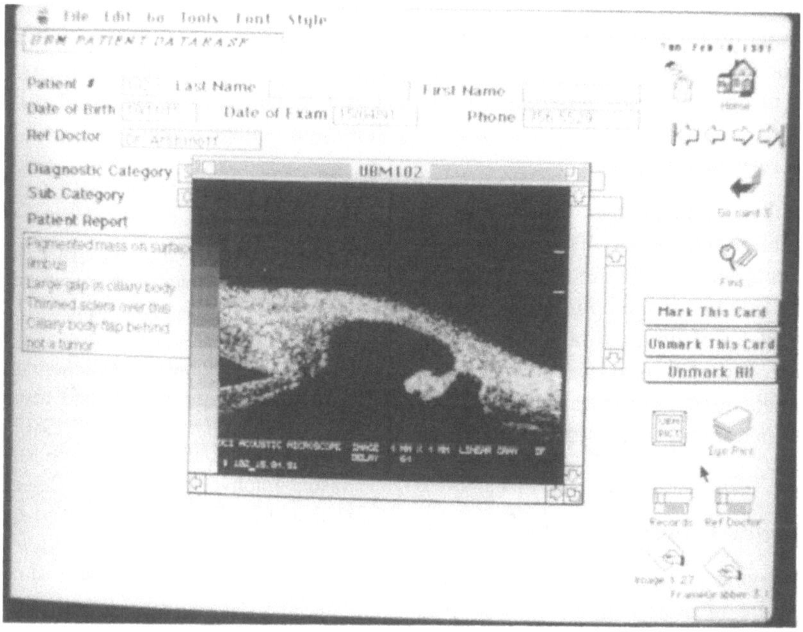

FIGURE 3.22. A database program that allows display of the patient's ultrasound biomicroscopic image as part of the patient record.

chamber depth, ultrasound biomicroscopy allows increased accuracy because of an improved ability to position the endpoints of the measurements. The section on normal intraocular structures contains a number of measuring techniques for anterior segment structures.

Speed of Sound in Tissue

For the measurements to be accurate, a knowledge of speed of sound in the tissues to be measured is required. All measurements in ultrasound basically consist of converting the time required for the sound to traverse the tissue and return to the transducer to distance using knowledge of the speed of sound in tissue. The speeds used in conventional ultrasound have been derived from a consensus based on numerous experimental observations. We have measured the speed of sound in ocular tissue at high frequencies using eye bank eyes [6]. Our results have been discussed in the chapter on basic physics and are outlined in Table 3.1.

The commercial version of the ultrasound biomicroscopic instrument uses a speed of 1530 m/s for all tissues. If one uses the internal measuring devices to measure a structure such as the sclera, which has a higher speed of sound, conversion is easily done by multiplying the measured distance (D_m) by a constant obtained by dividing the true speed of sound in the tissue in question by the speed of sound used by the machine. The formula for this would be as follows:

$$D = D_m \times (\text{true speed/speed used in machine})$$

For instance, a scleral measurement of 400 μm could be converted to the true distance presuming a speed in sclera of 1622 m/sec by the following calculation:

$$400 \times (1622/1530) = 424\ \mu\text{m}$$

Measurement Tools

Measurement of intraocular structures and distances between structures can be done in two ways. Measurements can be done using the integrated

TABLE 3.1. Measured speed of sound (m/s) in ocular structures using 60 MHz transducers.

Iris	1542
Ciliary body	1554
Cornea	1575
Sclera	1622

measurement tools in the instrument, or measurement can be done later by transferring the image to a computer and using an imaging program.

Using the Instrument Calipers

The commercial instrument has capabilities of measuring distances and angles. These are easily used on frozen images either at the time of examination or by bringing the image up from an internal storage device. If an external storage device that captures the video signal is used, these capabilities will not be available and a computer program will be required if measurement of stored images is desired.

Computer Imaging Programs

A number of imaging programs are available that allow measurement of stored images, as well as having various other capabilities such as histograms and image colorization. We have not found colorizing images to be particularly useful in diagnoses, but they do make pretty slides. Grayscale provides a continuous scale of sound intensity that is not present using color. We frequently use the program Image, which is a public domain program distributed by the National Institutes of Health. Using these programs to measure distances on images requires that the measuring tool be calibrated. This is done by using the rule that is present on the side of the image screen.

References

1. Pavlin CJ, Harasiewicz K, Foster FS. Ultrasound biomicroscopy of anterior segment structures in normal and glaucomatous eyes. *Am J Ophthalmol* 1992; 113:381–389.
2. Ossoinig KC. Standardized echography: Basic principles, clinical applications and results. Dallow RL, Ed. *Int Ophthalmol Clin* 1979;19:127–210.
3. Coleman DJ, Dallow RL, Smith ME. Immersion ultrasonography: Simultaneous A-scan and B-scan. Dallow RL, Ed. *Int Ophthalmol Clin* 1979;19:67–103.
4. Tello C, Potash S, Liebmann J, Ritch R. Soft contact lens modification of the ocular cup for high-resolution ultrasound biomicroscopy. *Ophth Surg* 1993;24: 563–564.
5. Byrne SF, Green RL. *Ultrasound of the Eye and Orbit*. 1992, pp. 21–27. Mosby-Year Book, St. Louis.
6. Ye SG, Harasiewicz KA, Pavlin CJ, Foster FS. Ultrasound characterization of ocular tissue in the frequency range from 50 MHz to 100 MHz. *IEEE Trans UFFC* (in press).

4
Ultrasound Biomicroscopic Anatomy of the Normal Eye and Adnexa

Before pathological conditions can be analyzed, it is necessary to have knowledge of the normal appearance of ocular anatomical structures as imaged by ultrasound biomicroscopy. It is important to emphasize that ultrasound biomicroscopy provides a view of subsurface structures in their normal relationships without the distortion that occurs with preparation of histological specimens. The resolution possible is similar to low-power light microscopy, but is not at a level that can differentiate individual cells. Because of the nature of the imaging modality (i.e., sound waves), some imaging features such as shadowing and backscatter patterns are unique to ultrasound.

Because a number of structures that we can image have not previously been imaged in their natural relationships in the living eye, we have found it useful to define a series of measurement parameters that can be used for future comparison between normal and pathological eyes. We fully expect modifications and additions will be necessary as this method is brought to bear on various ocular problems. We have attempted to define measurement sites in terms of fixed anatomical landmarks such as the scleral spur to allow reproducibility. Although the position of some of the structures will vary with internal dynamic changes such as those occurring with light exposure and accomodation, we have found reproducibility is good if repeated examinations are done under similar conditions, measurements taken in the same orientation, and careful technique used to produce good sections perpendicular to the structures being examined. The chapter on technique addresses issues of designating examination position, and acquiring examination skills. We will discuss ultrasound biomicroscopic appearance of normal anatomical features and also present results of measurements performed in normal eyes [1].

The Cornea

The superficial location of the cornea permits the use of higher frequency transducers, as depth of penetration is not as great a consideration. Higher frequency transducers allow a better definition of small distances such as epithelial thickness. With our original equipment we frequently do corneal studies with 75 to 100 MHz transducers. Even higher frequencies could be used for this structure.

A typical corneal cross section is shown in Figure 4.1. Corneal layers can be well differentiated. The reflection from the surface of the epithelium forms a smooth line in normal eyes that becomes more irregular in the presence of epithelial edema. The epithelial surface can be differentiated from Bowman's membrane, which forms a distinct, highly reflective line just below the reflection from the epithelial surface. The corneal stroma reveals a low, regular internal reflectivity. The endothelium cannot be differentiated from Descemet's membrane, but together they form a single highly reflective line at the posterior corneal margin.

The corneoscleral junction can be differentiated because of the lower internal reflectivity of cornea compared to sclera. This marked difference in backscatter coefficient has been confirmed by our studies in vitro [2], with scleral backscatter coefficients exceeding those of cornea by a factor of 4.6.

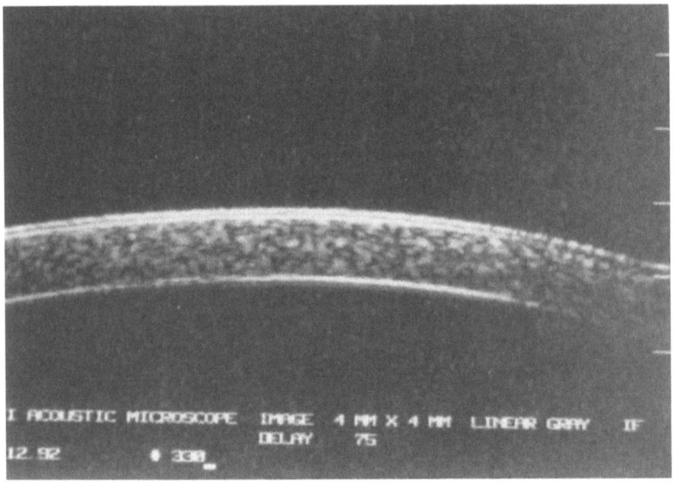

FIGURE 4.1. Ultrasound biomicroscopic image of normal cornea. The top echo is from the epithelial surface. The second echo just below this is from Bowman's membrane. The corneal stroma shows weak backscatter. The endothelium/ Descemet's layer provides a bright echo at the interface with aqueous. Reprinted with permission from the *Journal of Cataract and Refractive Surgery* 1994 in press.

This difference is most likely due to the difference in histological structure of these two regions. The smooth lamellae of the corneal stroma are less reflective than the irregular collagen bundles making up the sclera. Figure 4.2 shows a typical corneoscleral junction. The zone of change in reflectivity is not a clean line, but shows a gradual transition from the cornea to the sclera. This is similar to the gradual change that is seen histologically. The inner junction is generally referred to as Schwalbe's line. This junction is often not clearly defined on ultrasound biomicroscopy, but occasionally the inner line is hypertrophied (internal embryotoxin) and can be imaged as a highly reflective internal band, as seen in Figure 4.2. The surgical limbus as seen on examination of the external aspect of a normal eye is located approximately 1 mm anterior to the scleral spur. This represents the transition between conjunctival tissue and corneal epithelium.

Measurement of corneal thickness can be done by various methods as outlined in the techniques section. Great care must be taken to produce sections perpendicular to the corneal surfaces. This is done by maximizing the brightness of the signals from the epithelial and endothelial surfaces in a

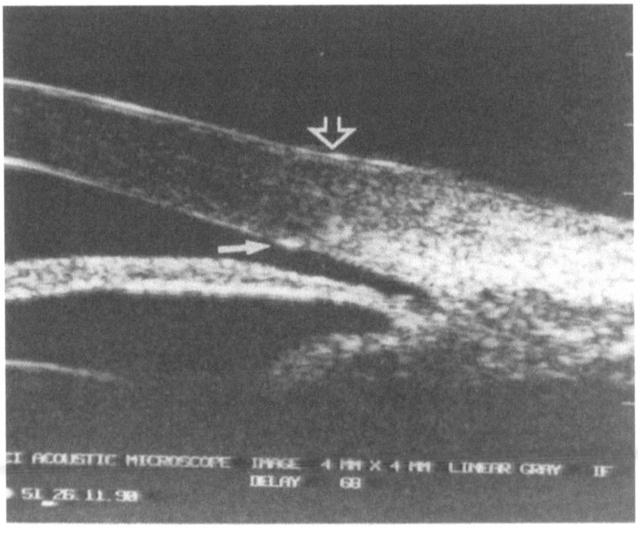

FIGURE 4.2. A cross section of the angle region showing a corneoscleral junction. The internal scleral reflectivity is much higher than that of the cornea. The internal corneoscleral junction is marked in this case by a distinctly reflective hypertrophied Schwalbe's line (closed arrow). The limbus (open arrow) is approximately 1 mm anterior to the scleral spur.

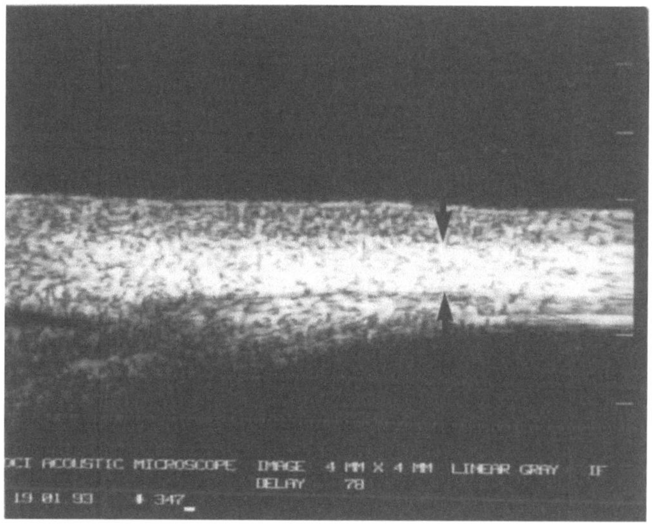

FIGURE 4.3. The high reflectivity of the sclera (arrows) allows it to be differentiated from overlying and underlying tissue. Published with permission from *The American Journal of Ophthalmology* (1993;116:628–635). Copyright by The Ophthalmic Publishing Company.

way similar to biometry techniques with conventional ultrasound. Measurement of small distances such as epithelial thickness requires special procedures [3].

The Sclera

The normal sclera has a relatively high reflectivity compared to the cornea. This high reflectivity allows definition of the corneoscleral junction and usually allows scleral tissue to be differentiated from the less reflective episcleral tissue and the less reflective ciliary body and peripheral choroid (Figure 4.3). It is essential to be as perpendicular as possible to the scleral surface for accurate measurement [4]. The sclera is generally thickest in the region of the scleral spur. The scleral spur forms an important landmark for orientation and measuring distances in the region. Figure 4.4 shows the corneoscleral junction with a clear view of the scleral spur. The insertion of muscle tendons into the sclera can be outlined as is noted in Figure 4.5. The sclera can be seen to be significantly thinned below the muscle insertion. Occasionally one can image large penetrating vessels through the scleral tissue

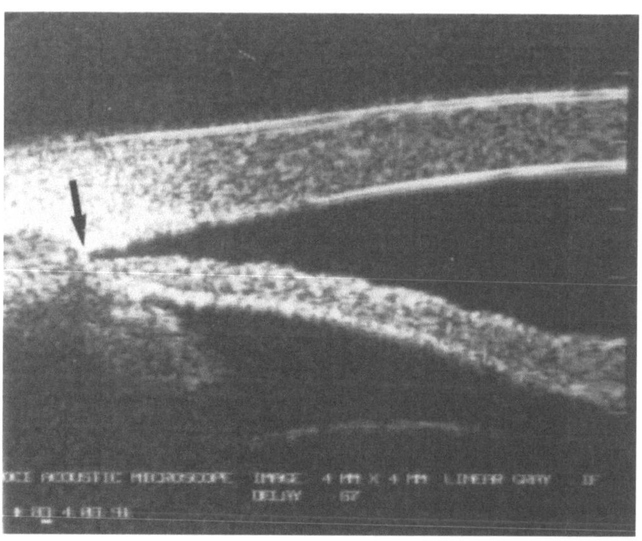

FIGURE 4.4. The corneoscleral junction can be clearly defined. The scleral spur (arrow) is an important landmark. Published with permission from *The American Journal of Ophthalmology* (1993; 116:628–635). Copyright by the Ophthalmic Publishing Company.

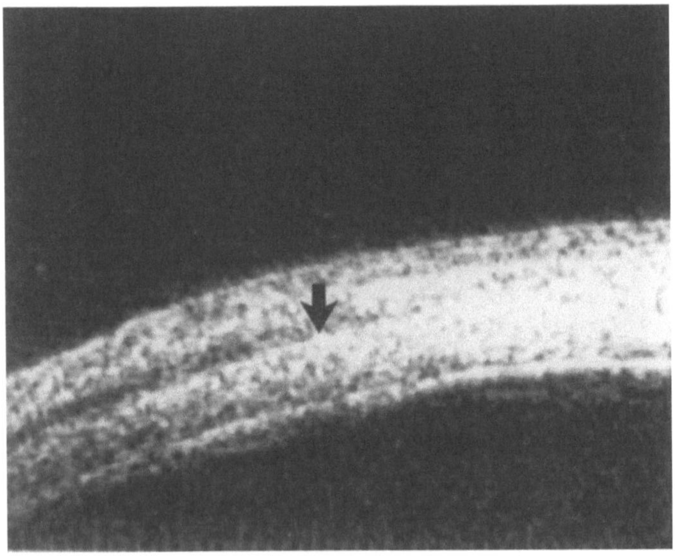

FIGURE 4.5. The sclera can be seen to be thinned posterior to the insertion of an extraocular muscle (arrow). Published with permission from *The American Journal of Ophthalmology* (1993;116: 628–635). Copyright by The Ophthalmic Publishing Company.

near the limbus (Figure 4.6). These are most likely anterior ciliary vessels.

Anterior Chamber

The central anterior chamber can be imaged from the internal cornea to the lens surface. Careful technique is required if measurement of axial anterior chamber depth is desired. This can be accomplished at the time of examination by careful attention to perpendicularity of the sound beam to the cornea and lens interfaces. Maximum brightness and a clean signal indicate perpendicularity. The iris margins provide orientation, and allow measurements to be done in the center of the pupillary space. An image such as that seen in Figure 4.7 is ideal for measuring axial anterior chamber depth in that it shows the central pupillary space with iris margins to each side, and bright corneal and lens echoes indicating perpendicularity.

Measuring the axial distance from the internal

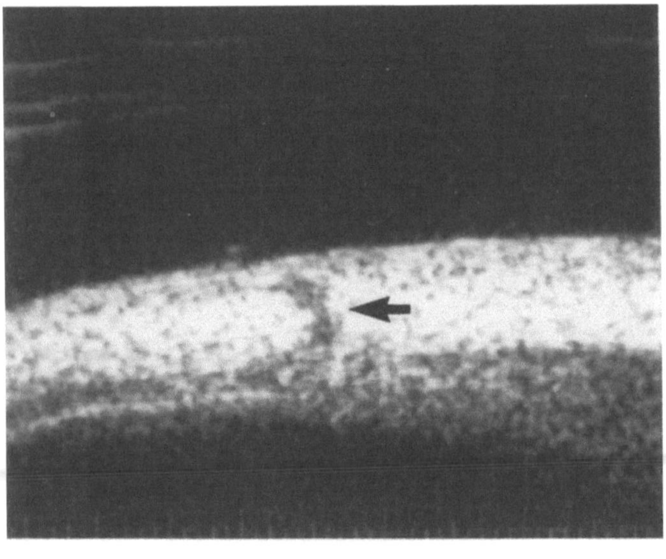

FIGURE 4.6. A vessel passing through scleral substance (arrow). Published with permission from *The American Journal of Opthalmology* (1993;116: 628–635). Copyright by The Ophthalmic Publishing Company.

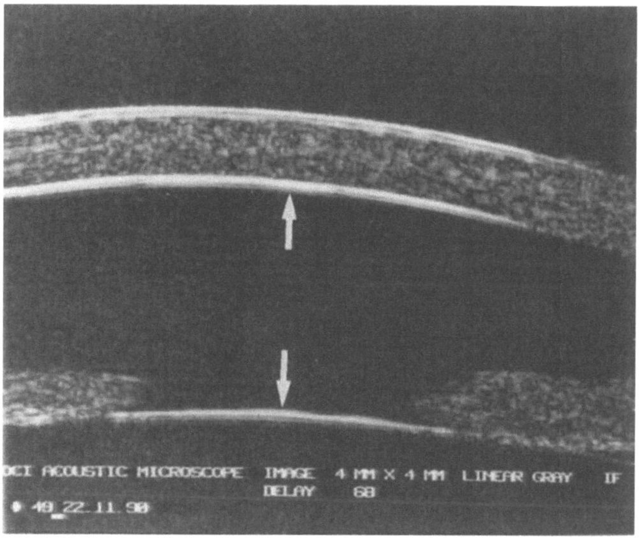

FIGURE 4.7. The central anterior chamber can be measured from the corneal endothelial surface to the lens surface (arrows). The bright reflection from the cornea and lens surface confirms perpendicularity and the presence of the iris margins confirms axial location.

corneal surface to the lens surface is facilitated by the ease of distinguishing the iris from the lens surface. This can be difficult in eyes with very small pupils using conventional ultrasound. Anterior chamber depth can be measured at points other than the axial position. The distance from the cornea to either the iris or lens can be determined at any of these points. In a series of normal eyes we found the average axial anterior chamber depth measurement to be 3128 ± 372 μm.

The Angle

Figure 4.8a represents a cross section through the angle region. This view is produced by orienting the probe in a radial fashion above the limbal region. The corneoscleral junction and scleral spur can be distinguished consistently with ultrasound biomicroscopy. These structures are important in maintaining orientation in the angle region. The scleral spur in particular is a very useful landmark presenting a constant reference point for measurement in the angle region. Figure 4.8b shows the location of the scleral spur in an open angle on gonioscopy.

Measurement of the degree of anterior chamber angle opening has generally been a qualitative estimate. Gonioscopy is used to estimate an angle of opening or to assign a number between one and four based on the amount of trabecular meshwork visualized. Methods have been used such as drawing intersecting lines on the inner corneal and iris surfaces of conventional ultrasound images to produce quantitative measurements [5,6]. These methods provide a gross estimate at best. Conventional ultrasound lacks the resolution required to appreciate the subtle variations in curvature of angle structures and fails completely in imaging very narrow angles.

We have previously presented techniques of quantifying angle measurements based on ultrasound biomicroscopy [1]. The first method consists of taking a point on the internal ocular wall 500 μm anterior to the scleral spur (which would fall on the anterior trabecular meshwork) and extending a line from this point perpendicular to the plane of the trabecular meshwork, to the opposing iris (Figure 4.9). The length of this line would then be measured. We call this measurement angle opening distance (AOD). Results of measurement in normal cases was 347±181 μm for AOD at 500 μm from the scleral spur.

Angular measurements in degrees are easily made but difficult to define because of anatomic variations in angle configuration. It is essential to designate the position of the apex, and to designate the points at which the arms of the angle touch the iris and inner corneoscleral wall. We have measured the angle formed with the apex at the iris recess, and the arms passing through the point on the meshwork 500 μm from the scleral spur and the

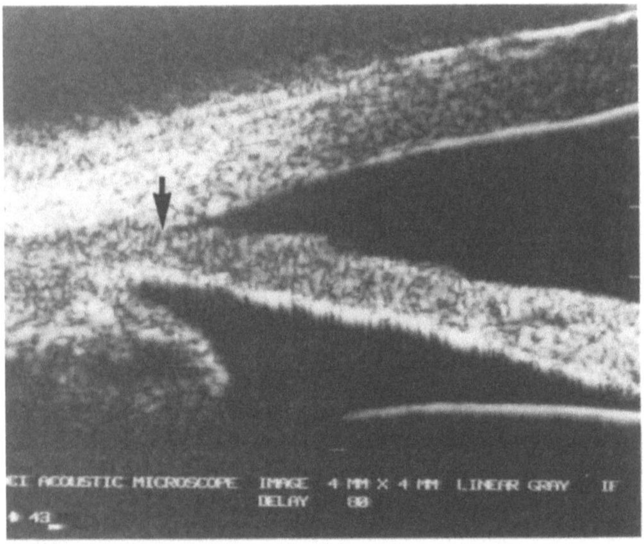

(a)

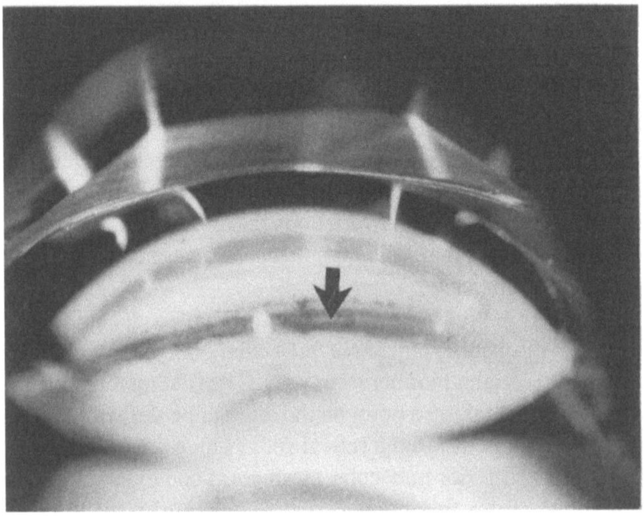

(b)

FIGURE 4.8 **(a)** A typical section through the angle. An arrow indicates the scleral spur. **(b)** Gonioscopy can be used to provide a qualitative estimate of angle opening. An arrow indicates the scleral spur. Published courtesy of *Ophthalmology* (1991;98:287–295).

point on the iris perpendicularly opposite (Figure 4.9), and termed this the trabecular-iris angle (θ1). This angle averaged 30±11 degrees in our series of normal eyes.

Measurements of angle opening can vary with change in the state of iris dilation. Subtle variations in iris curvature around the periphery will induce small differences in measurement at various locations. Reproducibility of measurement requires documentation of the precise radial position in which the measurement was made (usually designated in clock hours), and control of variables such as pupil dilation. With practice these measurements can be made with a reasonable degree of precision and reproducibility, allowing a quantitative approach to what has hitherto been a qualitative estimate.

The Iris

The iris is well imaged in cross section by ultrasound biomicroscopy (Figure 4.10). The iris recess varies in depth in normal eyes and can be outlined by ultrasound biomicroscopy. The iris and ciliary body converge in this region and insert into the scleral spur. The area under the peripheral iris and above the ciliary processes is defined as the ciliary

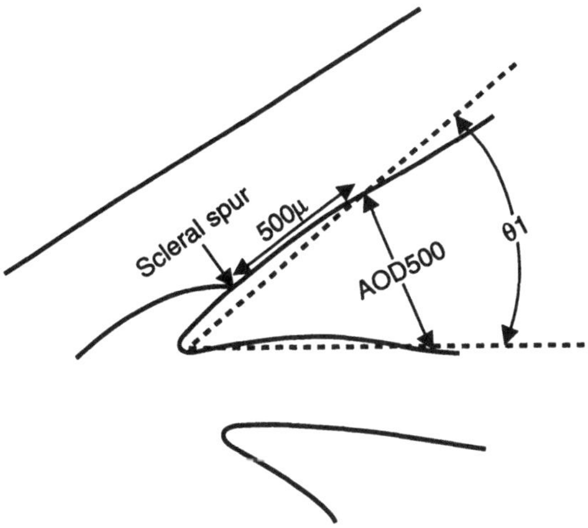

FIGURE 4.9. Quantitative angle measurement. Angle opening distance (AOD 500) is defined as the length of a perpendicular from the trabecular meshwork to the iris at a point 500 μm from the scleral spur. The trabecular/iris angle (θ1) is measured with the apex in the iris sulcus and the arms passing through the point 500 μm from the scleral spur and the point perpendicularly opposite on the iris.

sulcus. This is an important anatomical space, especially in relation to intraocular lens implantation. The iris shows subtle variations in surface curvature. The stroma shows a relatively low reflectivity. Occasional small spaces are seen in the iris stroma. The iris epithelium forms a constant, relatively thick, highly reflective layer on the posterior iris surface. This highly reflective line defines the posterior iris border and can be quite useful when one is differentiating intrairis lesions from lesions behind the iris. The epithelium can also be followed around the iris margin in cases of ectropion uvea.

Small indentations representing crypts (Figure 4.11) are frequently seen. The dilator muscle cannot be differentiated from surrounding tissue. The sphincter muscle is also difficult to detect routinely, but can frequently be imaged when a drug such as pilocarpine produces thickening of this muscle (Figure 4.12).

Figure 4.13 shows an interesting variation in iris structure with a more medial origin of the iris root. In this case the iris appears to take origin from the surface of the ciliary body. This configuration was present for the entire circumference of the iris. In this case there is a large ciliary sulcus behind the scleral spur.

The overall iris curvature can be clearly outlined by ultrasound biomicroscopy. We generally find a straight iris profile in normal patients. This contrasts with the anterior bowing seen in pupil block [1,7], and the posterior bowing seen in some patients with pigmentary glaucoma [8,9].

Measurement of iris thickness requires precise definition of measurement position. The iris normally shows variations in thickness in different regions. Histological studies show that it is generally thinnest at the iris root and thickest near the

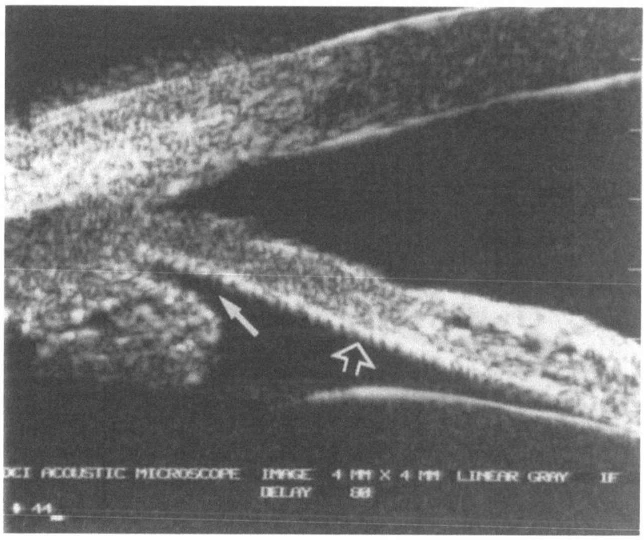

FIGURE 4.10. The normal iris. The stroma is relatively low in reflectivity and shows some small spaces. The iris epithelium forms a highly reflective line on the posterior iris surface (open arrow). The ciliary sulcus (closed arrow) is imaged between the peripheral iris and ciliary processes.

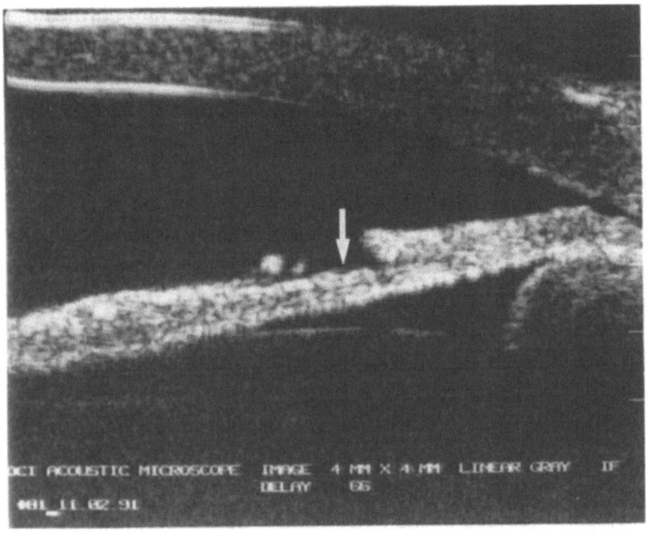

FIGURE 4.11. The iris surface frequently shows irregularities produced by iris crypts (arrow). Published with permission from *The American Journal of Ophthalmology* (1992;113:390–395). Copyright by The Ophthalmic Publishing Company.

pupillary margin. In addition there are variations in thickness depending on the presence of crypts, and the state of dilation or constriction. The pupil size is constantly variable within a small range in the absence of pharmacological agents.

The position of iris measurement can be defined with reference to the scleral spur. For example, in our previous study we picked three points to measure the iris. We ran a line from the point on the trabecular meshwork 500 μm from the scleral spur, perpendicularly through the iris, extended to the ciliary process. We termed this distance the trabecular-ciliary process distance (TCPD). Iris thickness along this line was designated ID1 (average thickness = 372 ±58 μm). The iris ciliary process distance that defines the ciliary sulcus depth can also be measured along this line. Other possible points of iris measurement include measurement 2 mm from the iris root (ID2; average thickness = 457±80 μm) and at its thickest point near the pupil (ID3; average thickness = 645 ±103 μm). Figure 4.14 shows these measurement positions. Measurements at other locations can be defined as required.

Other measurements that can be made include the zone of iris-lens contact (ILCD) (average distance in our normal eyes = 1388 ±370 μm) and

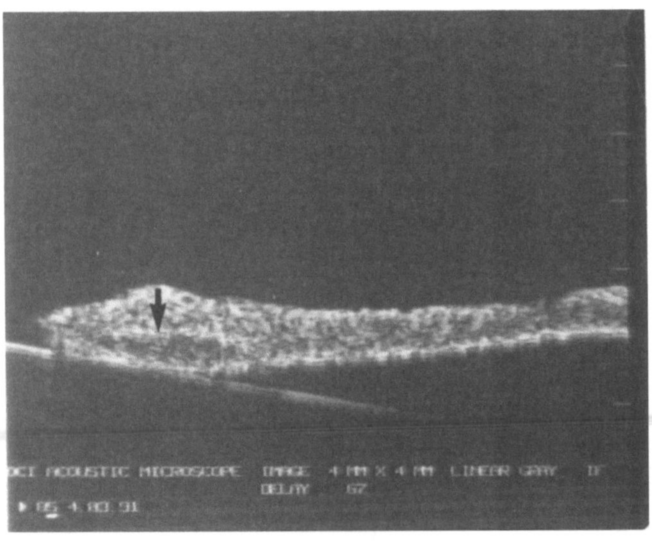

FIGURE 4.12. The iris sphincter (arrow) is imaged after pilocarpine administration.

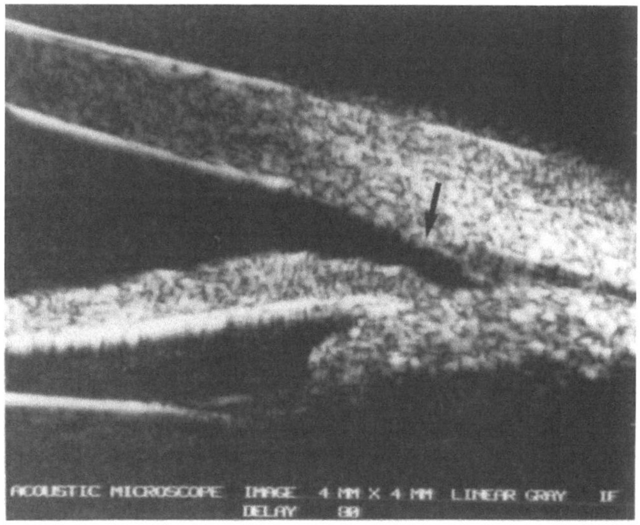

FIGURE 4.13. A variation in iris structure in which the root of the iris appears to arise from the surface of the ciliary body. The scleral spur is marked with an arrow, and a large iris recess is present. Published with permission from *The American Journal of Ophthalmology* (1992;113:381–389). Copyright by The Ophthalmic Publishing Company.

the angle at which the iris leaves the lens (θ2; average = 12±3°). The position of these measurements is defined in Figure 4.15. A typical image from which these measurements are taken is shown in Figure 4.16. Volumetric measurements are possible by tracing the iris profile on a computer and calculating the area of the iris. This can then be projected to a full 360°.

Another interesting measurement is the angle the iris makes to a tangent to the scleral surface (θ3). This measurement can have significance in regards to surgery that is done in a blinded manner below the iris such as transscleral intraocular lens fixation. This angle measured an average of 30±7° in our series of normal eyes. The angle the ciliary processes make to the scleral surface can also be defined (θ4; average = 52±18°). These measurements are also illustrated in Figure 4.15.

The Ciliary Body and Posterior Chamber

The Ciliary Body

The entire ciliary body can be clearly defined by ultrasound biomicroscopy from the ciliary processes to the pars plana. The ciliary processes can

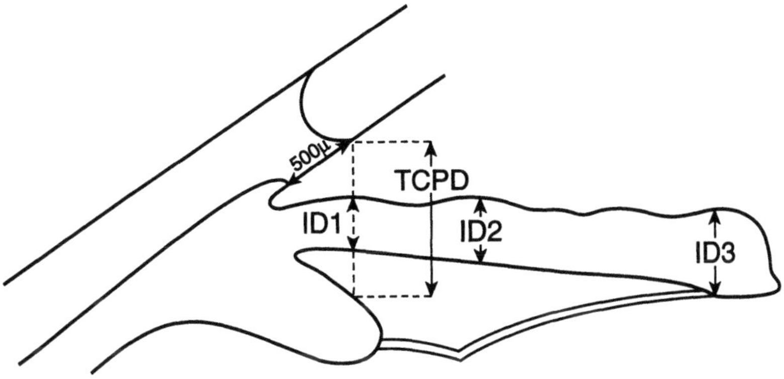

FIGURE 4.14. Diagram of measurement positions for the iris. The iris is measured at three points along its length. The first measurement (ID1) is located on a line perpendicular to the iris connecting a point on the trabecular meshwork 500 μm from the scleral spur to the ciliary process (trabecular-ciliary process distance, TCPD). The second (ID2) is measured 2 mm from the scleral spur. The third (ID3) is measured at the thickest point near the iris margin.

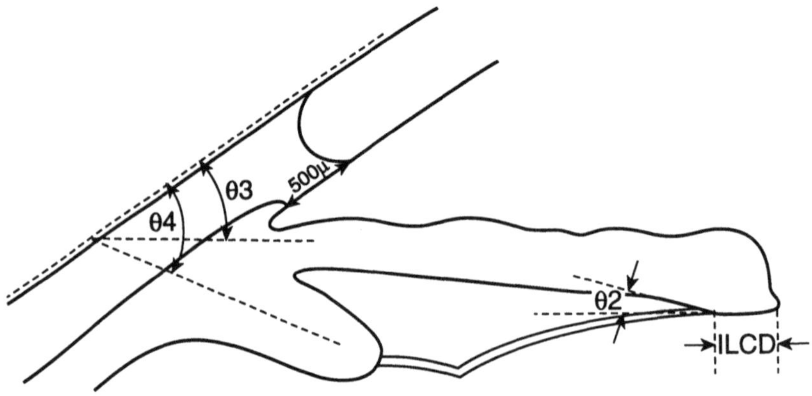

FIGURE 4.15. Diagram of the angle structures showing the zone of iris-lens contact (ILCD) and the angle the iris makes to the lens (θ2). The angles that the iris and ciliary body make to a tangent to the scleral surface (θ3 and θ4) can also be measured.

be quite variable in configuration and length. The appearance will vary depending on whether the section is passing through a process or valley between processes. During the examination one can produce either of these views as desired. The usual view shown in this book is taken radially through the tip of a ciliary process (Figure 4.17). This image shows the zonule extending from the ciliary process to the lens surface. Figure 4.18 shows a transverse image at right angles to the view shown in Figure 4.17 which displays the variable configuration of the ciliary processes and the valleys between them.

The distance between the anterior trabecular meshwork and the ciliary processes (TCPD; average distance = 1122 ± 232 μm) is an important measurement. We defined this distance above as the length of a line starting 500 μm from the scleral spur on the trabecular meshwork and extending perpendicularly through the iris to the ciliary process (Figure 4.14). This distance defines the port through which the iris must traverse and has implications as to the potential maximum angle opening.

The posterior ciliary body tapers off toward the pars plana (Figure 4.19). Not infrequently fine lines can be seen on the undersurface of the ciliary body in this position, most likely indicating zonular

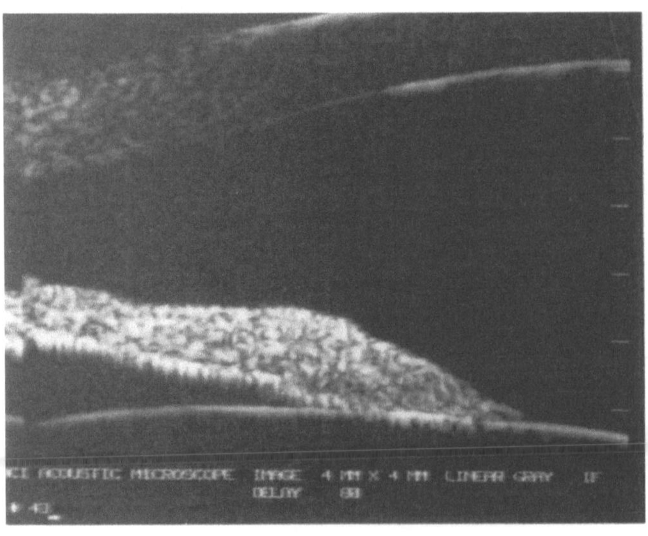

FIGURE 4.16. An image of the pupillary margin of the iris showing the zone of iris-lens contact. Published with permission from *The American Journal of Ophthalmology* (1992;113:381–389). Copyright by The Ophthalmic Publishing Company.

FIGURE 4.17. Image through a ciliary process (open arrow). The zonule can be seen extending from the ciliary process to the lens surface (closed arrow).

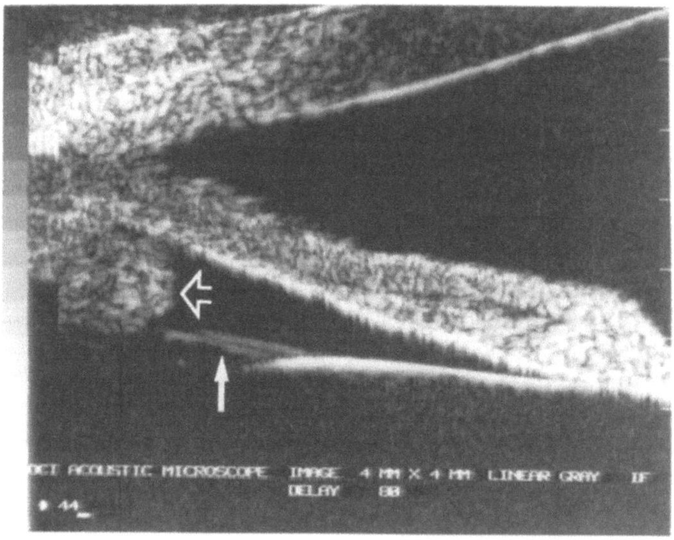

FIGURE 4.18. Transverse section through the ciliary processes shows variability in process configuration.

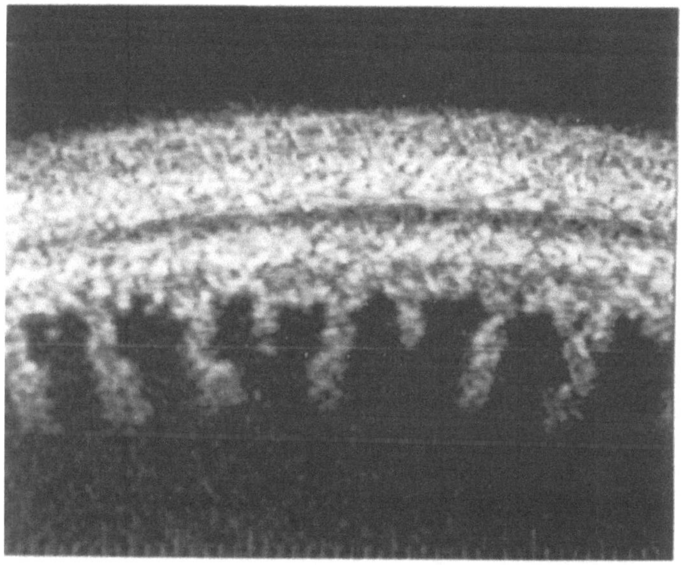

FIGURE 4.19. The posterior ciliary body tapers to the pars plana.

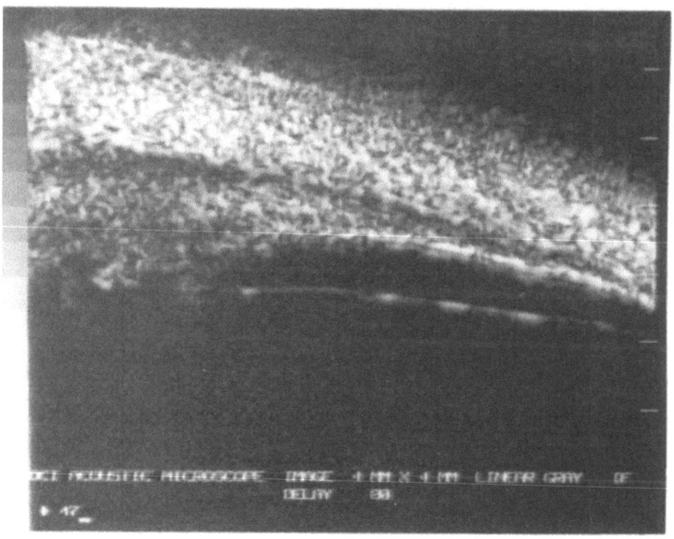

fibers in this region. The anterior vitreous face is occasionally visible.

The Zonule

The anterior zonular surface can be consistently imaged by ultrasound biomicroscopy. The appearance of the zonule is that of a medium reflective line extending from the ciliary process to the lens surface. The zonule tends to insert smoothly into the surface of the lens (Figure 4.17) but is occasionally more irregular, which may indicate the degree of zonular tension. Optimal visualization of the anterior zonule requires that the focal point of the transducer be in the zonular region. Cross sections of the angle above that do not show zonular fibers are generally sections with the focal zone at a more superficial depth.

The Zonule and Lens After Cycloplegia

Figure 4.20a shows the zonule and lens margin under the overlying iris. Figure 4.20b shows the same eye after instillation of cycloplegic drops. The zonule shows a greater degree of tension, lifting slightly off the lens surface. The lens margin shows a change in profile with a more squared-off

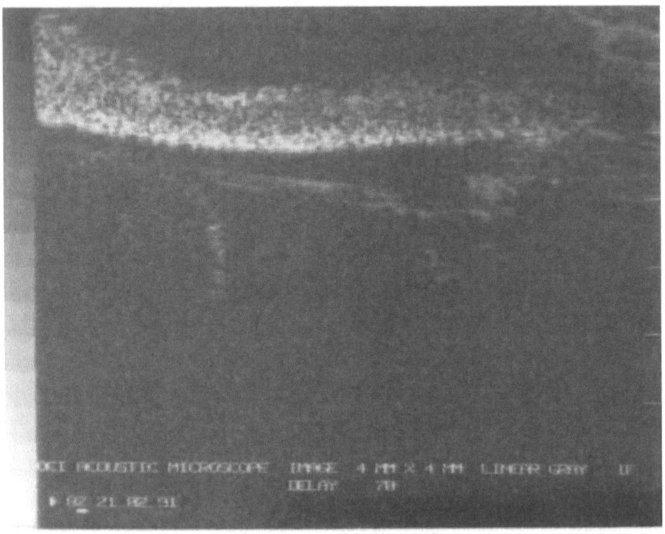

(a)

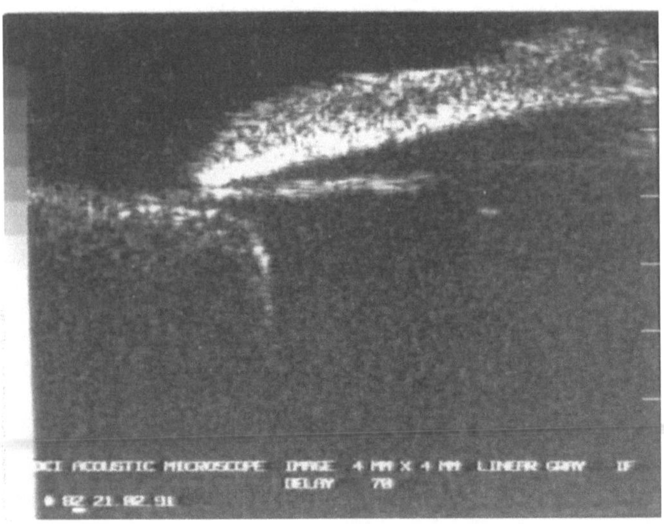

(b)

FIGURE 4.20. **(a)** Zonule inserting into the lens below the iris. **(b)** Postcycloplegia, the iris shortens, the zonule under increased tension lifts off the lens surface. The lens margin shows a more squared-off appearance.

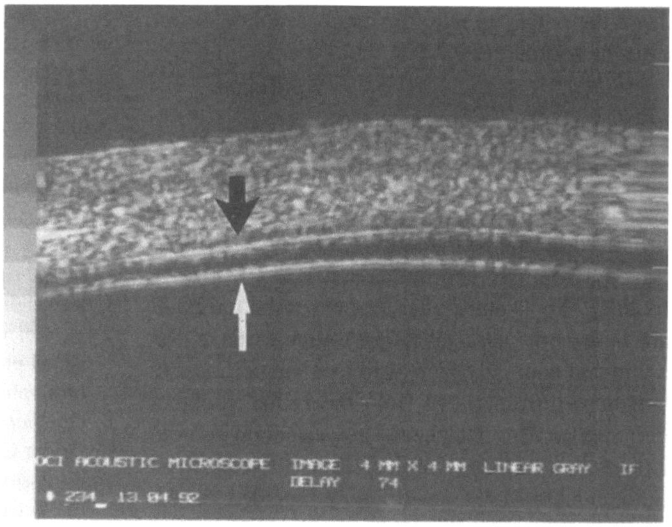

FIGURE 4.21. Region over peripheral retina shows the weakly reflective choroid (black arrow) bounded by the pigment epithelium. The retina is imaged as a single line that is slightly detached in this view (white arrow).

appearance. The margin of the dilated iris is observed at the edge of the lens.

The Posterior Chamber

The entire posterior chamber as defined as the space between the anterior vitreous face and the posterior iris cannot always be defined with ultrasound biomicroscopy. The posterior zonule and vitreous face can be resolved in some shallow chambered eyes, but not consistently in eyes with chambers of average or greater depth. It is also difficult to consistently image the lateral lens margin because of the curvature of this surface and its relationship to the incidence of the ultrasound beam. The region bounded by the posterior iris, ciliary body, and zonule/lens surface forms a distinct compartment that varies considerably in depth. We propose that this depth be defined quantitatively as the iris-zonule distance (IZD). In order to quantify this depth, measurement should be taken at a consistent position. This can be described as the distance between the iris and the anterior zonule at a position that just

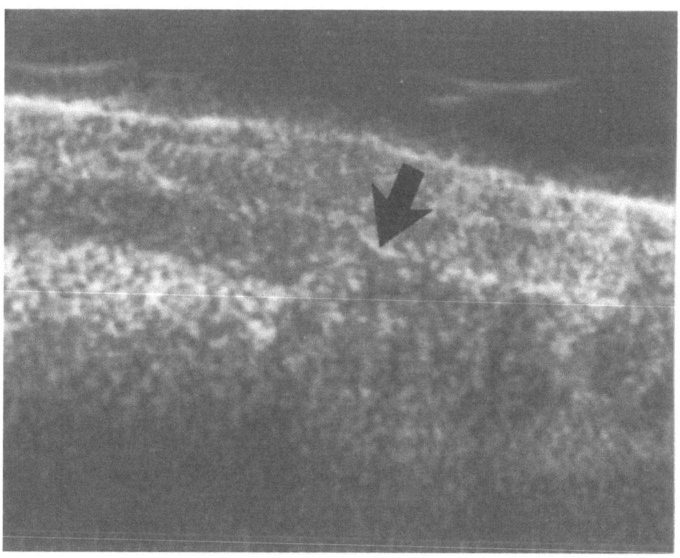

FIGURE 4.22. Cross section of the normal upper eyelid. The levator tendon can be noted inserting into the anterior tarsal surface (arrow).

clears the ciliary process (average distance in our series of normal eyes = 671 ± 124 μm).

The Peripheral Retina

The peripheral retina and pars plana region can be visualized as far peripherally as the probe can be moved before eye cup movement is prevented by the lids. This is somewhat farther on the temporal side than on the nasal side. The retina in this region is thin and generally is imaged as a single line that cannot be differentiated from the retinal pigment epithelium unless detached. The peripheral choroid appears as a thin zone of decreased reflectivity on the underside of the sclera. It is bounded on the internal surface by the highly reflective pigment epithelium and Bruch's membrane. It is not uncommon to find small areas of peripheral retinal detachment on routine examination (Figure 4.21).

Ocular Adnexa

Surfaces covered by skin present increased attenuation because of keratinized epithelium. Lid structure can be defined. Figure 4.22 shows a cross section of the lid with the tarsal plate differentiated from adjacent tissue. The levator tendon can be imaged inserting into the anterior tarsal surface. Lacrimal structures such as canaliculi are difficult to image unless dilated by fluid.

References

1. Pavlin CJ, Harasiewicz K, Foster FS. Ultrasound biomicroscopy of anterior segment structures in normal and glaucomatous eyes. *Am J Ophthalmol* 1992; 113:381–389.
2. Ye SG, Harasiewicz KA, Pavlin CJ, Foster FS. Ultrasound characterization of ocular tissue in the frequency range from 50 MHz to 100 MHz. *IEEE UFFC* (in press).
3. Reinstein DZ, Silverman RH, Trokel SL, Allemann N, Coleman DJ. High frequency ultrasound digital signal processing for biometry of the cornea in planning phototherapeutic keratectomy (Letter). *Arch Ophthalmol* 1993;111:430–431.
4. Pavlin CJ, Easterbrook M, Hurwitz JJ, Harasiewicz K, Foster FS. Ultrasound biomicroscopic assessment of anterior scleral disease. *Am J Ophthalmol* 1993;116:628–635.
5. Tane S, Ohba H, Komatsu A, Iguchi T. The quantitative biometry of the angle of the anterior chamber. *Acta Soc Ophthalmol JPN* 1979;83:1319.
6. Makabe R. Comparative studies of the anterior chamber angle width by ultrasonography and gonioscopy. *Klin Monatsbl Augenheilkd* 1989;194:6.
7. Anderson DR, Jin JC, Wright MM. The physiological characteristics of relative pupillary block. *Am J Ophthalmol* 1991;111:344.
8. Kavickhoff JR. Response to Fourman's Iridotomy in eyes with pigmentary glaucoma (letter). *Ophthalmic Surg* 1992;23:843–844.
9. Potash SD, Tello C, Liebmann J, Ritch R. Ultrasound biomicroscopy in pigment dispersion syndrome. *Ophthalmology* (in press).

Part 2
Ultrasound Biomicroscopy of Ocular Disease

5
Glaucoma

Several types of glaucoma are caused by structural abnormalities of the anterior segment of the globe. This is particularly true of angle closure glaucoma and infantile glaucoma. The ability of ultrasound biomicroscopy to image anterior chamber structures in depth at high resolution makes it a useful tool in glaucoma research and clinical practice. Although histological specimens are occasionally available in various glaucoma entities, these are usually obtained in the end stages of the disease process. Processing of sections suitable for optical microscopy invariably produces distortion of the relationships of intraocular structures. A good example of the problem of postmortem distortion is found in plateau iris syndrome. In a recent publication [1] we compared the histological findings in an enucleated eye with the findings in the remaining living eye and found very different features. The etiological role of the ciliary processes (see below) would have been entirely missed if only the histological specimen had been examined.

Ultrasound biomicroscopy, though lacking the resolution of optical microscopy, allows the relationship of anterior segment structures to be discerned in the living eye, in their actual state, at any stage of the disease process. Serial observations at different stages of the disease can be obtained and response of ocular structures to various forms of treatment ascertained. Some of the entities discussed in this chapter are still at the stage where mechanisms are being clarified, but are not completely elucidated. Ultrasound biomicroscopy is a helpful aid in this process and some of the new findings in these conditions are presented here.

Angle Closure Glaucoma

Ultrasound biomicroscopy is useful in analyzing angle closure glaucoma and the mechanisms that produce it. Angle opening can be measured quantitatively. Other ocular structures that may participate in the production of angle closure can be simultaneously imaged.

Phakic Pupil Block

In pupil block the iris assumes a convex profile due to the pressure differential between the posterior and anterior chambers. The gonioscopic appearance in a case of pupil block is shown in Figure 5.1a. Gonioscopically the status of the angle cannot be directly ascertained, because the convexity of the iris precludes a view over the crest of the hill. The ultrasound biomicroscopic image of this eye (Figure 5.1b) provides a cross section of the iris, and allows the full degree of angle opening to be appreciated. In spite of pupil block with marked iris convexity, the angle is still open in this view. This case illustrates the convex iris profile in pupil block and shows the relationship of the ciliary processes and zonule to the back of the iris. In the majority of these cases the ciliary sulcus is open, with a space between the ciliary processes and the back of the iris. The iris convexity increases the distance of the iris from the zonule and peripheral lens providing a margin of safety for Yag laser iridotomy.

Previous studies have been done to define iris profile. Tiedeman provided a theoretical analysis

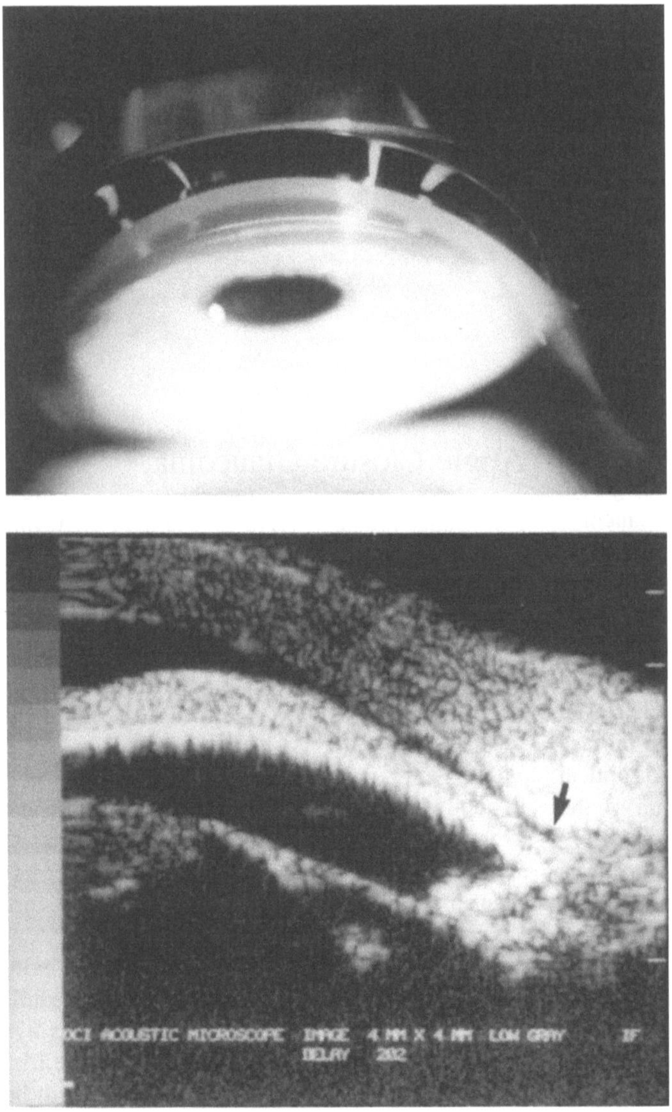

(a)

(b)

FIGURE 5.1. (**a**) Gonioscopic view of the angle in a patient with pupil block. The convexity of the iris precludes a view of the trabecular meshwork region. (**b**) Ultrasound biomicroscopic view of the same angle demonstrates that the angle is still open to the scleral spur (arrow). The anterior convexity of the iris is typical of pupil block. A space is present between the ciliary processes and posterior iris. Published courtesy of *Ophthalmology* (1991;98:287–295).

to predict iris profile [2]. Jin, Anderson, and Wright described an optical technique (Scheimpflug technique) to define iris profile in pupil block [3,4]. Ultrasound biomicroscopy presents a relatively easy method of accomplishing this task, and allows definition of the entire iris profile to the iris root. The most peripheral aspect of the iris is not clearly defined using optical techniques such as the Scheimpflug technique. Potash and colleagues presented a method of defining iris curvature using ultrasound biomicroscopy that involves drawing a line from the pupil margin to the iris root on the iris epithelial side and then designating the curvature as positive or negative [5]. Analysis of the actual curve is complex and requires sophisticated computer techniques.

The change in curvature following iridotomy can be defined by ultrasound biomicroscopy. Following iridotomy the profile changes from a convex configuration to a much straighter configuration as shown in Figures 5.2a and b, respectively. A forward bowing of the iris always implies a pressure differential between the two chambers. We have not seen this profile in normal patients [6]. Defining iris curvature variations could be useful in predicting potential angle closure and response to treatment.

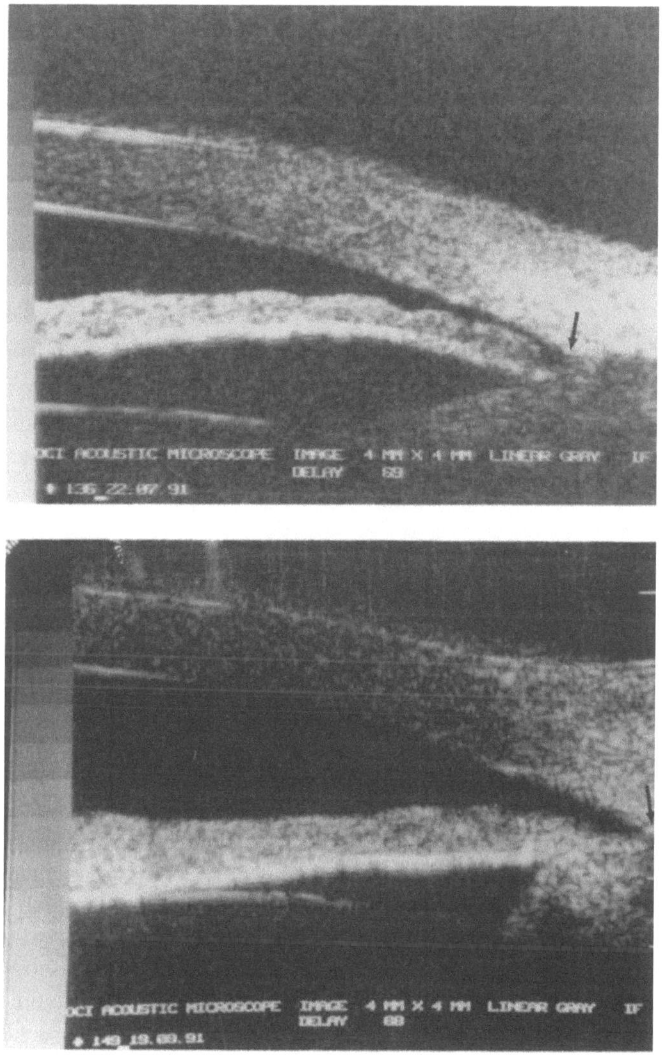

FIGURE 5.2. (**a**) A case of pupil block prior to iridotomy shows anterior iris bowing. The scleral spur is marked with an arrow. (**b**) Following iridectomy the iris profile becomes a straight line. The scleral spur is marked with an arrow. Published with permission from *The American Journal of Ophthalmology* (1992;113:381–389). Copyright by The Ophthalmic Publishing Company.

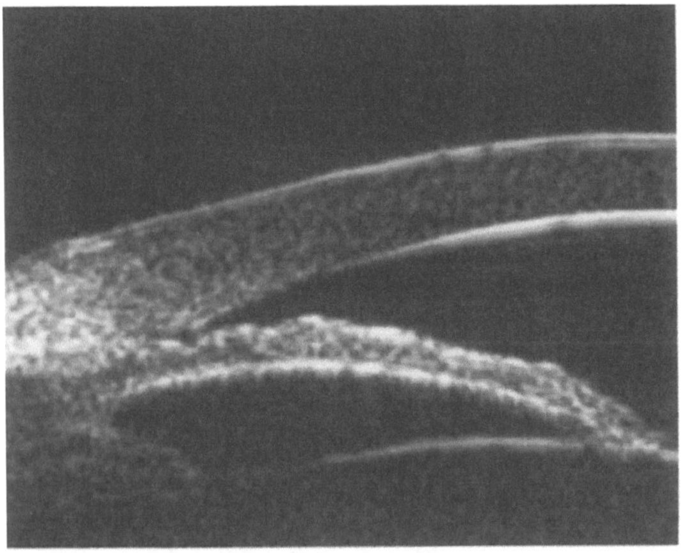

FIGURE 5.3. The area of contact of the pupil margin with the lens in pupil block is small.

Of interest is the very small zone of iris-lens contact seen in untreated angle closure glaucoma. Figure 5.3 shows the relationship of the iris to the lens surface in a typical case of angle closure with iris bowing. The anterior convexity of the iris lifts the iris off the lens surface, to the point where only the tip of the iris is lying against the lens surface. This amount of lens-iris contact is less than that seen in normal eyes. The continuing block thus does not appear to be related to the area of iris-lens contact, but rather to the internal iris dynamics that force the iris margin against the lens surface. The iris appears to be under tension related to the relative action of the sphincter and dilator muscles, and the structural anatomy that places the lens in a forward position. These forces keep the iris-lens junction relatively watertight in spite of increased pressure behind the iris.

Aphakic Pupil Block

Patients that have had intracapsular cataract surgery or dislocated lenses are also subject to pupil block glaucoma. In these cases the mechanism relates to the interface between the iris and the vitreous. The physician faced with a flat chamber in an aphakic eye may have difficulty determining the mechanism of the glaucomatous process. Aphakic malignant glaucoma may enter into the differential diagnoses. Figure 5.4a shows an example of pupil block occurring in a patient with a spontaneous lens dislocation. The lens was located in the inferior fundus and the patient had had recent signs of ocular inflammation before presenting with a flat anterior chamber and elevated pressures. Ultrasound biomicroscopy revealed that the iris was pushed forward and flattened against the internal cornea. The vitreous face was bowed posteriorly as shown in Figure 5.4b. Figure 5.4c shows that the vitreous face is adherent to the pupillary margin. The slight space noted between the iris margin and cornea on ultrasound biomicroscopy provided guidance to the surgeon regarding positioning laser treatment without corneal damage. This allowed the pupil block to be broken at the iris edge. Vitrectomy and lens removal were later required. This case illustrates the value of ultrasound biomicroscopy in the clinical setting. Ultrasound biomicroscopy can provide both diagnostic information and information that aids treatment decisions. Of interest is the posterior bowing of the vitreous face. It is apparent that aqueous did not misdirect into the vitreous itself despite considerable pressure.

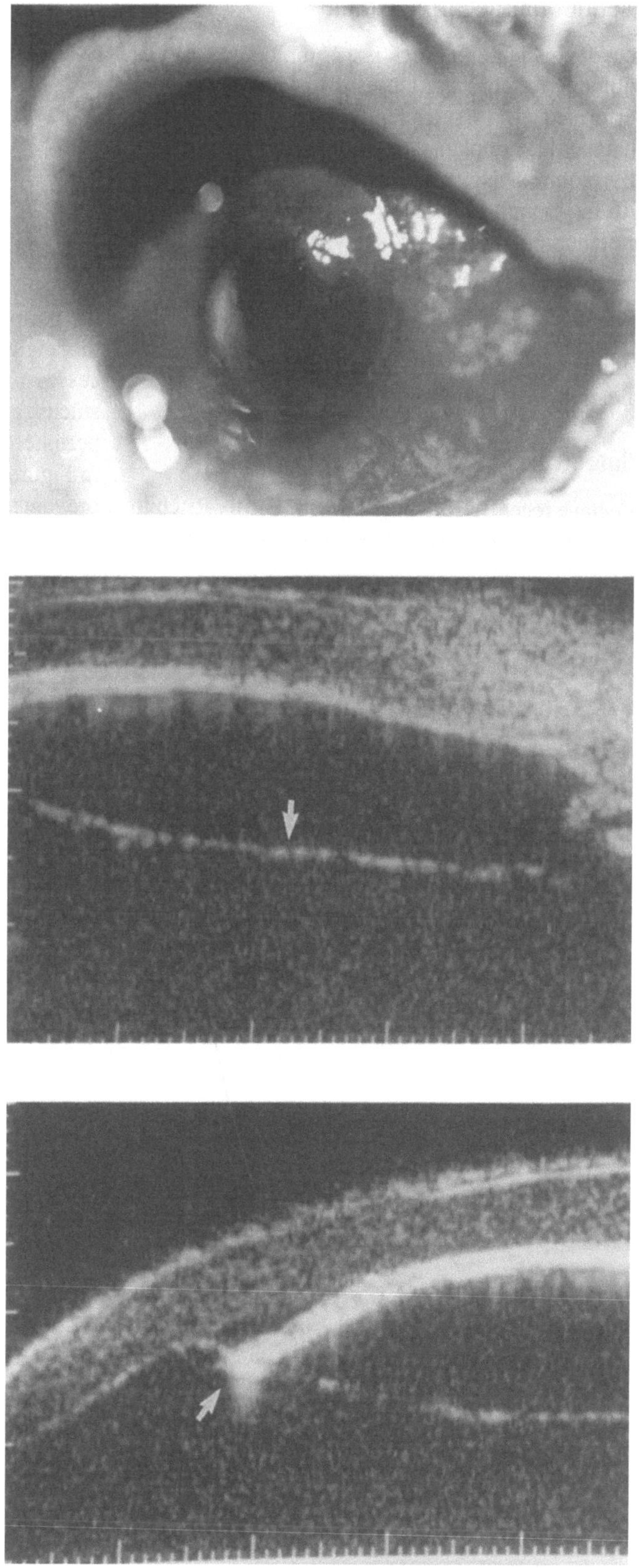

(a)

(b)

(c)

Figure 5.4. **(a)** Clinical photograph of an aphakic patient presenting with an inflamed eye, high pressure, and a flat chamber. **(b)** Ultrasound biomicroscopy images the iris pressed against the cornea. The vitreous face (arrow) is bowed backward. **(c)** The vitreous is adherent to the iris margin (arrow), and continues over the inner surface of the cornea.

Pseudophakic Pupil Block

Pseudophakic pupil block is a common occurrence with anterior chamber lenses if iridotomies are not performed. It is sufficiently rare with posterior chamber lens implants that iridotomies are not usually required. Nevertheless the occasional patient will have pupil block after posterior chamber lens implantation. Figure 5.5 shows anterior iris bowing in a case of pupil block secondary to an adhesion of the iris to a posterior chamber intraocular lens. The area of iris adhesion to the lens is well demonstrated and clarifies the etiology of this complication.

Plateau Iris

We have recently collaborated with Dr. R. Ritch to elucidate the etiology of plateau iris syndrome using ultrasound biomicroscopy [7]. In normal subjects, there is usually a distinct ciliary sulcus with ample room between the ciliary processes and the trabecular meshwork to allow the thickness of the iris to pass without angle narrowing. In pupillary block, there is anterior bowing of the iris caused by the pressure differential between the posterior and anterior chambers. The ciliary processes in most cases are positioned far enough posteriorly, so that loss of anterior bowing following iridotomy allows the peripheral iris to fall away sufficiently to open the angle. In plateau iris syndrome the ciliary processes are anteriorly located, closing the ciliary sulcus, and providing structural support behind the peripheral iris. This is illustrated diagrammatically in Figure 5.6. This position of the ciliary processes prevents the peripheral portion of the iris from falling away from the trabecular meshwork following

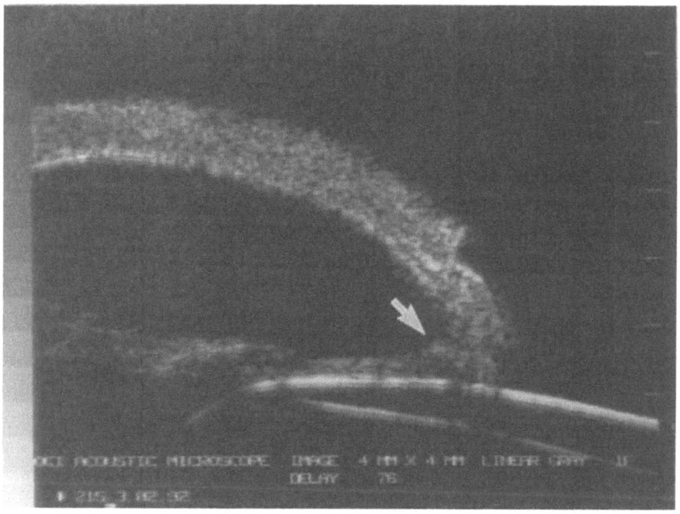

FIGURE 5.5. A case of pseudophakic pupil block shows the margin of the anteriorly bowed iris adherent to a membrane on the lens surface (arrow).

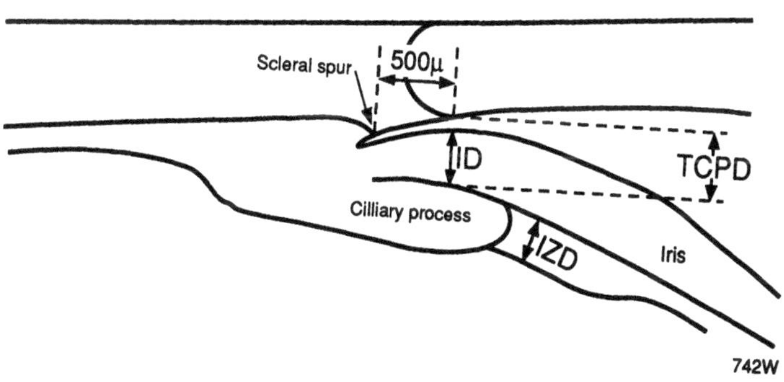

FIGURE 5.6. Diagrammatic representation of the relationships between the ciliary processes and the iris in plateau iris syndrome. The ciliary processes are located anteriorly supporting the peripheral iris. TCPD represents the trabecular-ciliary process distance at a point 500 µm from the scleral spur. ID refers to the iris thickness at this point, and IZD refers to the distance between the posterior iris and the zonule at a point just clearing the ciliary processes. Published with permission from *The American Journal of Ophthalmology* (1992; 113:390–395). Copyright by The Ophthalmic Publishing Company.

iridotomy. A good way of looking at this phenomenon is that the ciliary processes and the trabecular meshwork form a port through which the iris thickness must pass. The smaller this port and/or the thicker the iris in this region, the greater the degree of angle closure. Figure 5.7a through d illustrates some of the variations on this theme seen in clinical examples of plateau iris syndrome following iridotomy. We have found that the anterior chamber depth, trabecular-ciliary process distance, and iris zonule distance were all significantly smaller in plateau iris compared to normal eyes [7]. Iris thickness was not significantly different.

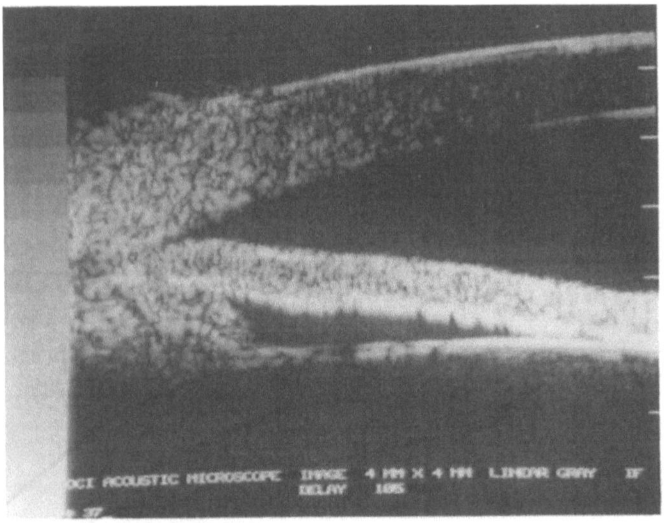

(a)

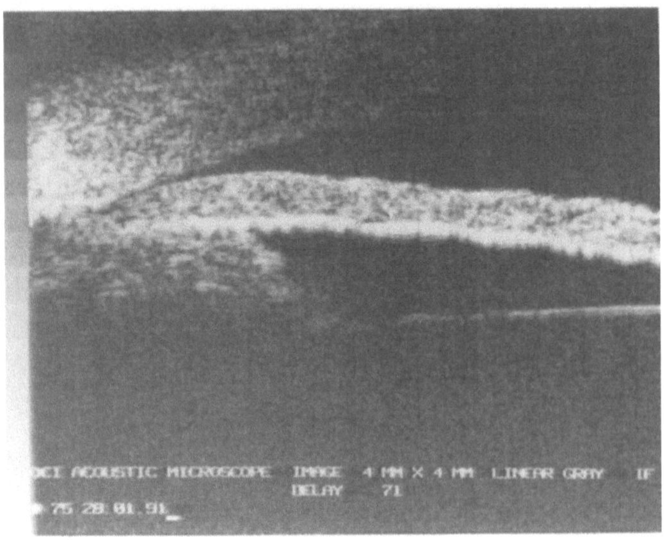

(b)

FIGURE 5.7. Four examples of plateau iris syndrome following iridotomy. All cases show the anterior location of the ciliary processes closing the ciliary sulcus, and preventing the peripheral iris from falling away from the trabecular meshwork. Published with permission from *The American Journal of Ophthalmology* (1992;113:390–395). Copyright by The Ophthalmic Publishing Company.

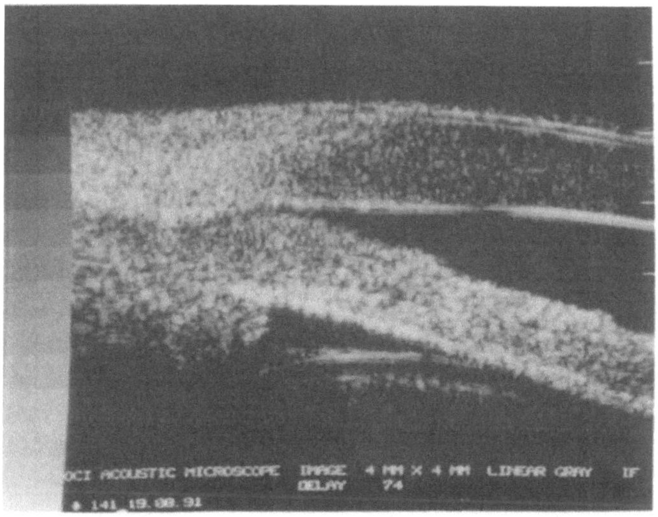
OCI ACOUSTIC MICROSCOPE IMAGE 4 MM X 4 MM LINEAR GRAY IF
DELAY 74
141 19.08.91

(c)

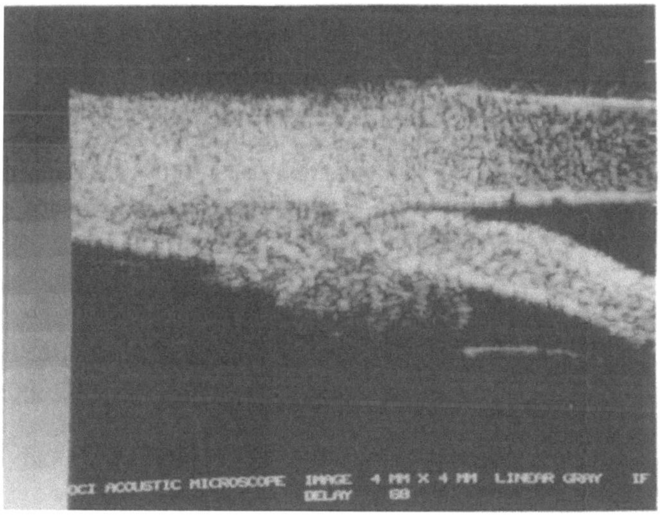
OCI ACOUSTIC MICROSCOPE IMAGE 4 MM X 4 MM LINEAR GRAY IF
DELAY 68

(d)

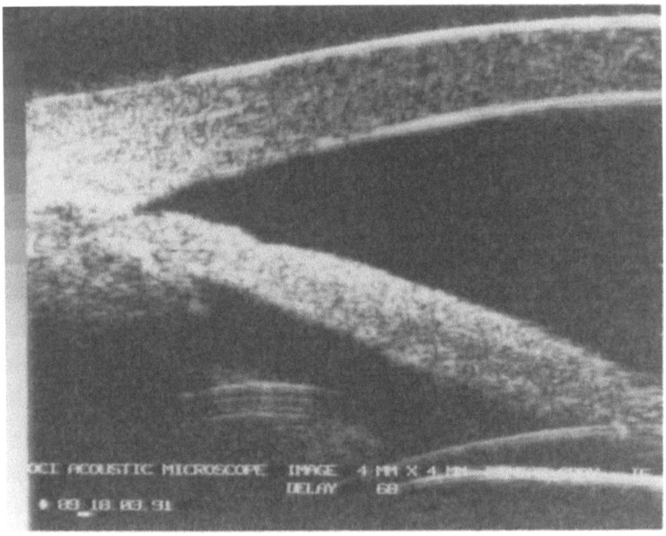

Figure 5.8. Patient with plateau iris syndrome following lens extraction. Despite the posterior movement of the iris, the most peripheral portion of the iris is still supported by the ciliary processes. Published with permission from *The American Journal of Ophthalmology* (1992;113:390–395). Copyright by The Ophthalmic Publishing Company.

This condition is most likely an anatomic variant. We have seen plateau configuration persist even after lens extraction (Figure 5.8), and have been able to diagnose the condition using ultrasound biomicroscopy prior to iridotomy. Figure 5.9 shows the appearance of a case of chronic angle closure before and after iridotomy. The plateau iris configuration in this case was present prior to iridotomy. The relationship of the ciliary processes to the peripheral iris showed little change after iridotomy, and the angle remained extremely narrow.

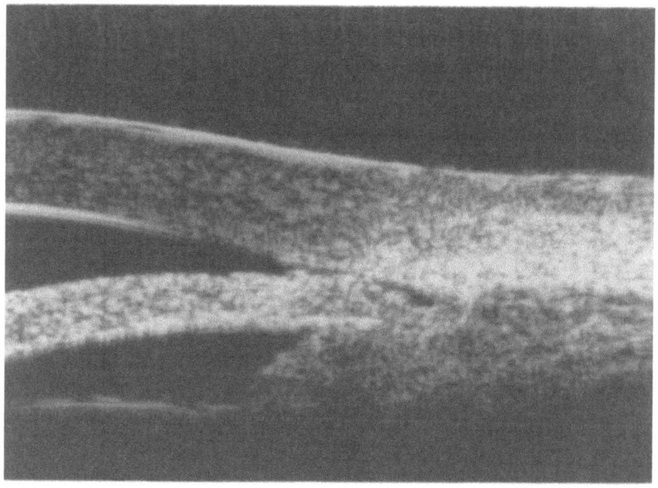

(a)

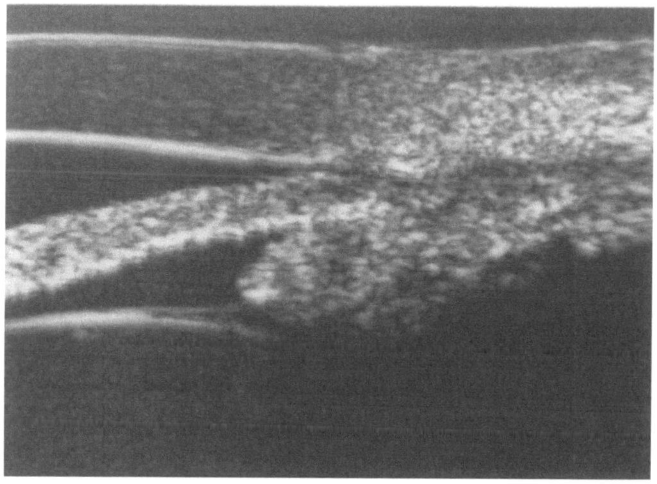

(b)

FIGURE 5.9. (**a**) Case of plateau iris syndrome prior to iridectomy. The ciliary processes are in the typical position that would prevent the peripheral iris from falling away following iridotomy. (**b**) Following iridotomy the angle remains very narrow due to the plateau configuration of the ciliary processes.

We have recently reported [1] with Dr. M. Wand the findings in the first case of plateau iris described by Dr. Chandler in 1955 [8]. This patient was recently located and examined with ultrasound biomicroscopy. Clinically the eye showed two patent iridectomies (Figure 5.10a) and a very narrow angle. Ultrasound biomicroscopy showed the typical appearance of anteriorly located ciliary processes (Figure 5.10b). The pathological findings in the fellow eye, which had been enucleated for glaucoma many years previously, were of interest. Pathology did not reveal any forward positioning of the ciliary processes (Figure 5.10c). Presuming that plateau iris is a bilateral phenomenon, this case illustrates the difference between the ability of ultrasound biomicroscopy to image structures in their normal anatomic relationships, and the distortion of these relationships that occurs following preparation of pathological specimens.

FIGURE 5.10. **(a)** Anterior segment photograph of the first patient with plateau iris presented in the literature. **(b)** Ultrasound biomicroscopy reveals the typical plateau iris configuration. **(c)** Photomicrograph of the previously enucleated fellow eye fails to show the plateau relationship between the ciliary processes and the peripheral iris. Reprinted with permission from reference [1].

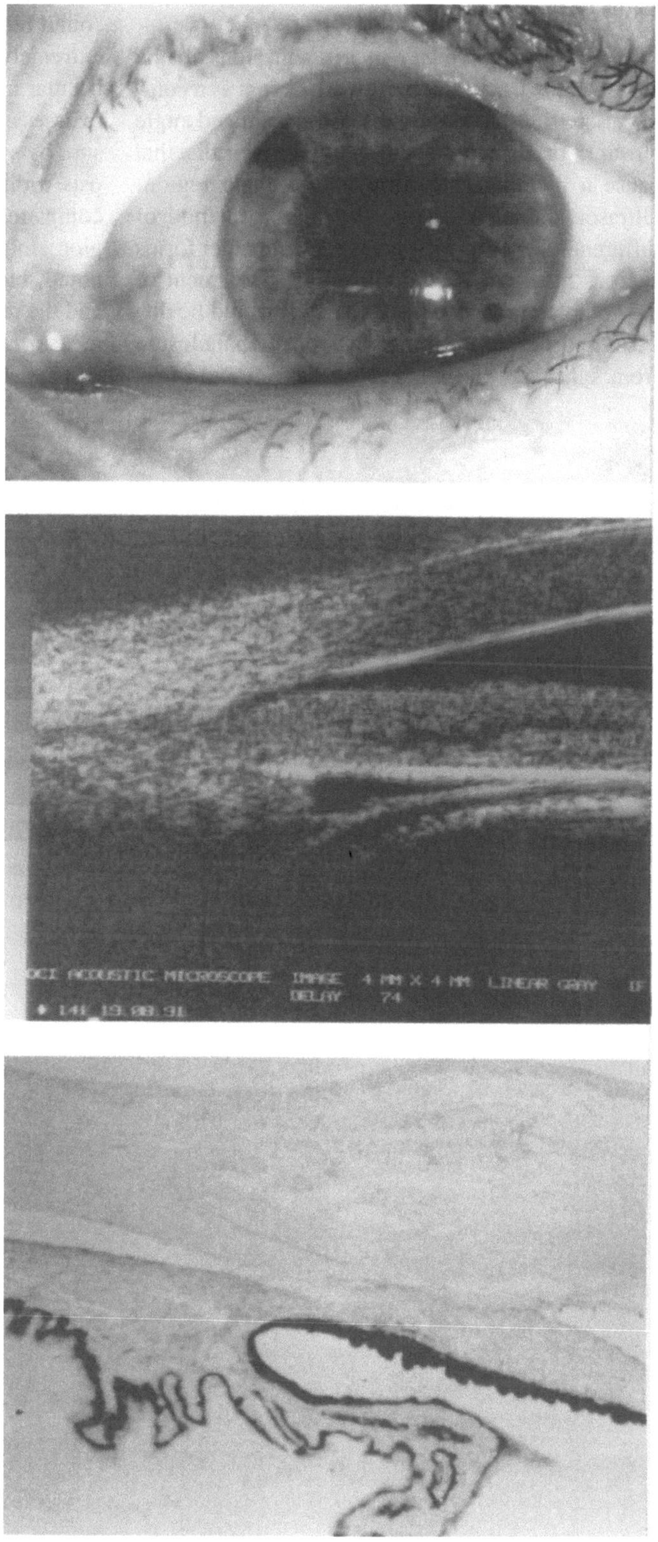

(a)

(b)

(c)

Anterior Synechia

Angle closure secondary to iris adhesions in the region of the trabecular meshwork occurs as a complication of inflammatory disease, prolonged angle closure, or diseases such as rubeosis iridis that cause a membrane to form in the angle region. Ultrasound biomicroscopy provides a method of differentiating this type of closure from other forms such as plateau iris, and allows an assessment of the completeness of angle closure. It would be difficult to differentiate complete appositional closure from synechial closure, but we have found ultrasound biomicroscopy to be capable of defining an extremely small split between the iris and the trabecular meshwork, which may improve our ability to assess prognosis in these cases. Total angle closure by synechiae is illustrated in the case of rubeosis iridis in Figure 5.11a. The peripheral iris is completely apposed to the trabecular meshwork region. In Figure 5.11b an anterior iris adhesion is noted, but a small space is noted between the iris and the region of the trabecular meshwork. In such a case the possibility exists that the meshwork is still capable of functioning.

FIGURE 5.11. **(a)** Complete occlusion of the angle due to anterior synechia in a case of rubeosis iridis. Published with permission from *The American Journal of Ophthalmology* (1992;113:381–389). Copyright by The Ophthalmic Publishing Company. **(b)** In another case with anterior synechia, a space is seen behind the synechia (arrow) that would not be noted gonioscopically.

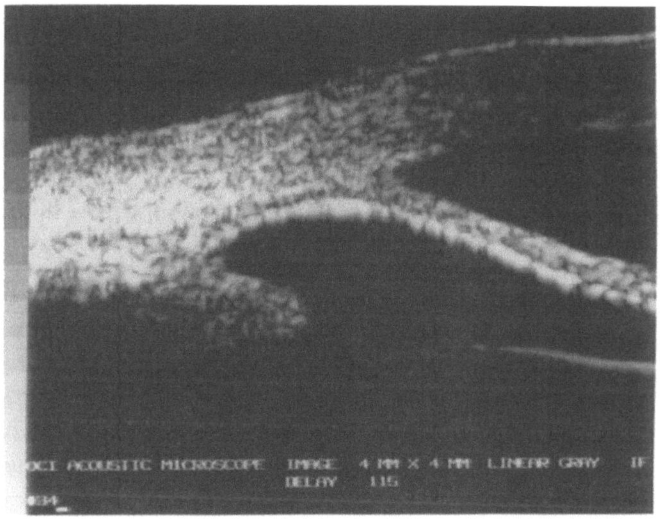

(a)

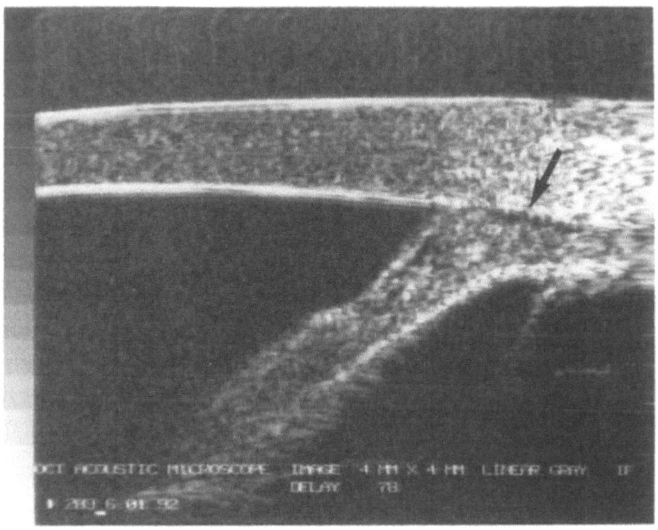

(b)

Ciliochoroidal Effusion

A number of conditions can result in angle closure glaucoma secondary to ciliochoroidal effusion. This complication has been described in relationship to uveal effusion, nanophthalmos, scleral buckling procedures, panretinal photocoagulation, central retinal vein occlusion, arteriovenous fistulas, uveitis, acquired immune deficiency syndrome, hemorrhagic choroidal detachments, and posterior scleritis [9]. The mechanism of angle closure glaucoma has been thought to be an anterior rotation of the ciliary body, or, in the case of massive choroidal hemorrhage or effusion, a direct displacement of the lens/iris diaphragm forward. Most of these cases have been noted to have choroidal detachments on ultrasound or by clinical examination of the fundus. We have found that a very small effusion over the ciliary body without clinically detectable choroidal detachment can be detected with ultrasound biomicroscopy.

The appearance of a supraciliary effusion is similar whether associated with a frank choroidal detachment or not. The ciliary body is detached almost to the scleral spur. The space is crossed by fine lines most likely representing cross sections of thin sheets that connect the ciliary body to the sclera. Figure 5.12a shows the clinical appearance of a case of angle closure secondary to a supraciliary effusion in a patient with IgA nephropathy [10]. On ultrasound biomicroscopy the chamber was shallow, and the ciliary processes were rotated forward producing direct angle closure in a manner similar to plateau iris (Figure 5.12b). A supraciliary effusion was present (Figure 5.12c). Following cycloplegia the ciliary processes had rotated back-

FIGURE 5.12. **(a)** Clinical photograph of a patient with IgA nephropathy presenting with spontaneous anterior chamber shallowing and angle closure. **(b)** Ultrasound biomicroscopy reveals a supraciliary effusion and anterior rotation of the ciliary processes closing the angle (arrow). **(c)** Area of supraciliary effusion. Strands cross the space representing cross sections of thin membranes attaching the ciliary body to the sclera. Published with permission from *The American Journal of Ophthalmology* (1993; 116:341–345). Copyright by The Ophthalmic Publishing Company.

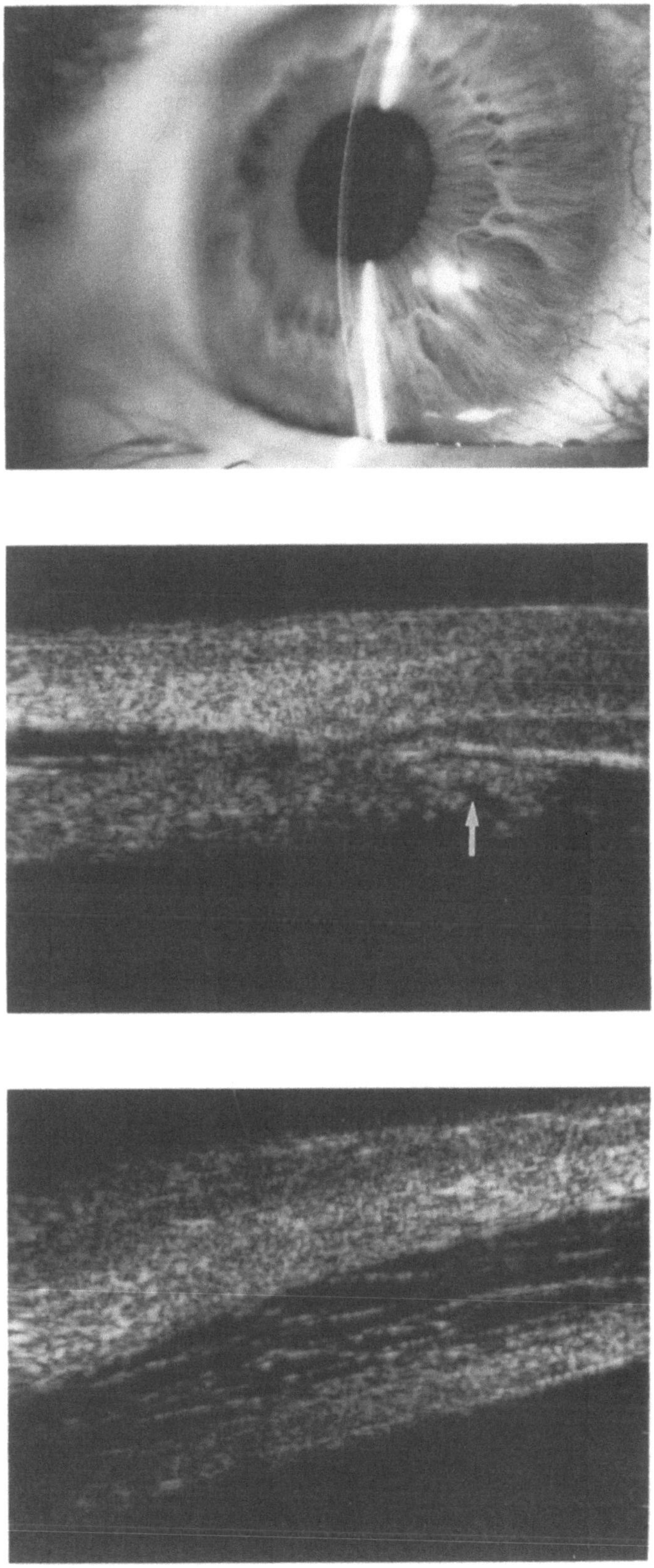

(a)

(b)

(c)

ward and the chamber had deepened (Figure 5.13a). The angle remained closed, however, secondary to a persistent element of pupil block, which is apparent from the anterior iris bowing. Supraciliary fluid was still present (Figure 5.13b). Iridotomy produced angle opening. The mechanism in this case appears to be a mixed one with direct angle closure secondary to rotation of ciliary processes and an element of pupil block secondary to anterior shift of the lens position. Figure 5.14 shows the open angle and the decrease in supraciliary fluid a few days later.

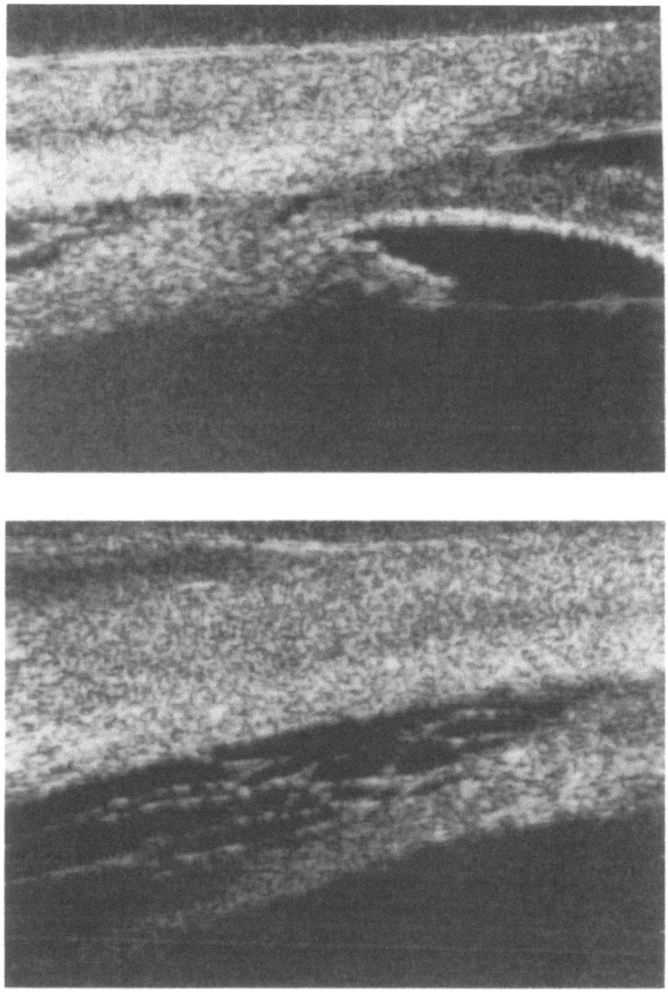

(a)

(b)

FIGURE 5.13. **(a)** Following cycloplegia, the ciliary processes move backward, but the angle remains closed secondary to pupil block with anterior iris bowing. **(b)** A significant amount of supraciliary fluid remains. Published with permission from *The American Journal of Ophthalmology* (1993;116:341–345). Copyright by The Ophthalmic Publishing Company.

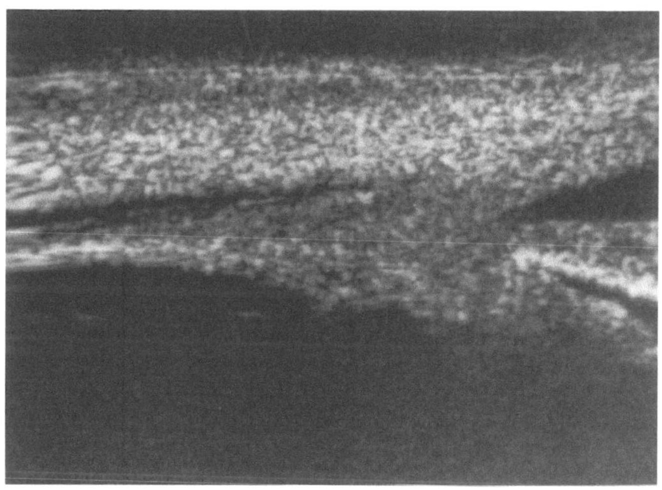

FIGURE 5.14. Ultrasound biomicroscopy shows a decrease in supraciliary fluid a few days later. Iridotomy had been performed. The angle is open. Published with permission from *The American Journal of Ophthalmology* (1993; 116: 341–345). Copyright by The Ophthalmic Publishing Company.

Malignant Glaucoma

Malignant glaucoma is defined as a condition in which shallowing of the anterior chamber with elevated pressure occurs in spite of a patent iridotomy, and in the absence of choroidal detachment. The condition frequently follows filtering surgery, especially in eyes with narrow angles. Various theories have been advanced to explain this phenomenon including posterior misdirection of fluid into the vitreous, and lenticular-ciliary block [11]. In two cases of phakic malignant glaucoma following filtering surgery examined by ultrasound biomicroscopy [12], we have found anterior rotation of ciliary processes to a position just behind the iris (Figures 5.15a and 5.16a), the presence of supraciliary fluid (Figures 5.15b and 5.16b), and closure of the trabeculectomy site by either the lens margin (Figure 5.15c) or ciliary processes (Figure 5.16c). In the case illustrated in Figure 5.16, the effusion was not detected on sclerotomy, which could be due to the small amount of effusion present or the

(a)

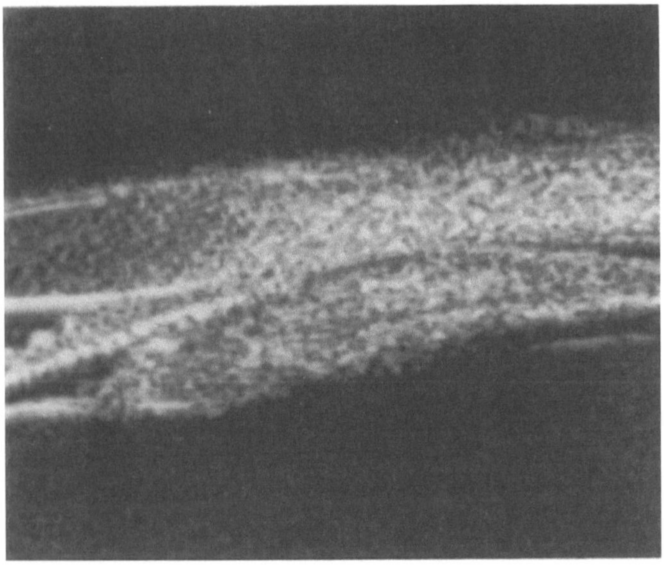

FIGURE 5.15. **(a)** Ultrasound biomicroscopy in a case of malignant glaucoma after 3 days of medical treatment reveals anterior displacement of the ciliary processes narrowing the angle. **(b)** A small amount of fluid is present over the ciliary body (arrow). **(c)** The iridectomy and trabeculectomy opening are closed by the margin of the lens (arrow). Reprinted with permission from reference [12].

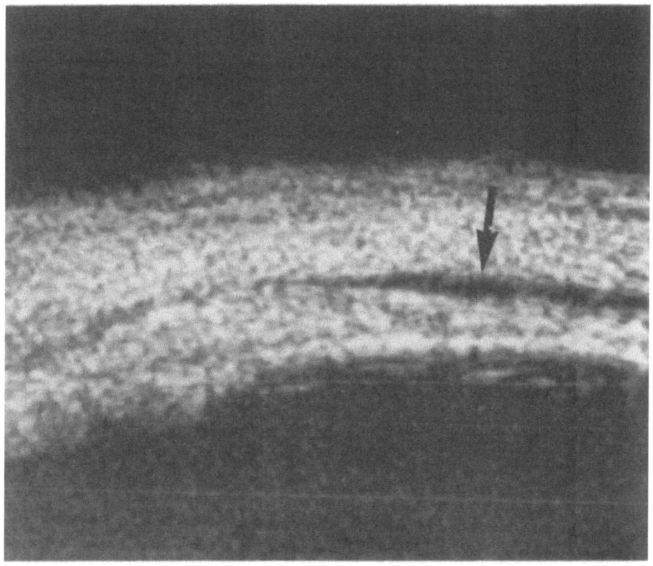

(b)

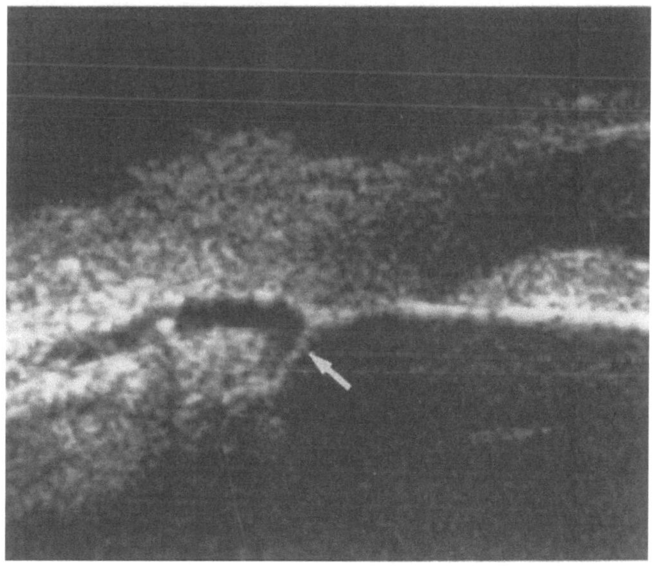

(c)

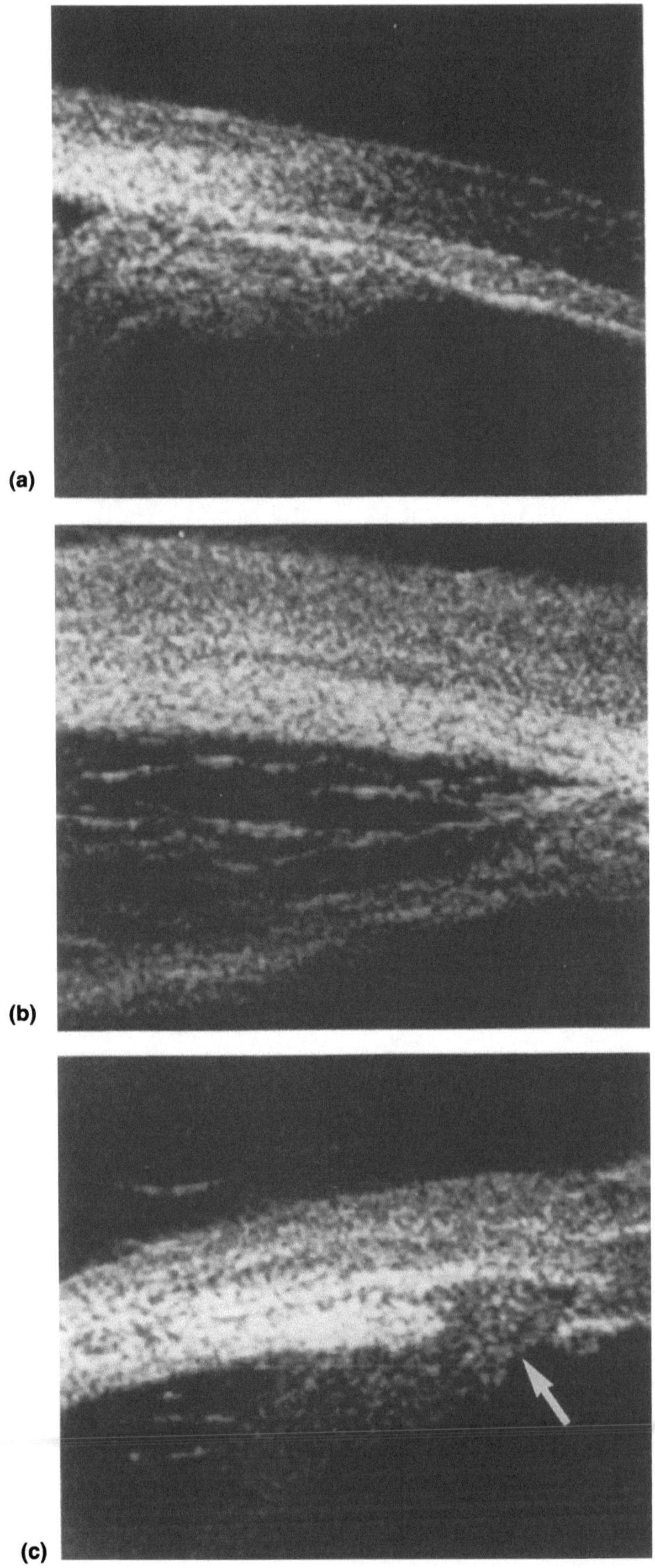

'IGURE 5.16. **(a)** A case of malignant laucoma following trabeculectomy. ınteriorly located ciliary processes ompress the peripheral iris. **(b)** A large ıpraciliary effusion is present. **(c)** The rabeculectomy opening is closed by cil-ıry processes (arrow). Reprinted with ermission from reference [12].

FIGURE 5.17. **(a)** Following vitrectomy in the case illustrated in Figure 5.16, the angle is open, and the trabeculectomy opening is clear. **(b)** The supraciliary effusion has now disappeared.

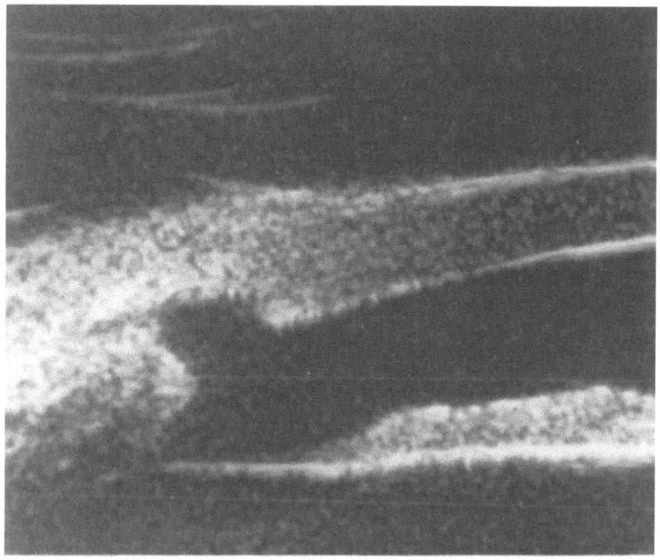

(a)

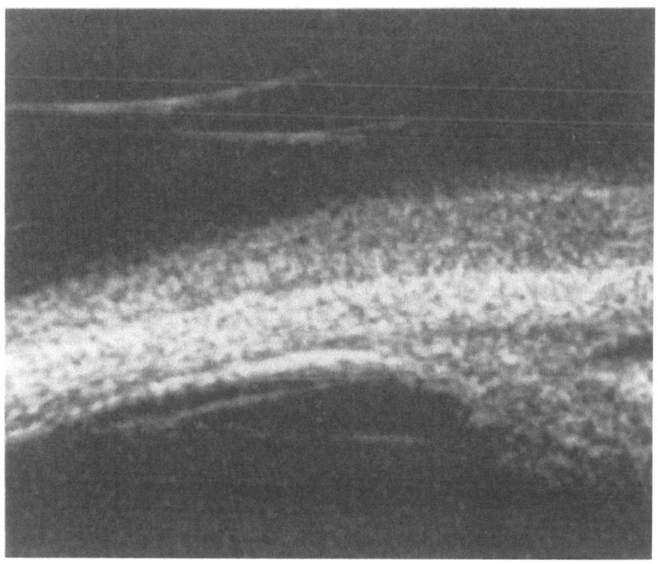

(b)

loculation of the fluid by the septa seen on ultrasound biomicroscopy. Figure 5.17a and b shows the ultrasound biomicroscopic findings following vitrectomy, and successful restoration of normal anatomy. The supraciliary fluid has disappeared at this stage. These findings bring up interesting questions regarding the possibility of undetected supraciliary effusion contributing to the etiology in at least some patients with malignant glaucoma. This could occur by ciliary process rotation closing the angle, bringing the lens forward, and closing the trabeculectomy site, with posterior aqueous diversion perpetuating this scenario. Tello and colleagues observed anterior ciliary process rotation in a case of pseudophakic malignant glaucoma, which improved after laser disruption of the vitreous face [13]. Supraciliary fluid was not observed in this case. Malignant glaucoma will require additional study before the etiology of this condition can be clarified. Ultrasound biomicroscopy should aid this process.

Cystic Angle Closure

An unusual variant of angle closure is due to the presence of multiple iris cysts that elevate the iris and produce varied angle narrowing. This condition has been described as a familial disease [14,15]. Ultrasound biomicroscopy of such a case is illustrated in Figure 5.18. Ultrasound biomicroscopy reveals these cysts to be thick walled and have multiple loculations. Loculations can be imaged behind the iris (Figure 5.18a) and at the pupil margin (Figure 5.18b). It is apparent that lasering a loculation through a widely dilated pupil may not affect the more peripheral loculation that is actually causing the angle closure. Figure 5.18c shows the collapse of some of these cysts following laser iridotomy. This condition is quite different to the iridociliary cysts that are seen as an occasional finding in individuals as described in the section on anterior segment tumors. Iridociliary cysts may cause localized angle narrowing, but are generally thin walled and confined to a small area.

FIGURE 5.18. **(a)** Multiple cystic angle closure. The cysts are thick walled and multiloculated (arrow). **(b)** Cyst at margin of the iris (arrow). **(c)** Laser iridotomy has collapsed some of the cysts.

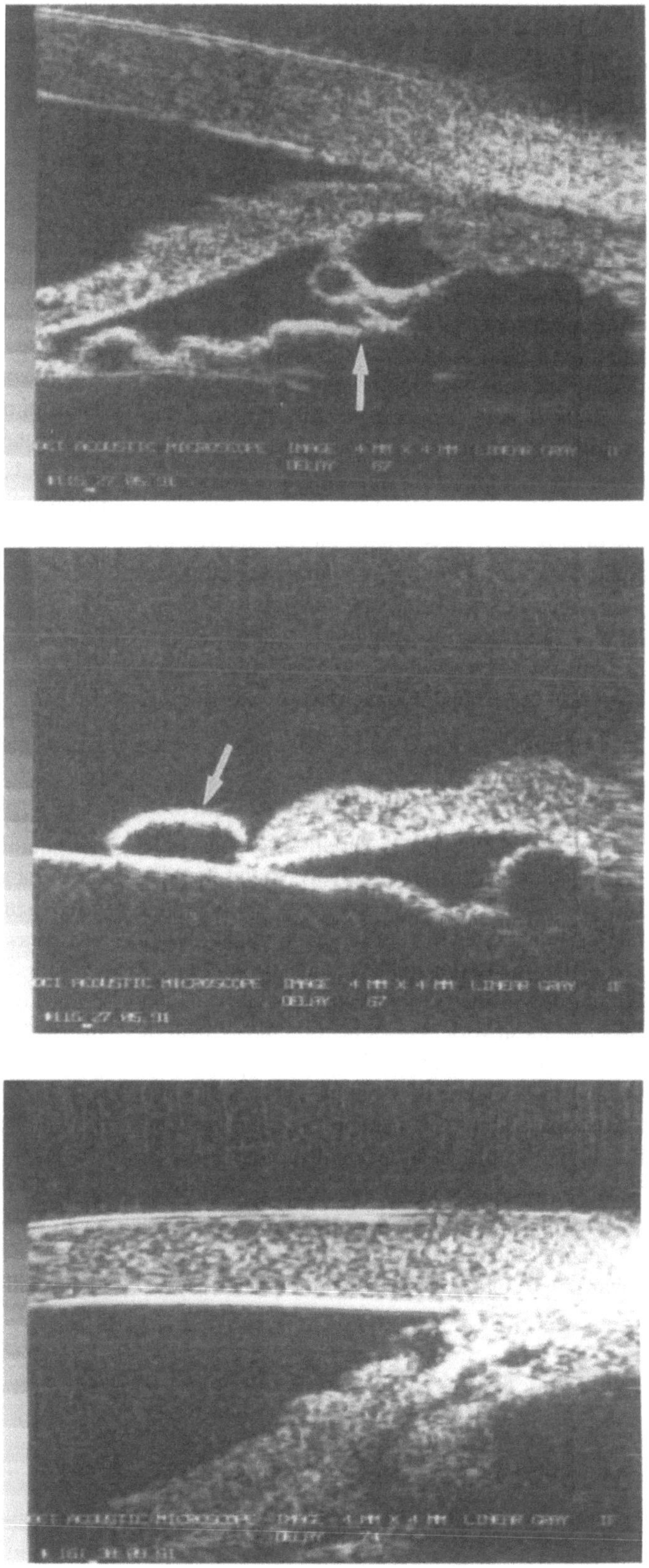

(a) **(b)** **(c)**

Open Angle Glaucoma

Various types of open angle glaucoma have been examined by ultrasound biomicroscopy. Open angle glaucoma is not as productive a field as angle closure because many of the changes taking place in open angle glaucoma occur at a level beyond the current resolution of ultrasound biomicroscopy. Although the trabecular meshwork position can be easily defined in reference to the scleral spur, the actual meshwork itself cannot be differentiated from inner sclera. Schlemm's canal is occasionally imaged, but not consistently. This most likely relates to the degree of opening of this structure. On histology Schlemm's canal is usually flattened in profile. In this situation the opening may not be large enough to be defined by ultrasound biomicroscopy. Nevertheless, ultrasound biomicroscopy should be a useful tool in providing various anatomical measurements that might differentiate populations with glaucoma from those without. In certain open angle variants such as pigmentary glaucoma, ultrasound biomicroscopy can play a much greater role.

Pigmentary Dispersion Syndrome

Pigmentary glaucoma is a variant of open angle glaucoma that occurs in a relatively young population, primarily young male myopes [16]. Clinical manifestations include radial transillumination defects of the midperipheral iris, and the finding of pigment deposition on the lens, iris, cornea, and trabecular meshwork. The collection of pigment in the trabecular meshwork is felt to cause decreased outflow and glaucoma. Patients can display the features of pigment dispersion without elevated pressures. The disease is generally progressive in the early stage, but often stabilizes or improves with passing time.

A theory as to the cause of pigment loss first put forward by Campbell [17] is that the posterior surface of the iris rubs on the zonular fibres near their attachment to the lens. This theory would be consistent with the radial pattern of iris transillumination defects. Recently Karickhoff [18] and others have postulated that posterior iris bowing allowing such contact is caused by a reverse pupil block. This theory implies that peripheral iridotomy could produce equalization of pressure in the two chambers, and allow the iris to come forward. It has been observed clinically [18] and by ultrasound biomicroscopy [19,20,21] that the iris concavity decreases following peripheral iridotomy.

Ultrasound biomicroscopy provides a method of determining iris curvature, defining the relationship of the undersurface of the iris to the zonule and lens, and documenting changes that take place after therapeutic intervention. In our experience with ultrasound biomicroscopy of pigment dispersion syndrome, two variations have been noted. One group shows no obvious concavity of the iris, as illustrated in Figure 5.19. The anterior chamber is deep, but the iris profile is straight, and the zone of iris lens touch is quite small (Figure 5.19b). It is possible that these examinations are taking place at a time when the forces that produce posterior iris bowing are not acting, or have ceased to act.

The second group that shows concavity of the peripheral iris on slit lamp examination has a quite different appearance on ultrasound biomicroscopy. The posterior concavity of the iris is quite apparent on ultrasound biomicroscopy and tends to vary slightly on repeated examinations. The iris is draped over the lens margin creating a greater area of iris–lens contact than in normals. The posterior iris surface is often very close to the zonule and in a number of cases the appearance is consistent with zonular fibres touching the posterior iris. Figure 5.20 shows the posteriorly curved iris and the proximity of the zonular fibres to the posterior iris surface, as well as the increased amount of lens iris contact. These examinations are done with the patient lying in the supine position.

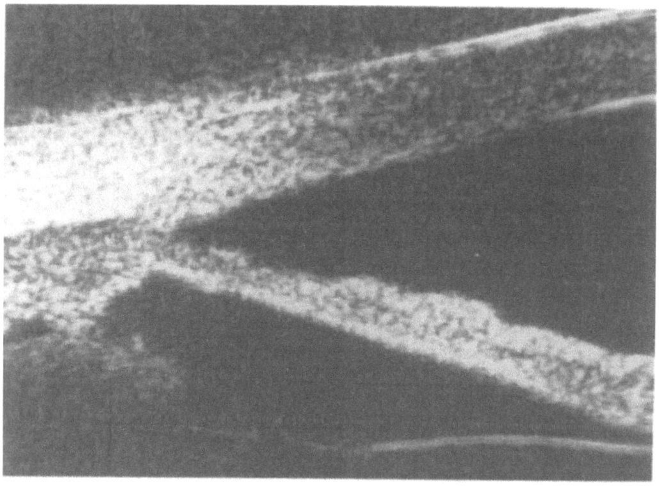

(a)

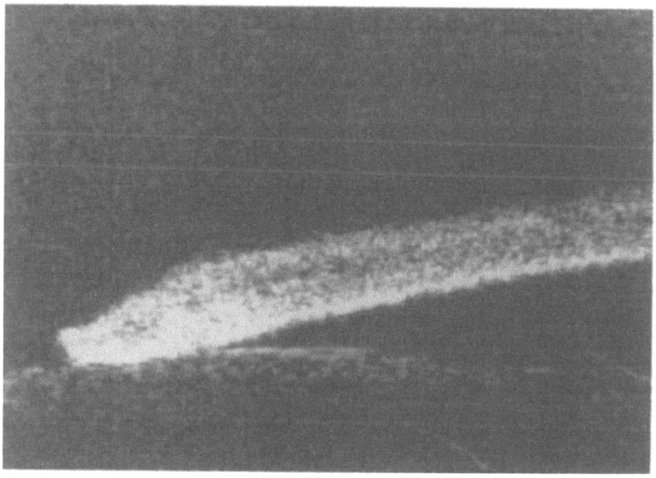

(b)

FIGURE 5.19. (**a**) Patient with pigment dispersion without iris concavity. A large ciliary sulcus is present. (**b**) The iris-lens contact zone is small in this patient.

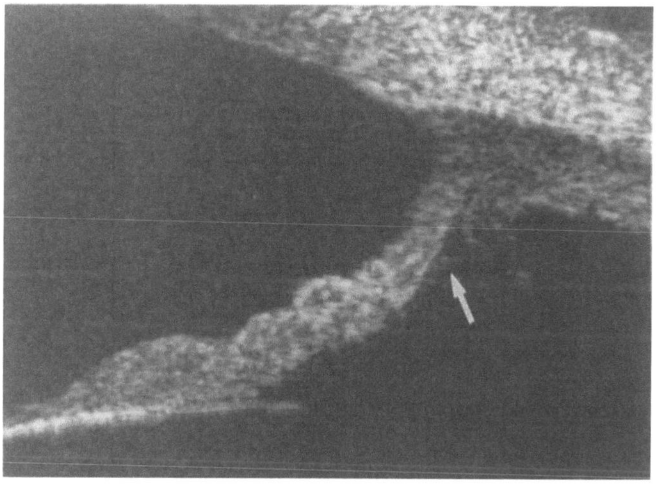

FIGURE 5.20. Marked posterior bowing in a patient with pigment dispersion syndrome. The ciliary process is immediately behind the peripheral iris, and the zonule is likely in contact with the iris pigment epithelium (arrow).

Peripheral iridotomy in these patients has been observed to produce a flattening of the iris profile on slit lamp examination [18]. We have been able to demonstrate this change in iris profile following iridotomy using ultrasound biomicroscopy in patients with a pre-operative posteriorly bowed iris profile. In Figure 5.21a the clinical appearance of posterior iris bowing inferiorly is noted on slit lamp examination. Ultrasound biomicroscopy (Figure 5.21b) shows the posterior bowing in profile. Figure 5.21c shows the straightened iris profile imaged in the same location as Figure 5.21b. This change in iris profile from a concave to a straight line following iridotomy is consistent with the theory of reverse pupil block.

FIGURE 5.21. **(a)** Clinical photograph shows the posterior bowing of the inferior iris in a patient with pigment dispersion. **(b)** Ultrasound biomicroscopy shows the posterior bowing of the iris in this patient. **(c)** Ultrasound biomicroscopy following laser iridotomy shows straightening of the iris profile.

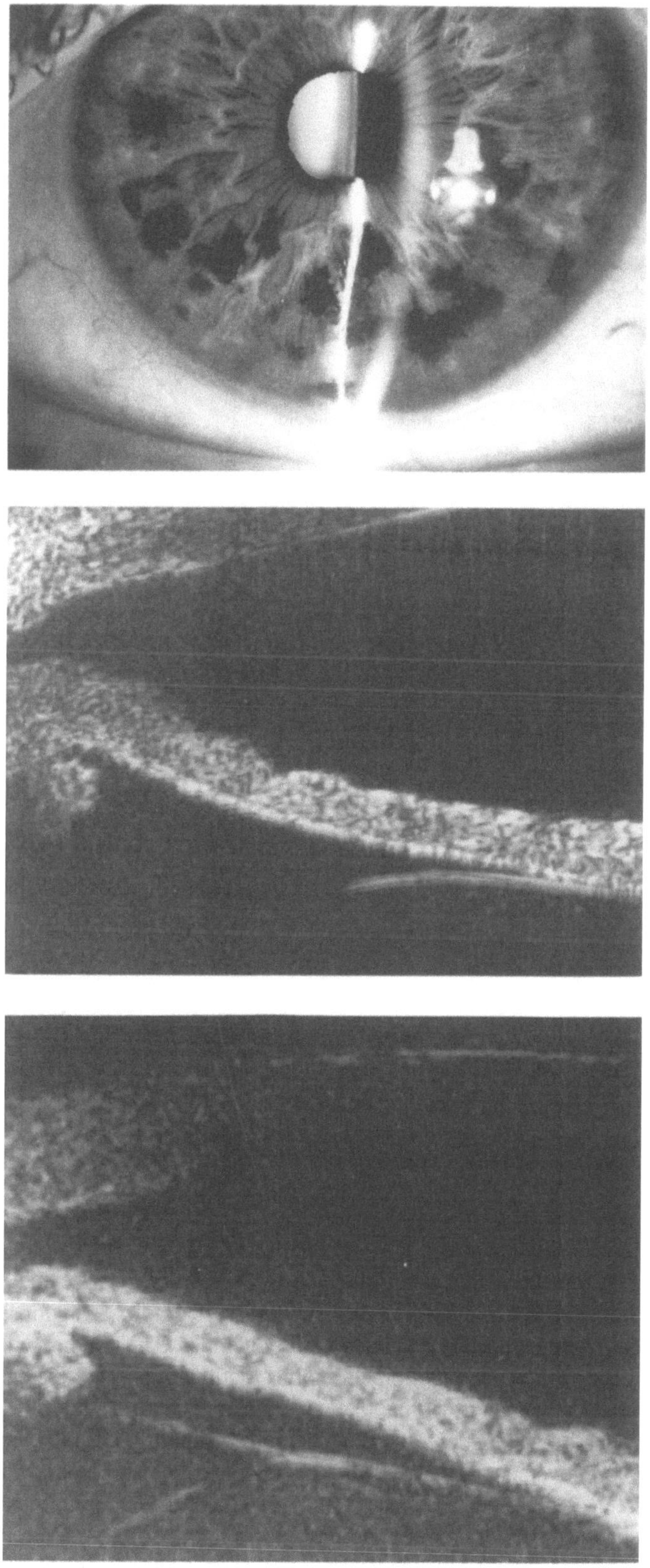

(a)

(b)

(c)

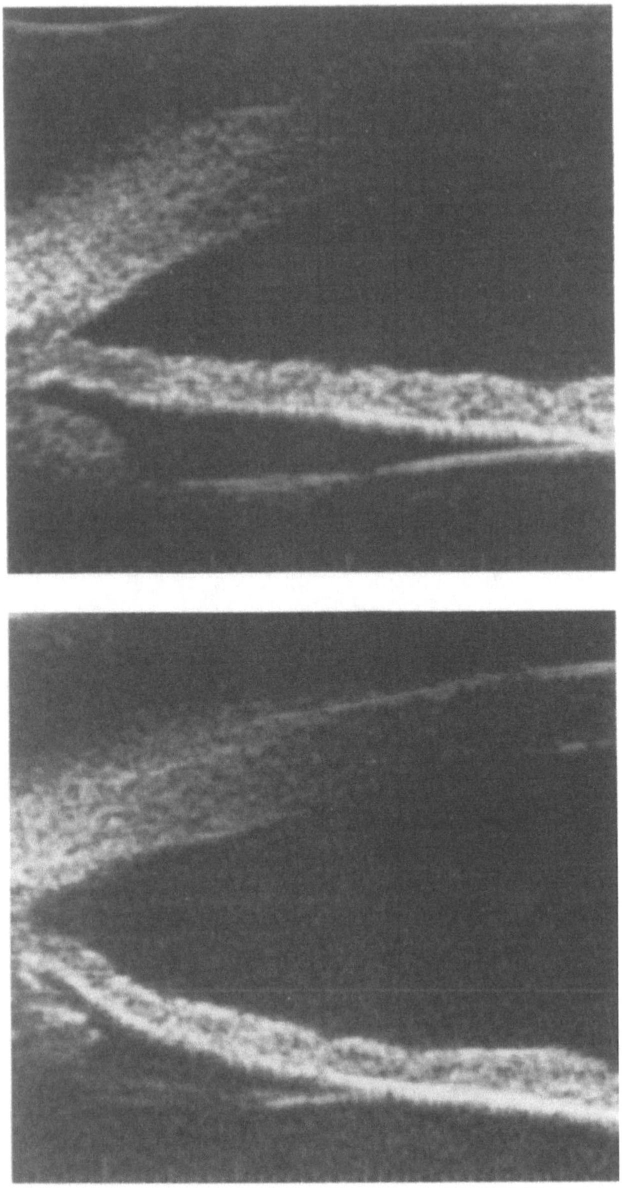

(a)

(b)

FIGURE 5.22. **(a)** Ultrasound biomicroscopic image of the angle structures and iris on distance fixation. The iris displays a straight profile. **(b)** Ultrasound biomicroscopic image of the angle structures and iris on near fixation. The iris assumes a posteriorly bowed profile. From Reference 22. Published with permission from *The American Journal of Ophthalmology*. Copyright by The Ophthalmic Publishing Company.

A remaining question is the nature of the process that produces a reversal of the usual pressure gradient from the posterior to the anterior chamber. The theory of reverse pupil block implies that the pressure in the anterior chamber at least transiently exceeds that in the posterior chamber. Blinking, eye movement, and vascular pulse waves have been suggested. McWhae and Crichton have shown posterior iris bowing with accommodation in normal patients using ultrasound biomicroscopy. We have been able to demonstrate posterior iris bowing in pigment dispersion occurring synchronous with accommodation and forward movement of the anterior lens surface (Figure 5.22) [22]. The anterior lens movement could increase the pressure in the anterior chamber. Slow outflow through the trabecular meshwork and the inability to equalize pressure with the posterior chamber due to the flap valve formed by the iris–lens interface, could result in this increased pressure producing posterior iris

FIGURE 5.23. **(a)** Surgical iridectomy shows sharp margins in the iridectomy site. Reproduced with permission from Reference [1]. **(b)** Yag laser iridotomy shows irregular iris stromal disruption.

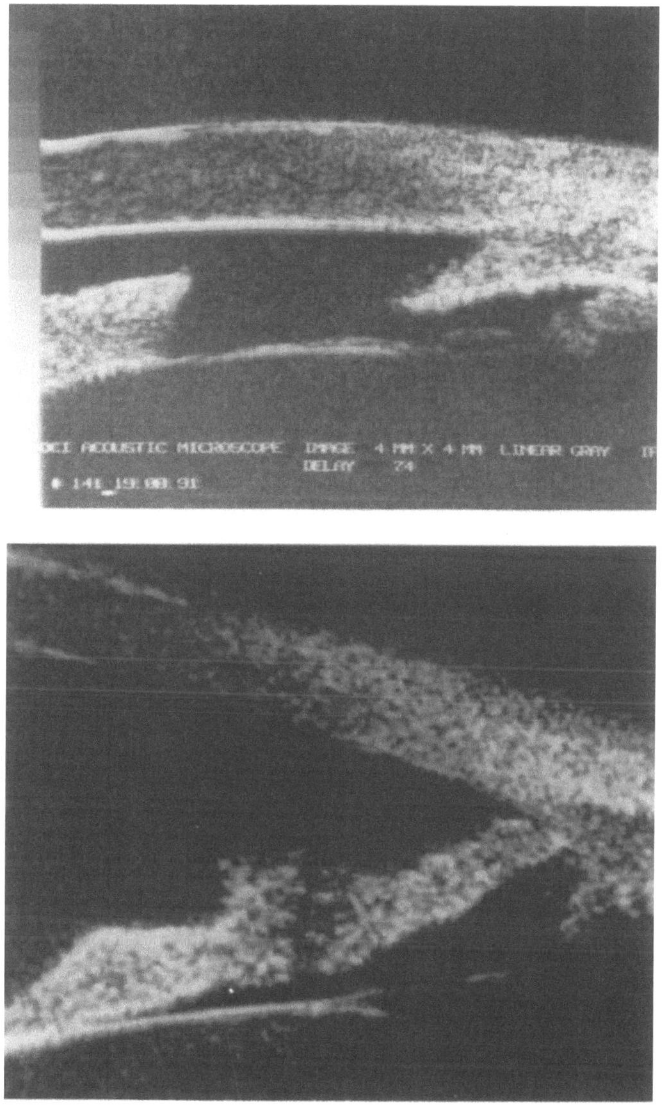

(a)

(b)

bowing. We have observed that the phenomenon of posterior iris bowing with accommodation disappears after iridotomy.

Pigment dispersion syndrome and pigmentary glaucoma are excellent examples of conditions that are in the process of evolution as far as our understanding of disease mechanisms and possible introduction of new treatment modalities. Ultrasound biomicroscopy is proving a valuable tool in aiding our understanding of this disease.

Glaucoma Surgery

Iridectomy

Surgical iridectomy sites generally show a smooth-edged gap in the iris on ultrasound biomicroscopy as illustrated in Figure 5.23a. Yag laser iridotomy, in contrast, is imaged as a much more irregular opening, with stromal disruption as illustrated in Figure 5.23b.

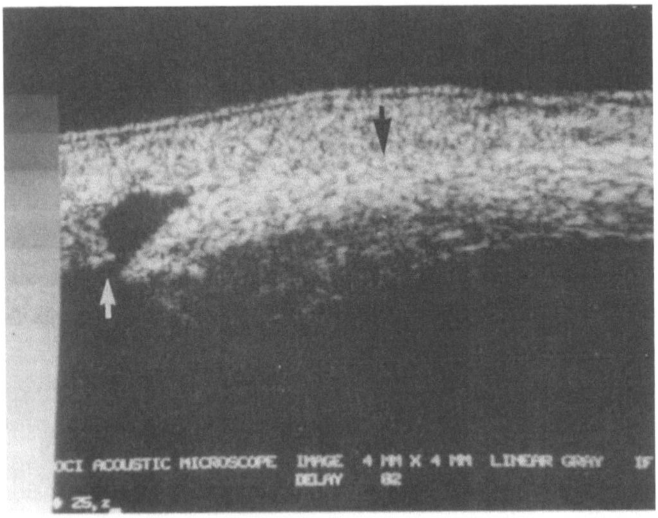

(a)

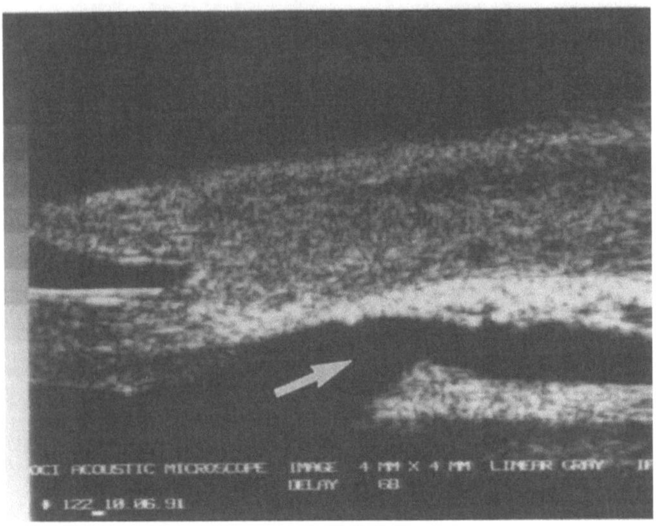

(b)

FIGURE 5.24. **(a)** Failed trabeculectomy procedure. Ultrasound biomicroscopy shows a patent opening (white arrow), but no space at the scleral dissection site (black arrow), and no bleb. **(b)** Functioning trabeculectomy procedure. The opening into the anterior chamber (arrow) is continuous with a patent intrascleral pathway, and a filtering bleb is present. Published with permission from *The American Journal of Ophthalmology* (1992;113:381–389). Copyright by The Ophthalmic Publishing Company.

Trabeculectomy

Ultrasound biomicroscopy can image a very small surgical opening. This attribute makes it a useful tool for the examination of filtering techniques and causes of failure. The internal surgical opening can be consistently visualized and the state of the filtering bleb assessed. Figure 5.24 illustrates the ability of ultrasound biomicroscopy to analyze the state of filtering procedures. Figure 5.24a shows the internal ostium in a nonfunctioning case with close apposition of the scleral incision and no functioning bleb. Figure 5.24b, in contrast, shows a patent opening continuous with a distinct scleral split and a functioning bleb. Our findings show the internal structure of filtering blebs to show variable internal reflectivity. This most likely depends on the distribution of fluid in the episcleral tissue. A clear fluid space is found occasionally. Figure 5.25 shows a filtering bleb with a mixture of clear fluid spaces and spongy episcleral tissue.

Molteno Implants

Molteno implants and other procedures involving stents also lend themselves to analysis using ultrasound biomicroscopy. Figure 5.26 shows the ultrasound biomicroscopic appearance of the tube in the anterior chamber of a patient with a Molteno implant.

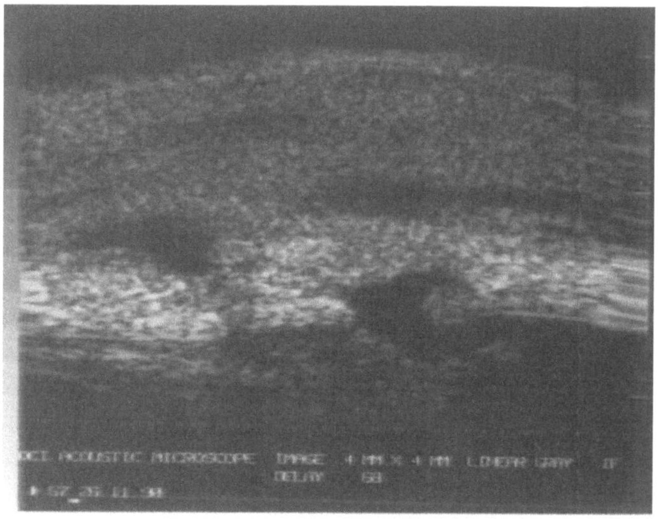

FIGURE 5.25. A functioning filtering procedure. The bleb shows occasional open fluid spaces, but mostly consists of low-reflective, spongy episcleral tissue.

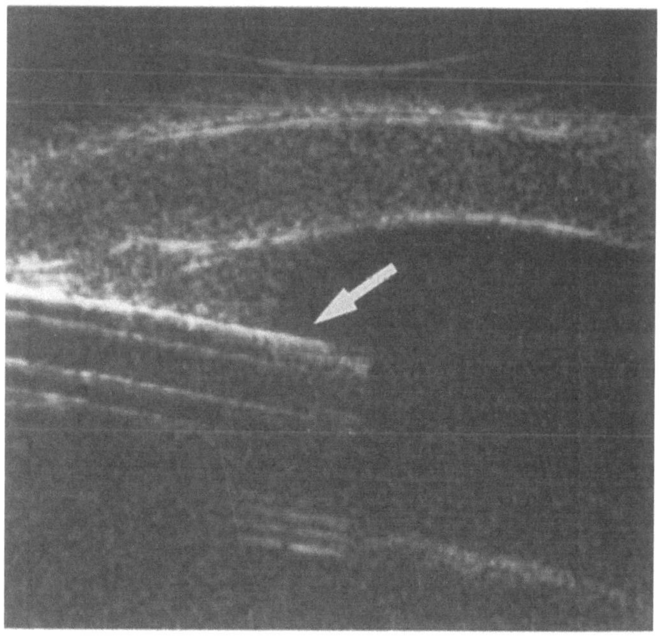

FIGURE 5.26. Molteno implant. The position of the tube is imaged in the anterior chamber (arrow).

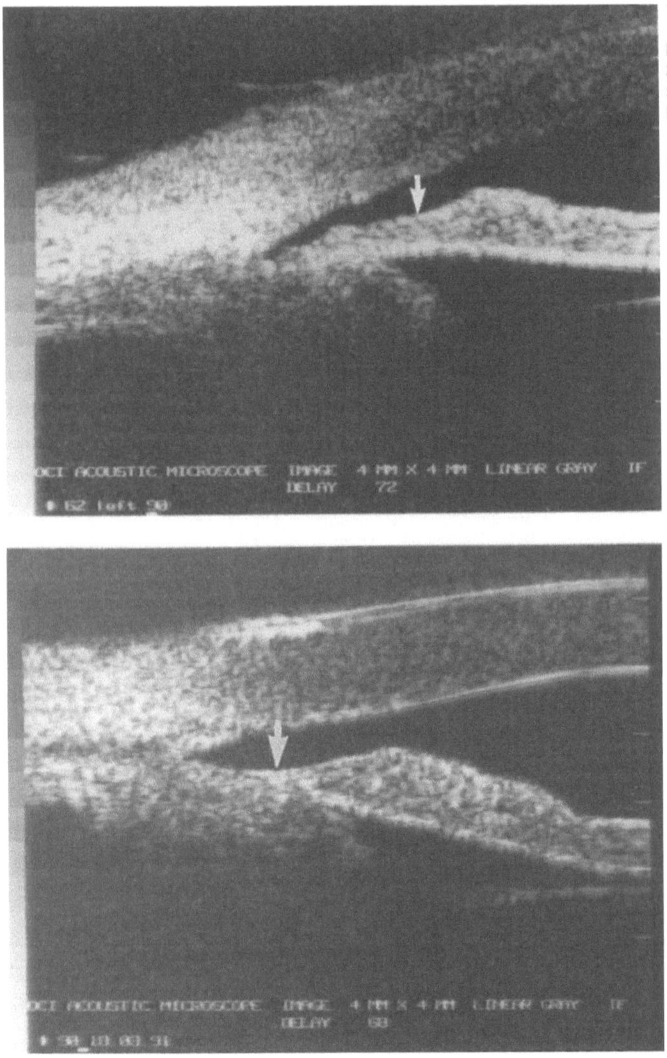

(a)

(b)

FIGURE 5.27. **(a)** Laser iridoplasty (arrow) shows partial opening of the angle. **(b)** Iridoplasty in more peripheral location (arrow) shows a wider angle opening. Published with permission from *The American Journal of Ophthalmology* (1992;113:390–395). Copyright by The Ophthalmic Publishing Company.

Laser Iridoplasty

Laser iridoplasty is used to produce flattening and thinning of the peripheral iris in conditions such as plateau iris. Figure 5.27a shows the appearance of the iris following iridoplasty in a case of plateau iris. The angle is partially opened. More peripheral burns as illustrated in Figure 5.27b produce greater angle opening.

Summary

The glaucomas constitute a wide variety of disease entities. Some of these are well understood and some remain enigmas. Ultrasound biomicroscopy is an imaging tool that could aid in resolving some of these enigmas. Plateau iris syndrome, supraciliary effusions, malignant glaucoma, and pigmentary glaucoma are just some examples of entities in which useful information has been gained by using this tool. In addition to its value as a clinical research device, ultrasound biomicroscopy has value in clinical assessment and guiding treatment in difficult glaucoma cases.

References

1. Wand M, Pavlin CJ, Foster FS. Plateau iris syndrome: Ultrasound biomicroscopic and histological study. *Ophthalmic Surg* 1993;24:129–131.
2. Tiedeman JS. A physical analysis of the factors that determine the contour of the iris. *Am J Ophthalmol* 1991;111:338.
3. Jin JC, Anderson DR. The effect of iridotomy on iris contour. *Am J Ophthalmol* 1990;110:260.
4. Anderson DR, Jin JC, Wright MM: The physiological characteristics of relative pupillary block. *Am J Ophthalmol* 1991;111:344.
5. Potash SD, Tello C, Liebmann J, Ritch R. Ultrasound biomicroscopy in the pigment dispersion syndrome. *Ophthalmology* 1994;101:332–339.
6. Pavlin CJ, Harasiewicz K, Foster FS. Ultrasound biomicroscopy of anterior segment structures in normal and glaucomatous eyes. *Am J Ophthalmol* April 1992;113:381–389.
7. Pavlin CJ, Ritch R, Foster FS. Ultrasound biomicroscopy in plateau iris syndrome. *Am J Ophthalmol* April 1992; 113:390–395.
8. Wand M, Grant W, Simmons RJ, Hutchinson BT. Plateau iris syndrome. *Trans Am Acad Ophthalmol Otol* 1977;83:122.
9. Fourman S. Angle closure glaucoma complicating cilio-choroidal detachment. *Ophthalmology* 1989; 96:646–653.
10. Pavlin CJ, Easterbrook M, Harasiewicz K, Foster FS. An ultrasound biomicroscopic analysis of angle-closure glaucoma secondary to cilio-choroidal effusion in IgA nephropathy. *Am J Ophthalmol* 1993;116:341–345.
11. Luntz MH, Rosenblatt M. Malignant glaucoma. *Surv Ophthalmol* 1987;32:73–92.
12. Trope G, Pavlin CJ, Bau A, Baumal C, Foster FS. Malignant glaucoma: clinical and ultrasound biomicroscopic characteristics. *Ophthalmology* (in press).
13. Tello C, Chi T, Shepps G, Liebmann J, Ritch R. Ultrasound biomicroscopy in pseudophakic malignant glaucoma. *Ophthalmology* 1993;100:1330–1334.
14. Chandler PA, Braconier HE. Spontaneous intra-epithelial cysts of iris and ciliary body with glaucoma. *Am J Ophthalmol* 1958;45:64–74.
15. Vela A, Rieser JC, Campbell DG. The heredity and treatment of angle-closure glaucoma secondary to iris and ciliary body cysts. *Ophthalmology* 1984; 91:332–337.
16. Sugar HS. Pigmentary glaucoma: A 25 year review. *Am J Ophthalmol* 1966;62:499–507.
17. Campbell DG. Pigmentary dispersion and glaucoma: A new theory. *Arch Ophthalmol* 1979;97: 1667–72.
18. Karickhoff JR. Pigmentary dispersion syndrome and pigmentary glaucoma: A new mechanism concept, a new treatment, and a new technique. *Ophthalmic Surg* 1992;23:269–277.
19. Karickhoff JR. Response to Fourman S. Iridotomy in eyes with pigmentary glaucoma (Letter). *Ophthalmic Surg* 1992;23:843–844.
20. Potash SD, Tello C, Liebmann J, Ritch R. Ultrasound biomicroscopy in pigment dispersion syndrome. *Ophthalmology* 1994;101:332–339.
21. Pavlin CJ, Macken P, Trope G, Feldman F, Havasiewicz K, Foster FS. *Can J Ophthalmol* (in press).
22. Pavlin CJ, Havasiewicz K, Foster FS. Accommodation produces posterior iris bowing in pigmentary dispersion syndrome. *Am J Ophthalmol* (in press).

6
Anterior Segment Tumors

We have found ultrasound biomicroscopy to be a useful adjunct in the diagnosis and management of anterior segment tumors [1]. A combination of standardized ultrasound, clinical observation, and fluorescein angiography has proven very accurate in the diagnosis of posterior uveal melanomas [2], but many anterior segment lesions still present problems in differential diagnoses. Clinical observation remains the main method of differentiating and following these lesions, with little help from diagnostic testing. The small size of these lesions makes them difficult to image with conventional ultrasound, although water bath techniques can improve definition of larger lesions [3,4]. Anterior segment fluorescein angiography has been found to be of limited accuracy in differentiating iris tumors [5].

Most iris lesions are currently followed by slit lamp observation, looking for change in surface characteristics. Ultrasound biomicroscopy adds the dimension of depth. The ability to measure these lesions accurately adds a quantitative aspect to demonstrating tumor change. Ultrasound biomicroscopy allows accurate assessment of tumor margins and definition of which ocular structures are involved. Internal reflectivity patterns add diagnostic information. The most significant limitation of ultrasound biomicroscopy is limited penetration of large lesions. In such cases conventional ultrasound may be more helpful in measuring tumor thickness.

Iris Tumors

Iris tumors are common, but the majority of tumors confined to the iris tend to show less aggressive characteristics. As a result, the majority of iris lesions are observed for long periods of time and only removed if they have an ominous clinical appearance or are demonstrably changing. This factor makes it difficult to have extensive clinical-pathological correlation between ultrasound biomicroscopic findings and the pathology of lesions. In past studies, tumors diagnosed as melanomas have been extensively reclassified as benign lesions both from clinical observation [6], and from pathological review [7]. This difficulty in diagnosing malignant versus benign pathology even on histological examination points out the difficulty of doing the same on the basis of clinical or ultrasound appearance. Nevertheless, certain patterns emerge on ultrasound biomicroscopy that can be helpful in classifying these lesions.

Iris Nevi

The majority of solid lesions that occur on the iris are nevi. These lesions are benign, but malignant change cannot be excluded. We have found certain ultrasound biomicroscopic features commonly present in lesions that are clinically believed to be nevi.

FIGURE 6.1. (**a**) Clinical appearance of a highly pigmented iris nevus. (**b**) Ultrasound biomicroscopy shows a low-reflective surface layer (arrow), with diffuse iris thickening below.

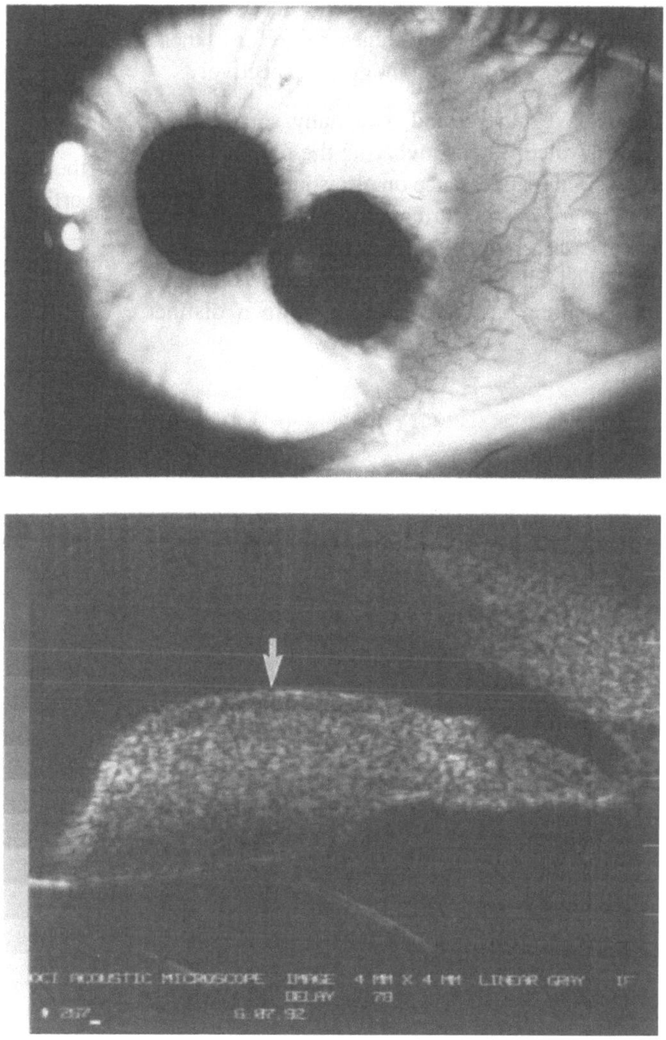

(a)

(b)

Surface Plaques

Surface plaques are commonly found in histological studies of iris lesions [7]. These consist of superficial layers of pure tumor cells, frequently accompanied by more diffuse involvement of underlying iris stroma. The presumed ultrasound biomicroscopic counterpart is a superficial layer of low reflectivity. Figure 6.1a shows the clinical appearance of an eye with an iris nevus. Ultrasound biomicroscopic appearance in Figure 6.1b shows a low reflective surface plaque overlying an area of iris thickening. Surface plaques are frequently seen and are often very thin (50 to 150 μm). Underlying iris stroma can be thickened, but it is often difficult to tell whether this is a contraction phenomenon, or actual tumor involvement of the iris stroma.

Morphology

The presence of a typical morphological appearance on ultrasound biomicroscopy could be helpful as a diagnostic sign. A number of these appearances are repetitive and could be helpful in differential diagnoses of these lesions.

Of Mice and Moguls

Two of the more common shape variations encountered are fusiform thickening of lesions of the central iris and a bowed appearance of lesions at the iris root. In our clinic we sometimes refer to these lesion shapes as mice and moguls, respectively.

Moguls. We have found that many small, minimally elevated lesions involving the peripheral iris have a similar appearance on ultrasound biomicroscopy (Figure 6.2a through c). They uniformly share the ultrasound biomicroscopic appearance of small, moderately thickened peripheral iris lesions, not extending past the iris root, with a distinct anterior convex bowing. There is usually a hypoechoic layer on the surface of these lesions, possibly indicating that the superficial layer is involved with a tumor plaque. It is interesting to speculate on the cause of this curvature. The bowing forward of the peripheral iris may relate to contraction of superficial tumor tissue as compared to normal iris. This would put tension on the iris, and in combination with a fixed point of attachment of the iris root, may cause it to arch.

FIGURE 6.2. **(a)**–**(c)** Examples of peripheral iris lesions that present with a bowed appearance, often with a surface plaque. Figure **(c)** published courtesy of *Ophthalmology* (1992;99:1220–1228).

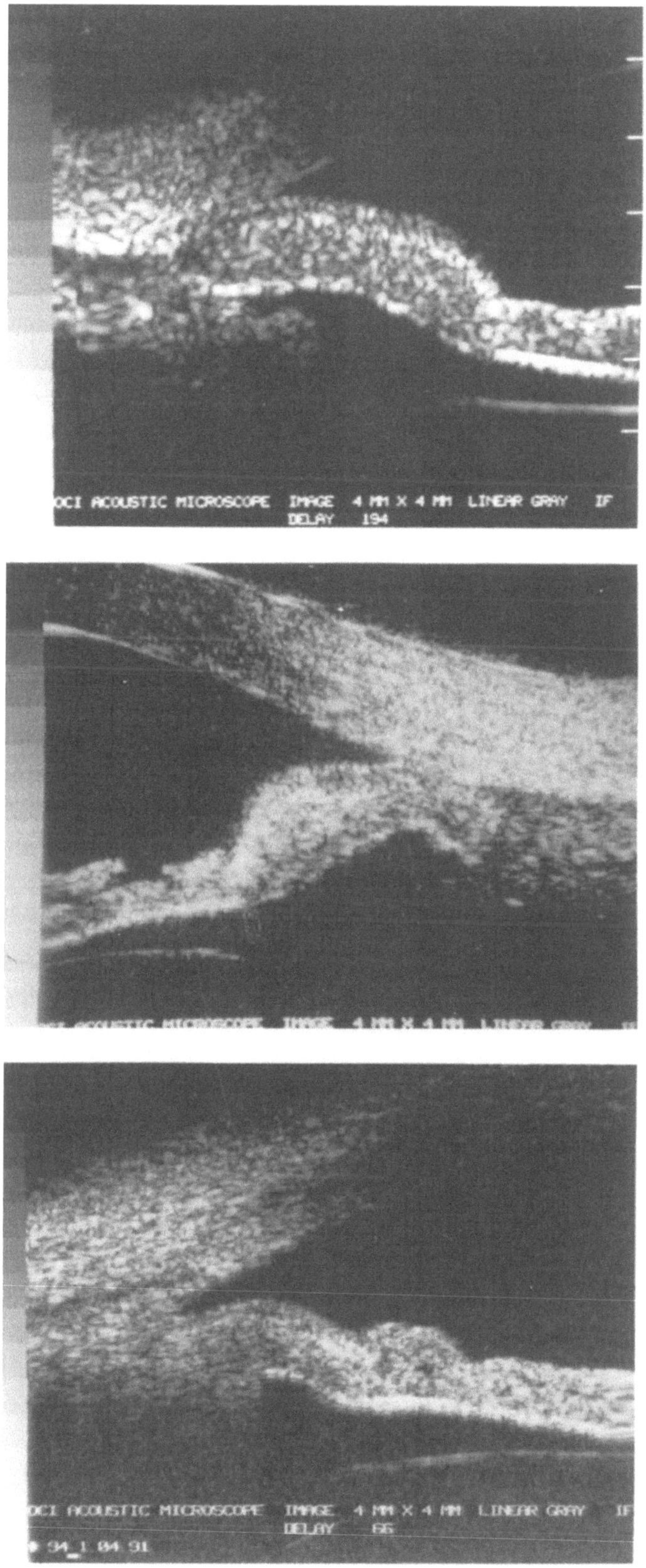

(a)

(b)

(c)

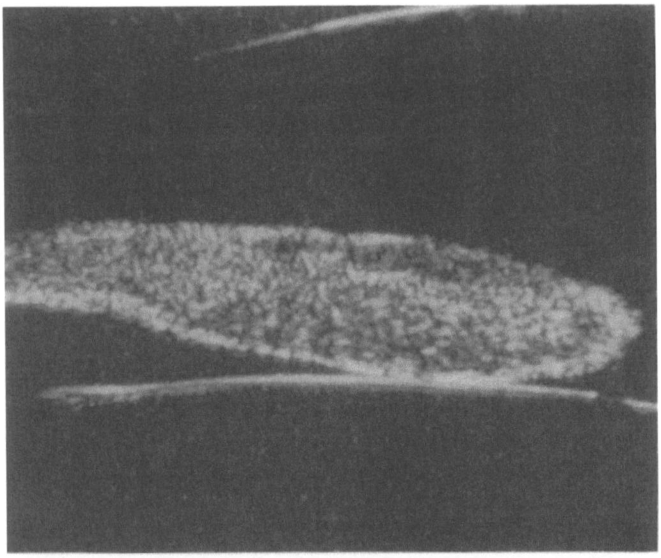

(a)

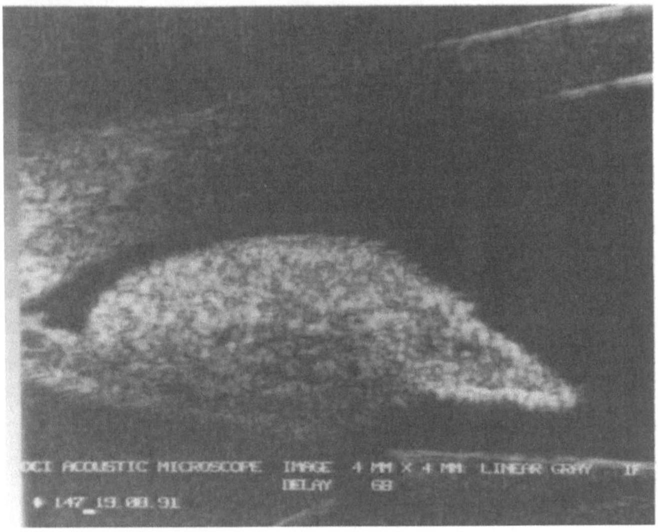

(b)

FIGURE 6.3. **(a)–(d)** Examples of more central iris lesions that usually produce a fusiform thickening without iris bowing. Figure **(a)** published courtesy of *Ophthalmology* (1992;99:1220–1228).

Mice. Similar lesions located more centrally do not show convex bowing, but rather thickening of the iris in a fusiform fashion and occasional ectropion uveae (Figure 6.3a through d). In these cases there may be a similar tension phenomena occurring on the surface that manifests differently because of the lack of a fixed point of attachment.

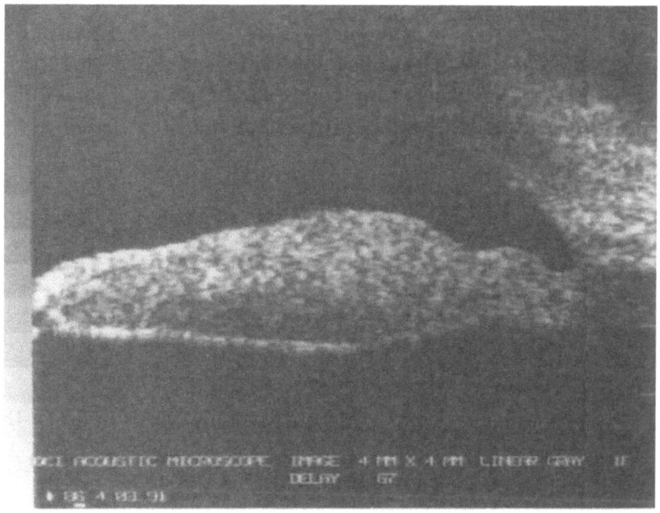

(c)

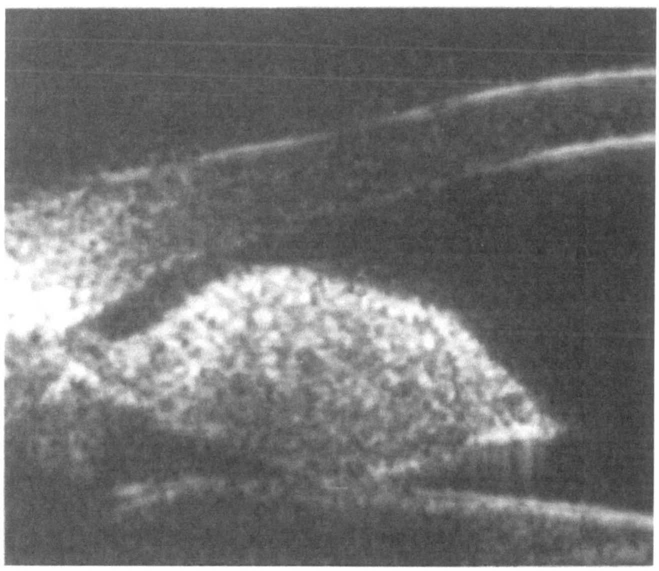
(d)

Other Morphological Appearances

Elongated Thickening. Diffuse thickening of the iris structure can occur with widespread iris lesions. Not infrequently it is difficult to detect a division between tumor tissue and iris tissue on ultrasound biomicroscopy. Figure 6.4a and b shows the clinical and ultrasound biomicroscopic appearance of such a lesion.

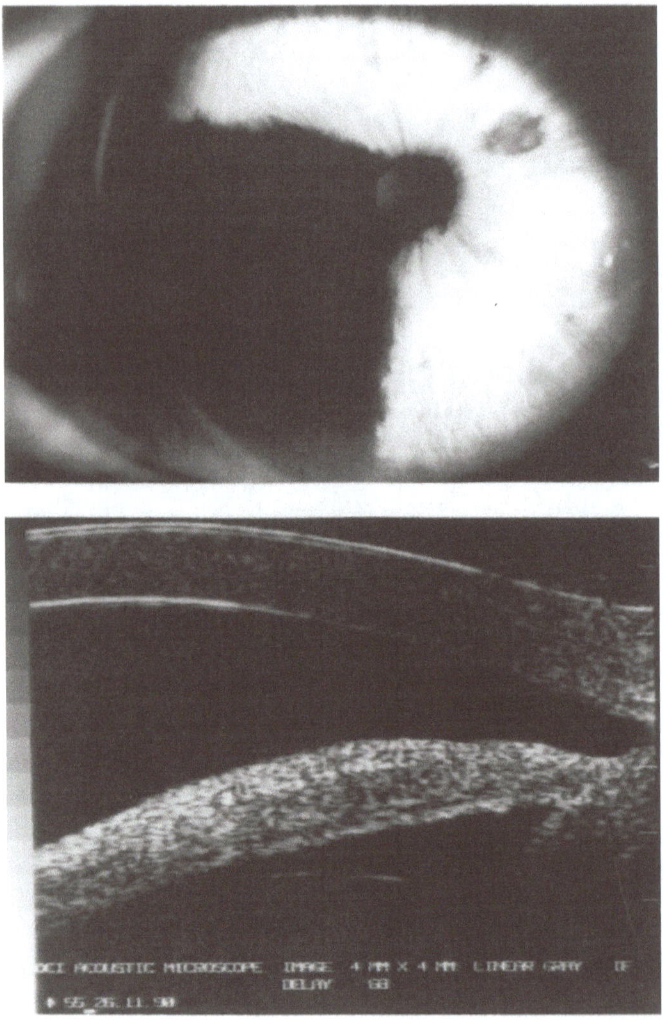

(a)

(b)

FIGURE 6.4. **(a)** Clinical appearance of a diffuse iris tumor. **(b)** Ultrasound biomicroscopy displays uniform thickening with an uncertain margin between tumor and iris tissue.

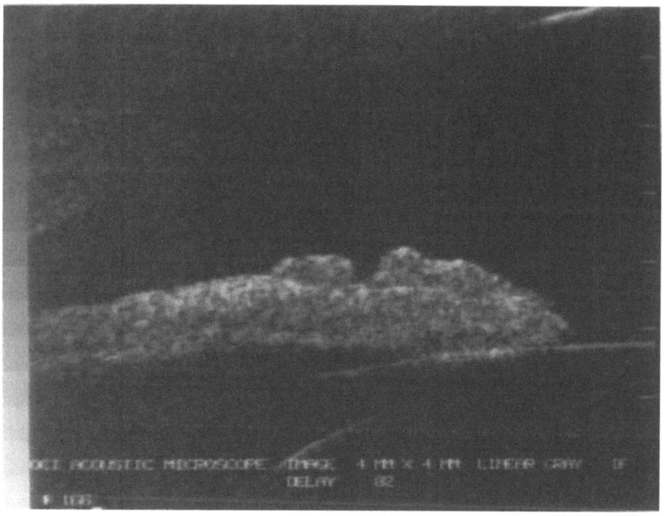

FIGURE 6.5. A tumor near the iris margin with a "stuck on" appearance.

"Stuck on" Appearance. Some iris lesions show an irregular "stuck on" appearance with a distinct border between the lesion and iris tissue on ultrasound biomicroscopy. Figure 6.5 shows such a lesion. These lesions can be measured separately from the total iris thickness. It is usually wise to measure both the lesion and the total iris thickness because the degree of involvement of iris stroma cannot be ascertained with certainty.

Pedunculated Masses. Occasionally tumors appear in cross section as pedunculated masses on the iris surface. These lesions have a smaller base, and a larger top. Figure 6.6 shows an example of such a tumor.

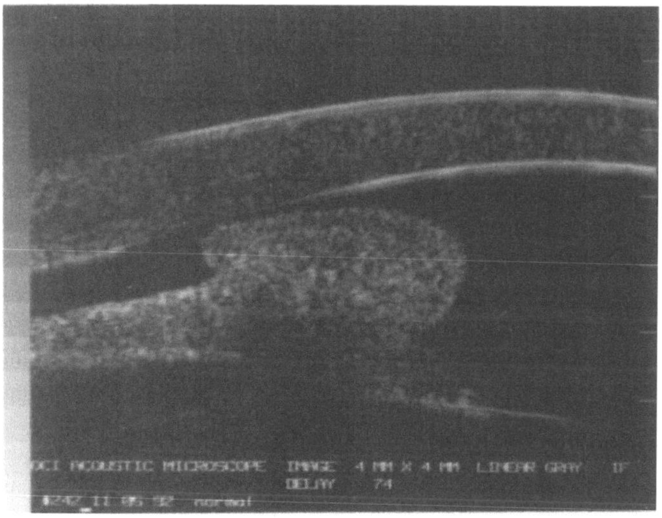

FIGURE 6.6. Pedunculated iris mass with the base smaller than the top of the lesion.

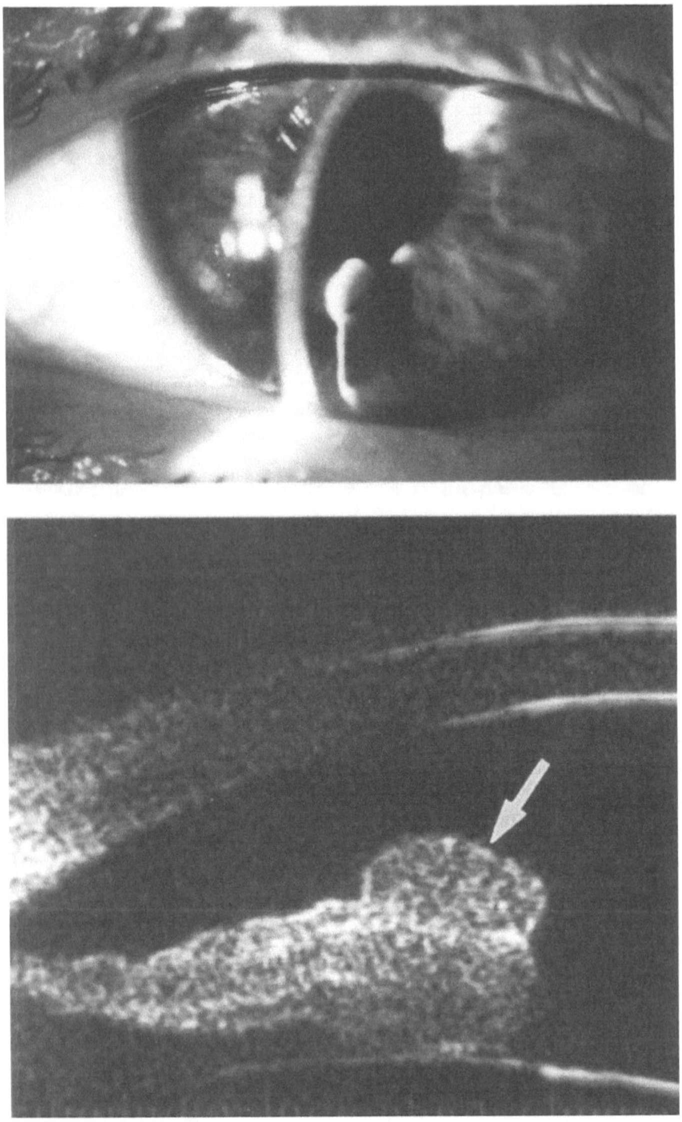

(a)

(b)

FIGURE 6.7. **(a)** Clinical photograph of an iris lesion that shows a "collar button" shape. **(b)** The nodule on the surface (arrow) shows a lower internal reflectivity than the rest of the lesion.

Collar Button Shape. Some lesions show a collar button shape (Figure 6.7a and b) similar to that seen with choroidal tumors breaking through Bruch's membrane. The significance of this appearance is uncertain.

Tumor Boundaries

One of the major values of ultrasound biomicroscopy is an improved ability to define tumor boundaries, and an ability to determine whether iris tumors extend beyond the iris root to involve the ciliary body. Such observations have significant value in planning surgical removal should such be contemplated, and allows more precise classification of iris versus iridociliary tumors. The tumor borders cannot be resolved on a cellular level, but very frequently the change in shape and reflectivity allows reasonably accurate posterior boundary determination, such as the boundaries between the ciliary body and iris tumors as shown in Figure 6.2. Cross-sectional views as shown in Figure 6.8 allow an estimate of lateral extent. Tumors of the peripheral iris that extend high enough to touch the cornea preclude a view of the peripheral iris beyond them by gonioscopy. Ultrasound biomicroscopy allows an estimate as to whether there is uninvolved iris remaining between the tumor margin

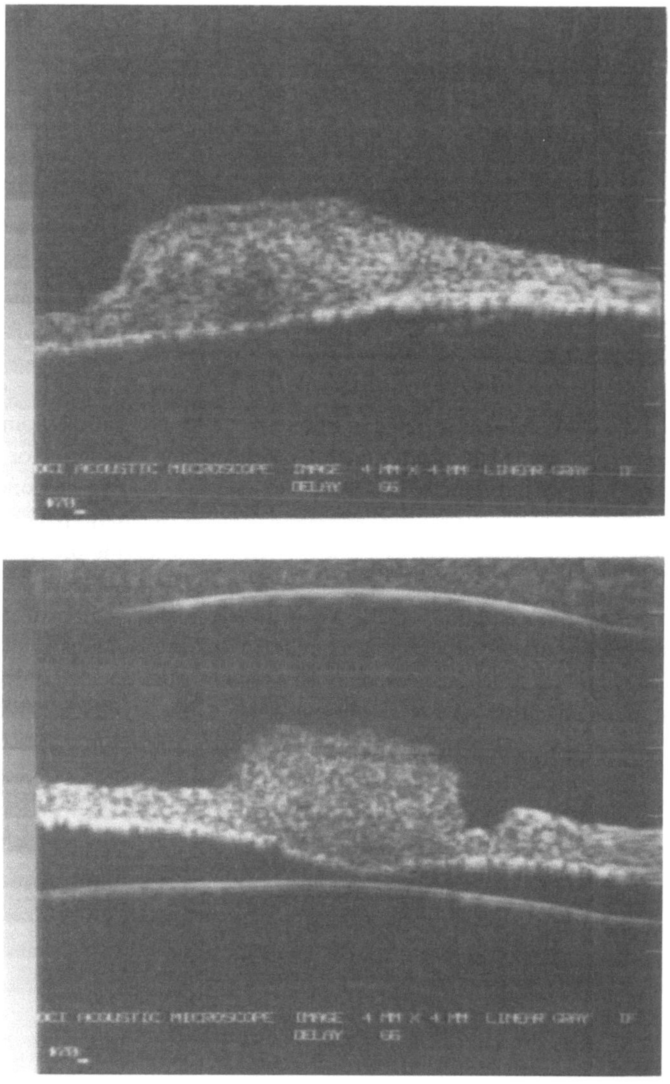

(a)

(b)

FIGURE 6.8. **(a)** Iris lesion in radial section, the most common view seen in this chapter. **(b)** Same iris lesion in cross section. The lateral margins are discernible from the iris by a change in reflectivity.

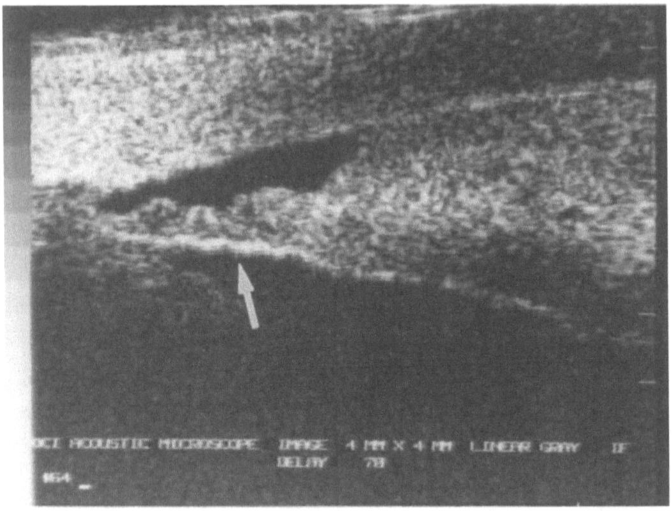

FIGURE 6.9. A peripheral iris lesion extends to the inner corneal surface. Uninvolved iris can be imaged peripheral to the mass (arrow).

and the iris root, as illustrated in Figure 6.9. Occasionally a tumor can extend laterally beneath the iris, as shown in Figure 6.10.

Monitoring Tumor Change

Traditionally, detection of change in iris lesions has been a matter of defining change in surface characteristics or surface extent as observed on slit lamp examination or serial photographs. Ultrasound biomicroscopy adds a new dimension to our criteria for defining change. Depth measurement can be done with high accuracy. Defining change requires careful judgment regarding duplication of the previous measurement location. Generally one will scan the tumor in a radial fashion until the region of greatest thickness is on the screen. The image is then frozen and a measurement vector is placed through the greatest depth on the screen image. The easiest method is to measure the total

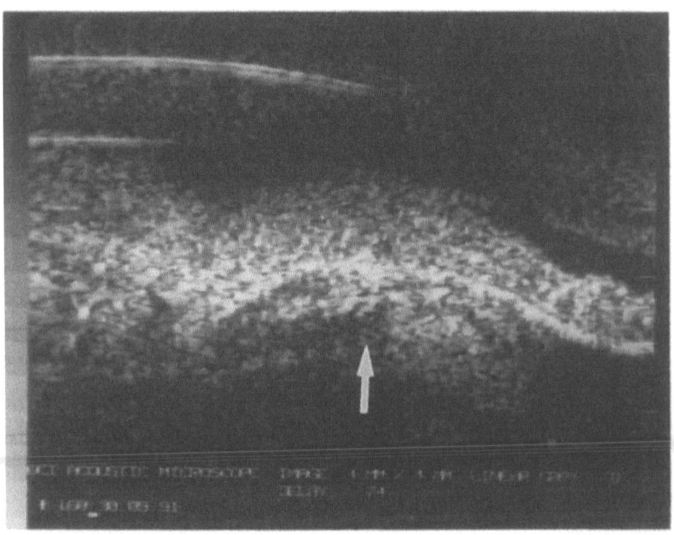

FIGURE 6.10. A large iris tumor shows extension under adjacent normal iris (arrow).

FIGURE 6.11. (**a**) Iris lesion in radial section shows fusiform shape. (**b**) Follow-up examination reveals a small projection on the posterior aspect (arrow).

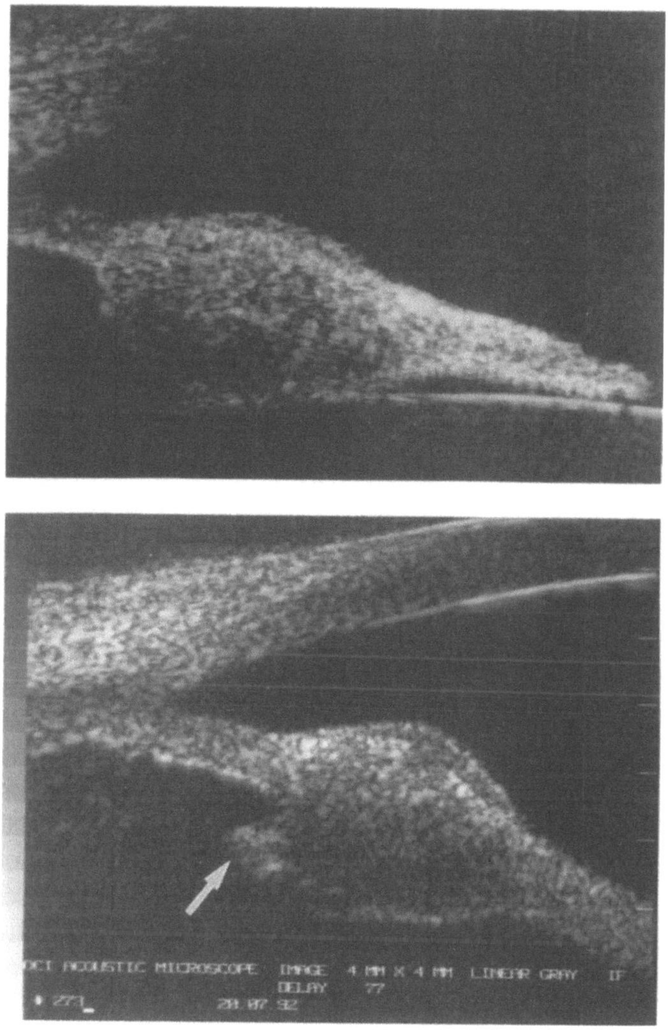

(a)

(b)

depth to the posterior iris surface. It is frequently impossible to tell exactly how much of the iris thickness is involved even in the presence of apparent layering. Layering usually presents on ultrasound biomicroscopy as a low-reflective surface region with a variable thickness of underlying iris stroma. The low-reflective region may imply a surface plaque, but the underlying iris stroma may also be involved. If the layering is distinct, a separate measurement can be made of the surface layer.

A change in profile may also be an indication of growth. The posterior margin of iris tumors cannot be visualized by slit lamp examination, but can be easily defined by ultrasound biomicroscopy. In the example shown in Figure 6.11a the posterior margin of the tumor is smooth. Follow-up examination (Figure 6.11b) revealed the new finding of a projection on the posterior surface.

A change in internal characteristics can also be important. In the example given in Figure 6.12 the tumor was observed to increase in area. Ultrasound biomicroscopically, the relatively smooth surface of the tumor in Figure 6.12b is seen to change to an irregular shape (Figure 6.12d) over several months of observation. The internal reflectivity in the superficial aspect of the tumor is seen to change to an irregular linear pattern that has similarities to the pattern seen in the region of pure tumor cells of the histologically confirmed iris melanoma shown in Figure 6.13.

(a)

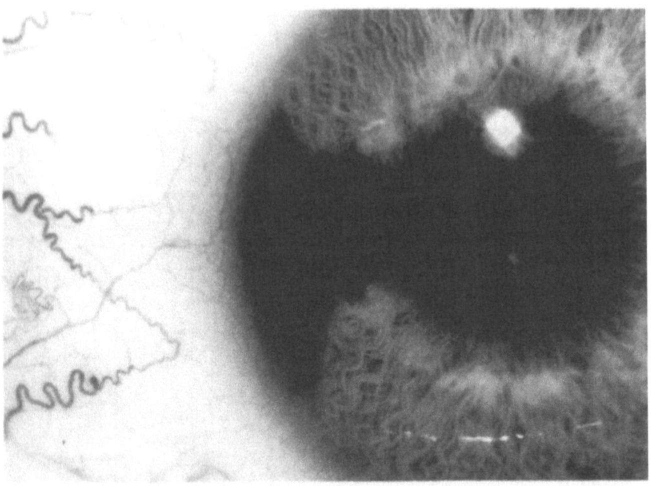

(b)

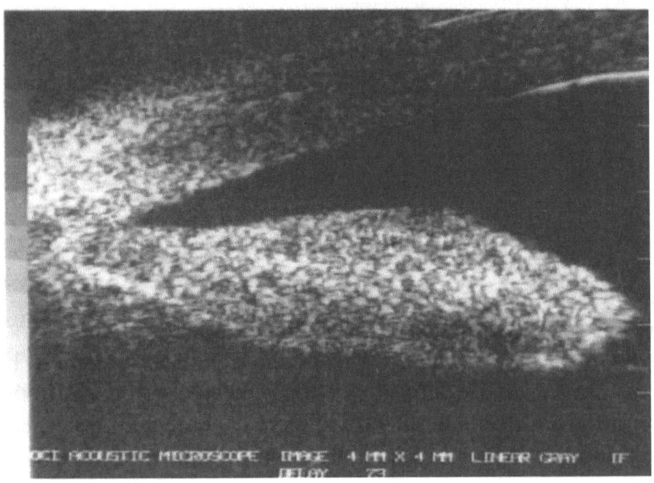

FIGURE 6.12. **(a)** Clinical photograph of a pigmented iris lesion. **(b)** Ultrasound biomicroscopy shows a relatively smooth surfaced fusiform lesion. **(c)** Clinical photograph shows slight increase in the size of the lesion. **(d)** Follow-up ultrasound biomicroscopy shows thickening, and a change in profile of the lesion. The internal aspect shows a superficial linear pattern.

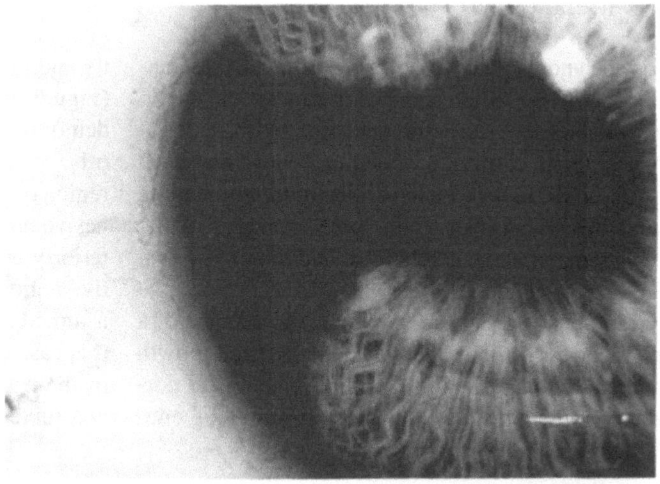

(c)

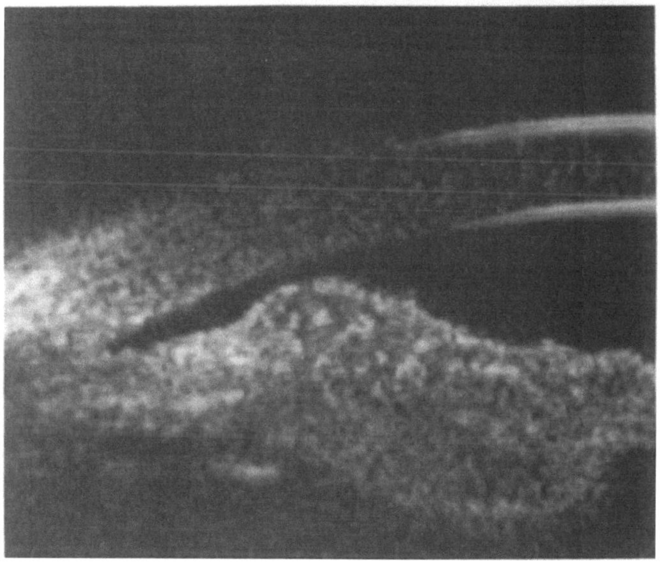

(d)

Iris Melanomas

Iris melanomas can have varied clinical presentations. Differentiation between melanomas and nevi can at times be difficult, and may require serial observation. Ultrasound biomicroscopy may have a role in defining characteristics more compatible with melanoma than nevi. Some examples of iris melanoma in patients that have had tumor removal are presented here.

Figure 6.13a shows the clinical appearance of a pigmented iris tumor that had demonstrated growth and caused unilateral glaucoma. Pathological correlation was possible in this lesion following enucleation. On ultrasound biomicroscopy a variable internal reflectivity is noted with a higher reflectivity and linear pattern in the more superficial tumor (Figure 6.13b). Histopathology (Figure 6.13c) demonstrated poorly cohesive tumor cells anteriorly corresponding to the more highly reflective region on ultrasound biomicroscopy, with more cohesive tumor cells interspersed with iris tissue posteriorly corresponding to the more weakly reflective region. Weaker echoes in the deeper aspect of a tumor can relate to absorption of sound, but in this case the pattern did appear distinctly different in these two regions. The pathological diagnosis was mixed cell melanoma.

FIGURE 6.13. (**a**) Clinical appearance of a pigmented iris melanoma that had increased in size and caused glaucoma. (**b**) Ultrasound biomicroscopy shows higher reflectivity superiorly with a linear pattern. (**c**) Histological specimen shows a region of pure tumor cells superiorly with more diffuse involvement of the iris stroma inferiorly. Published courtesy of *Ophthalmology* (1992;99: 1220–1228).

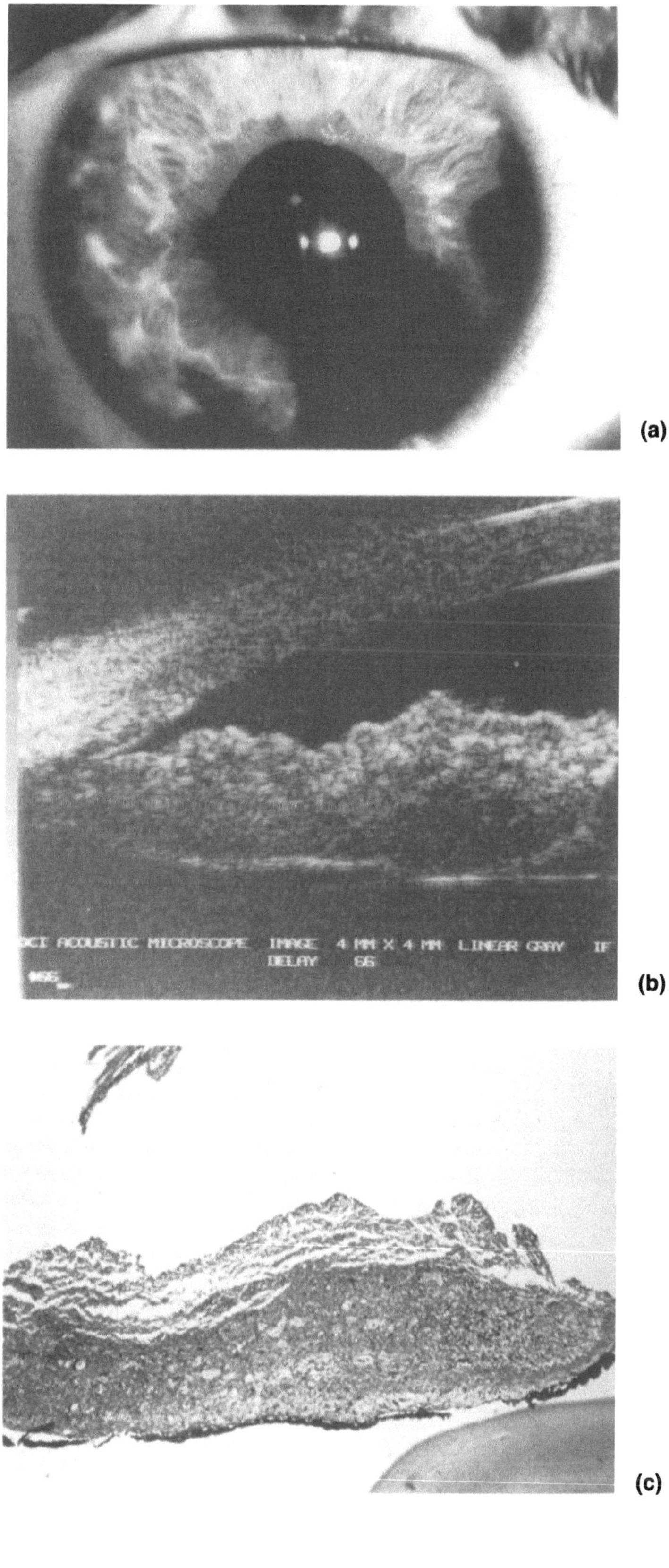

Figure 6.14a shows an amelanotic lesion with a lobulated appearance clinically. Ultrasound biomicroscopy displays this lobulated appearance extending through the substance of this medium reflective tumor (Figure 6.14b). An iridocyclectomy specimen shows the lobulated appearance with the lobules shrunken down secondary to fixation artifact (Figure 6.14c). The pathological diagnosis was spindle cell melanoma.

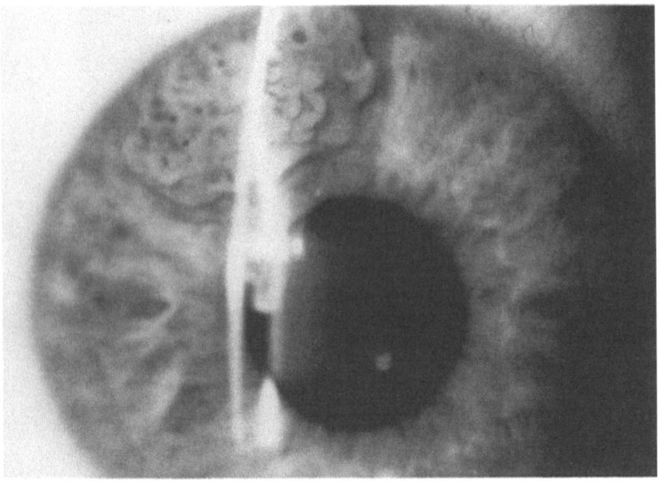

(a)

FIGURE 6.14. **(a)** Clinical appearance of an amelanotic lobulated iris melanoma. **(b)** Ultrasound biomicroscopy shows the internal lobulated appearance. **(c)** Histological specimen shows a lobulated spindle cell melanoma. Published courtesy of *Ophthalmology* (1992;99: 1220–1228).

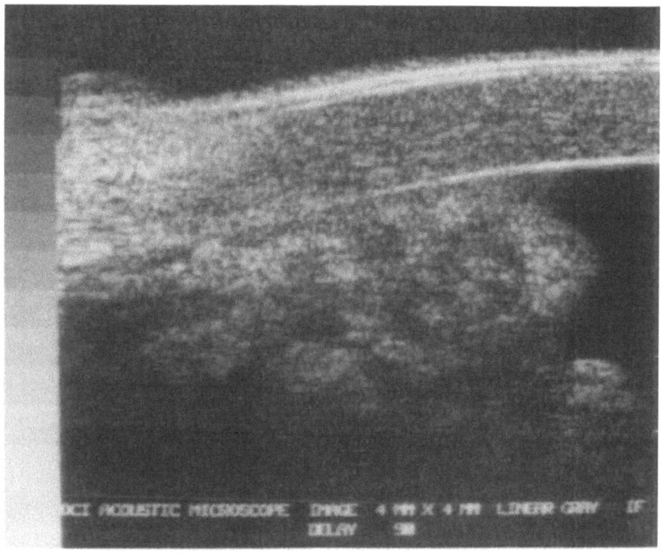

(b)

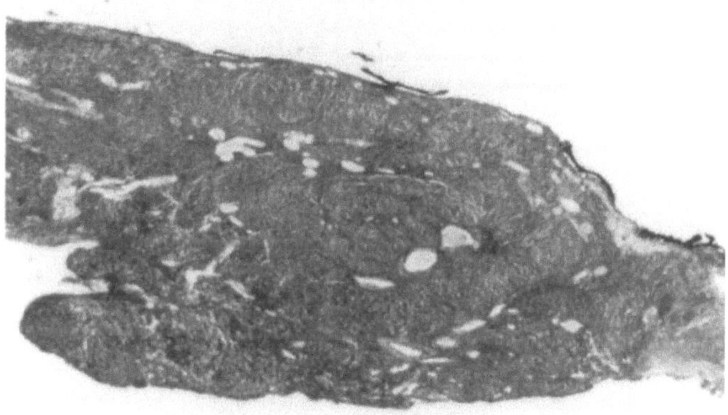

(c)

Figure 6.15a shows the clinical appearance of an amelanotic mass lesion that appears vascularized. Ultrasound biomicroscopy reveals a relatively highly reflective superior aspect to the tumor with spaces that could correspond to blood vessels (Figure 6.15b). Pathology of the iridocyclectomy specimen (Figure 6.15c) shows a spindle cell melanoma with pure tumor cells anteriorly and large blood vessels.

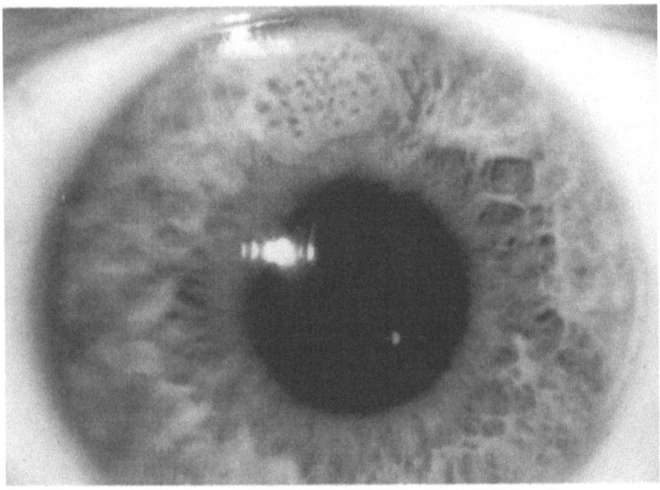

(a)

FIGURE 6.15. **(a)** Clinical appearance of an amelanotic vascular melanoma. **(b)** Ultrasound biomicroscopy shows higher reflectivity superiorly and cystic spaces. **(c)** Histological specimen shows a spindle cell melanoma with pure tumor cells anteriorly and vascular channels. Published courtesy of *Ophthalmology* (1992;99:1220–1228).

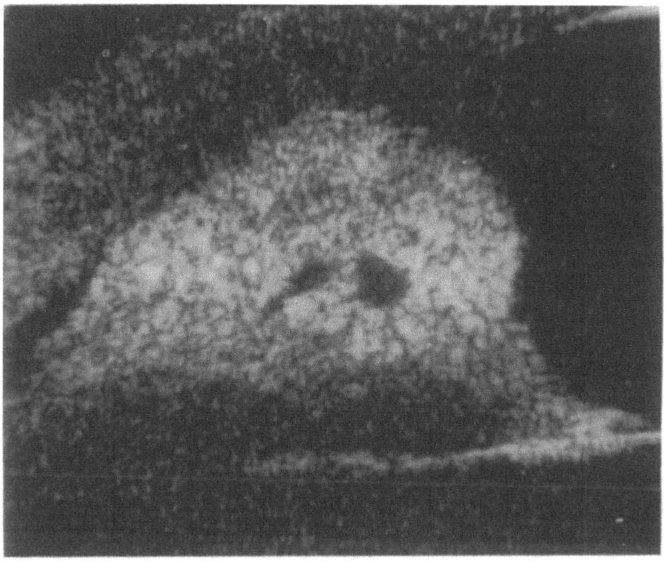

(b)

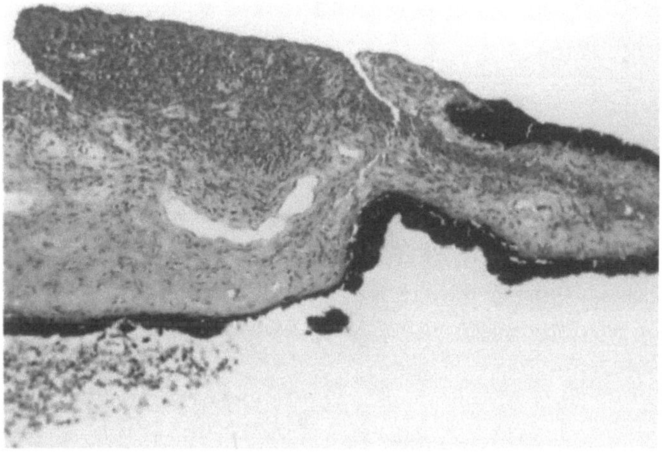

(c)

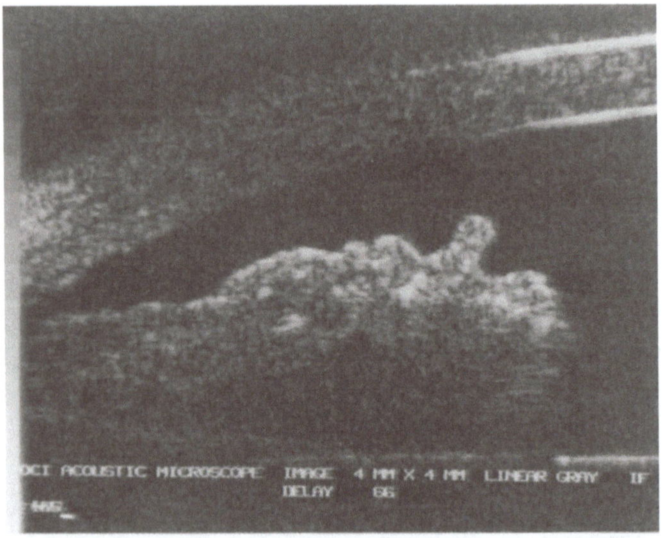

(a)

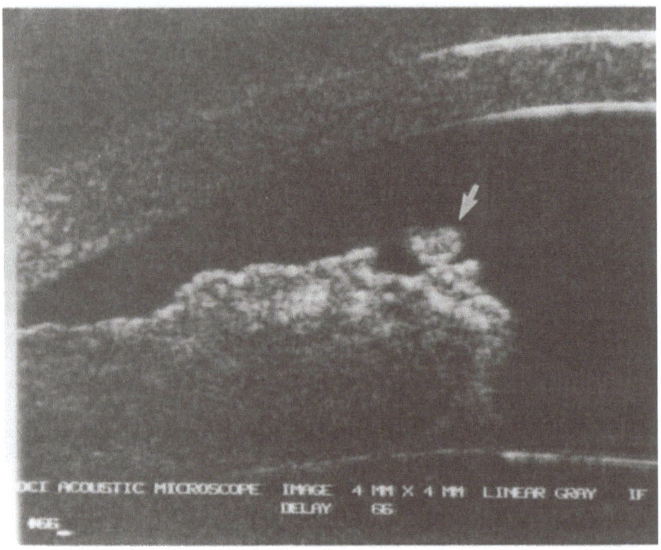

(b)

FIGURE 6.16. **(a)** Ultrasound biomicroscopic image of an iris melanoma shows surface projections. **(b)** A small projection (arrow) is tenuously attached to the main tumor. **(c)** A small satellite lesion (arrow) seeded in the angle with no connection to the main tumor. Published courtesy of *Ophthalmology* (1992;99: 1220–1228).

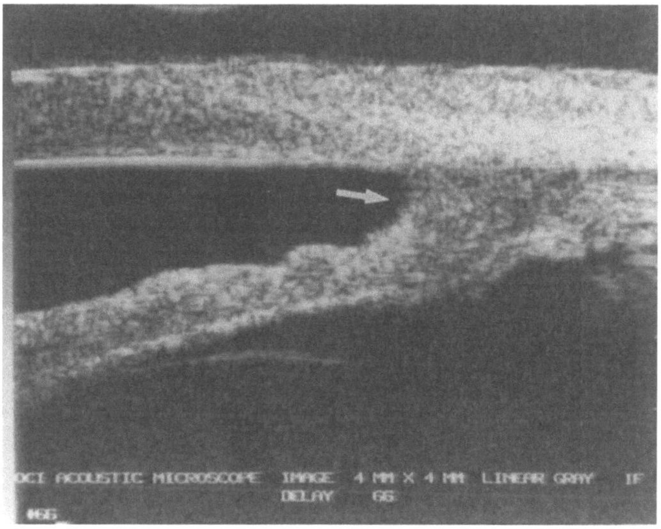

(c)

Local Tumor Spread

An example of a tumor associated with local seeding in the anterior chamber is shown in Figure 6.16. A suspected satellite lesion could be seen in the opposite angle on gonioscopy. An ultrasound biomicroscopic image of the main tumor (Figure 6.16a) shows an irregular surface with occasional projections. Another region of the same tumor showed a small extension tenuously attached to the main tumor (Figure 6.16b). These phenomena are most likely a precursor to development of satellite lesions. Ultrasound biomicroscopy demonstrated a small lesion unconnected to the main tumor mass involving the opposite angle (Figure 6.16c). These findings add insight into this type of spread.

Ciliary Body Tumors

Ciliary body tumors are in a region that can be easily assessed by ultrasound biomicroscopy. Ultrasound biomicroscopy allows differentiation of ciliary body tumors with a peripheral iris component from pure iris tumors. Ultrasound biomicroscopy gives information on the internal reflectivity patterns of the superficial aspect of the tumor that may be helpful in differential diagnoses. Clarification of the dividing line between ciliary body tumors and peripheral choroidal tumors is aided. Boundaries of ciliary body tumors, both posterior and lateral, can be detected, which can be very helpful information if surgical procedures such as iridocyclectomy are contemplated. Small ciliary body tumors can be detected and followed at a much smaller height than with conventional ultrasound, allowing therapeutic decisions to be made earlier. Large tumors (>4 mm in depth) are frequently incompletely imaged by ultrasound biomicroscopy because of sound attenuation. In this type of tumor, measurement of depth is better done with conventional ultrasound using a water bath technique.

Iris Tumors Versus Ciliary Body Tumors

As discussed in the section on iris tumors, a peripheral tumor on the iris surface involving the angle can frequently not be classified as purely iris, or mixed ciliary body-iris on the basis of its appearance by slit lamp or gonioscopic appearance. If the ciliary body component is small, even indirect ophthalmoscopy with wide dilation or conventional ultrasound can miss this component. Ultrasound biomicroscopy images this transition zone clearly and can aid in determining the portion of the tumor that involves ciliary body. This can frequently be the basis of reclassifying a tumor as iris or ciliary body origin, depending on the relative amount of tumor in each structure.

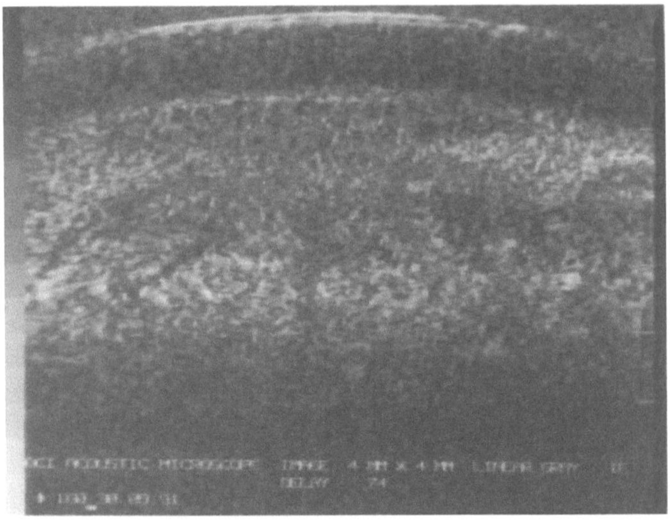

FIGURE 6.17. Ultrasound biomicroscopy of the superficial aspect of a ciliary body melanoma. The lesion displays a medium reflectivity, with occasional irregular areas.

Reflectivity Patterns

As in iris tumors, relatively small ciliary body tumors tend to be observed, and correlation between ultrasound biomicroscopic and pathological changes are not always available. Ciliary body tumors tend to be medium reflective with occasional irregular areas. Figure 6.17 shows the superficial region of a ciliary body tumor felt to be a ciliary body melanoma. The reflectivity pattern shows a generally regular medium reflectivity with some more irregular areas.

Determining Tumor Margins

The ability to define boundaries of ciliary body tumors is important if surgery such as iridocyclectomy is contemplated. The anterior margin is usually obvious. Figure 6.18 shows the anterior border of a ciliary tumor indenting the peripheral margin of the lens. The posterior margin is usually detectable by a change in profile and frequently by a change in reflectivity from the tumor to normal

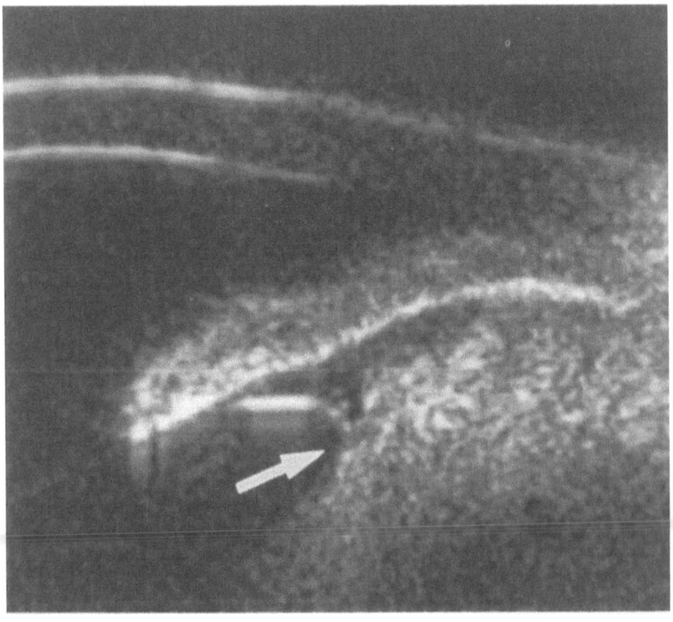

FIGURE 6.18. The anterior margin of a ciliary body tumor is noted to be indenting the lens (arrow).

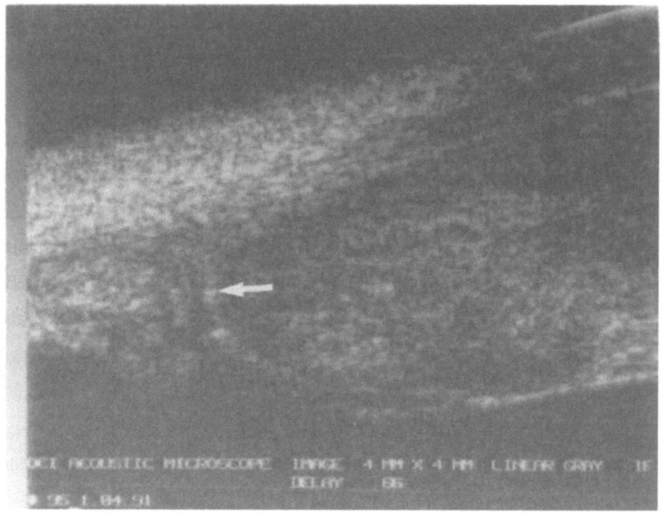

FIGURE 6.19. The posterior margin of a ciliary body tumor (arrow) is detected by a change in reflectivity and profile. Published courtesy of *Ophthalmology* (1992;99:1220–1228).

ciliary body. This is illustrated in Figure 6.19. It is important to be able to define the posterior margin in terms of external landmarks as a guide to the operating surgeon. This can be accomplished with reference to fixed points such as the scleral spur, which is generally slightly less than 1 mm posterior to the limbus. The lateral margins can be defined by holding the axis of the probe tangential to the limbus and assessing the change from tumor tissue to normal ciliary body structures. Figure 6.20 shows the lateral margin between tumor tissue and normal ciliary body processes. One must be careful to make a note of the precise probe position, usually defined as the clock hour position of the center of the probe.

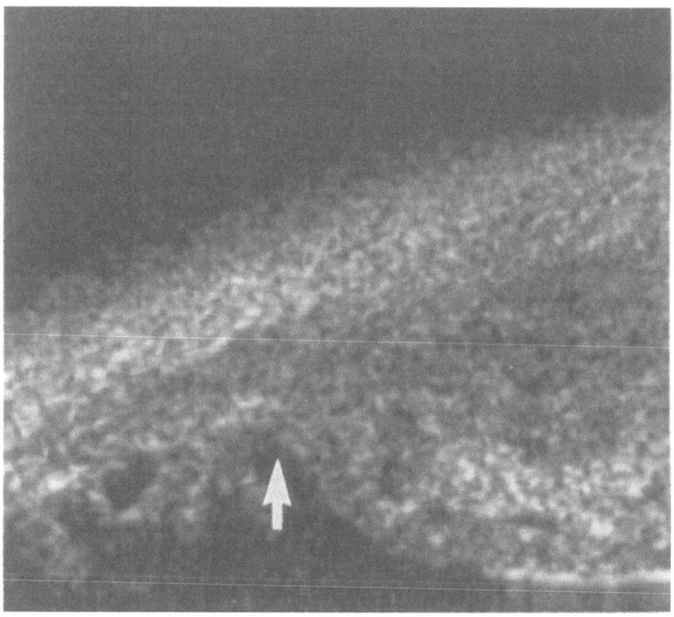

FIGURE 6.20. The lateral margin of a ciliary body tumor shows a transition to normal ciliary body appearance (arrow).

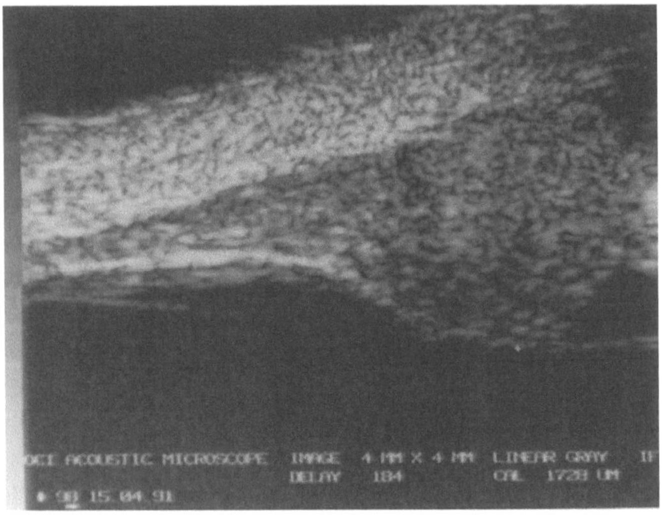

FIGURE 6.21. A small ciliary body tumor that could only be imaged by ultrasound biomicroscopy. Published courtesy of *Ophthalmology* (1992;99:1220–1228).

Following Small Tumors

The ability to define very small tumors in the ciliary body is exemplified by the example in Figure 6.21. Attention is usually drawn to lesions of this sort by the presence of some discoloration in the peripheral iris. The differential diagnoses would be between a peripheral iris tumor or the margin of a ciliary body tumor breaking through into the angle. This lesion was undetectable by conventional B-scan ultrasound. On ultrasound biomicroscopy this lesion was shown to be a small ciliary body tumor. It measured 1608 μm in A-P diameter on ultrasound biomicroscopy and has not increased in size on two follow-up examinations. The inability to detect a lesion of this size with conventional B-scan ultrasonography relates to the fact that it cannot be differentiated from the normal ciliary body tissue in which it is embedded. The ability to detect and follow a very early ciliary body lesion is unique in imaging and could result in the ability to define change and institute appropriate therapeutic measures such as iridocyclectomy at a much earlier stage in this type of patient.

FIGURE 6.22 (**a**) An iridocyclectomy site shows the internal scleral surface with no tumor tissue (arrow). (**b**) Lateral margin of the iridocyclectomy site shows the transition from sclera to normal ciliary body (arrow).

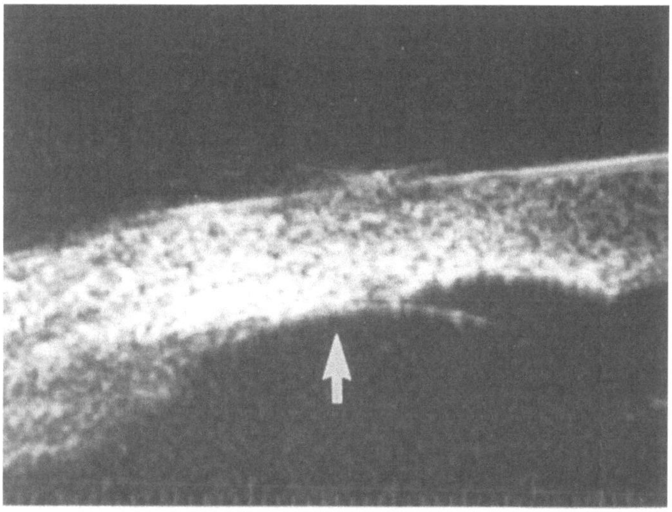

(a)

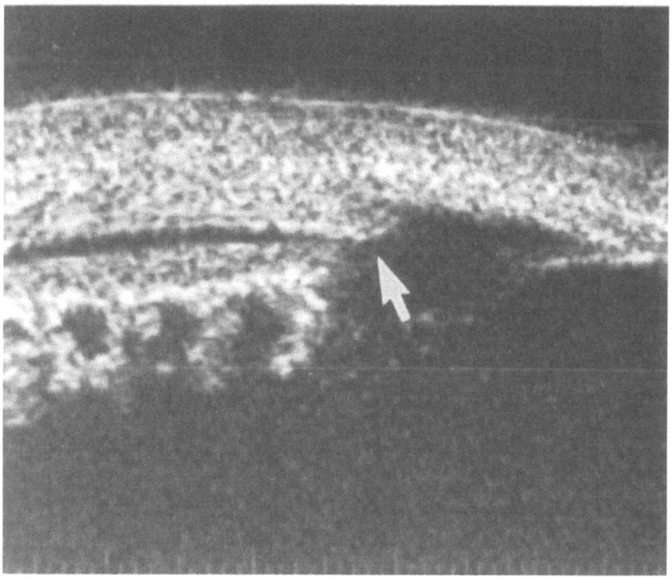

(b)

Monitoring Iridocyclectomy Sites

After iridocyclectomy, ultrasound biomicroscopy provides a method of monitoring the iridocyclectomy site for recurrence. This is particularly important if incomplete removal is indicated on histological examination. Figure 6.22a shows the appearance of the site of tumor removal following iridocyclectomy for a ciliary body melanoma. Figure 6.22b shows the lateral margin of the iridocyclectomy site. In this case, the site shows scleral tissue with minimal tissue internal to the sclera and no evidence of recurrence.

Cysts

Cysts can be found in various locations throughout the anterior segment and can have varied etiologies. Those secondary to trauma or surgery are discussed in the section on trauma. Spontaneously occurring cysts are usually found in relationship to the iris or ciliary body. These cysts are most commonly found at the iridociliary junction [8], but can be found at other locations in relationship to the iris and iris epithelium.

Iridociliary cysts usually present as small localized elevations of the iris, as illustrated in Figure 6.23. The margins of these lesions can often be seen if the pupil is widely dilated and a three-mirror lens is used. They cannot always be imaged in this way, however. Ultrasound biomicroscopy is excellent at imaging the iridociliary region in the posterior chamber and essentially eliminates any difficulty in determining if there is an abnormality in the region. Ultrasound biomicroscopy is diagnostic for cysts in this region, and clearly displays these lesions as thin-walled cysts, with no internal reflectivity, and occasional multiloculations. Figure 6.24a through c shows some variations of iridociliary cysts. The total lack of internal reflectivity indicates a fluid-filled cyst and this feature eliminates any possibility of confusion with a solid lesion.

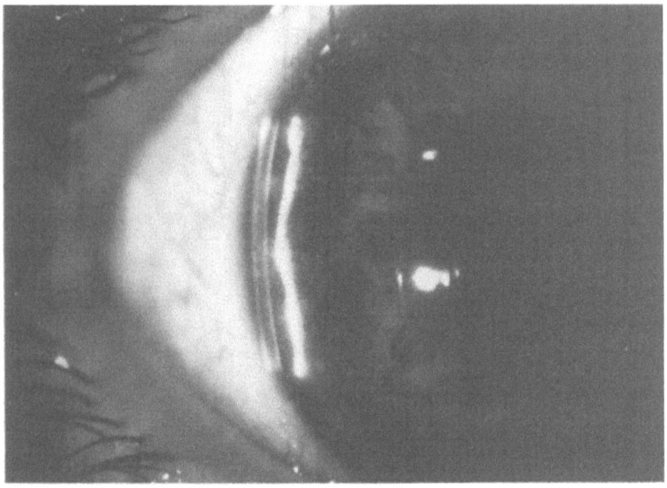

FIGURE 6.23. Typical clinical appearance of an iridociliary cyst with iris elevation without visible involvement of the iris tissue.

FIGURE 6.24. **(a)** Ultrasound biomicroscopy of a cyst at the iridociliary junction. A small loculation is on the anterior border. **(b)** A larger cyst shows distinct iris elevation. **(c)** Cross section of a cyst under the iris.

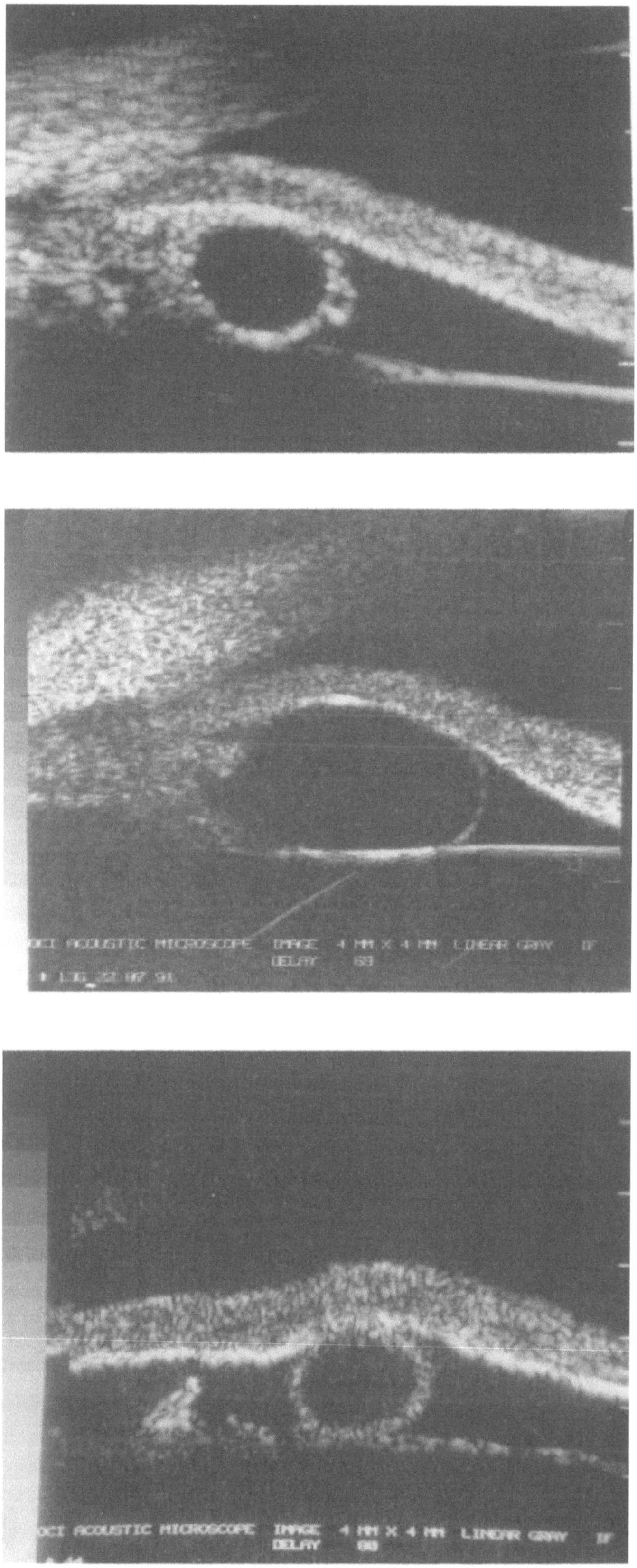

(a)

(b)

(c)

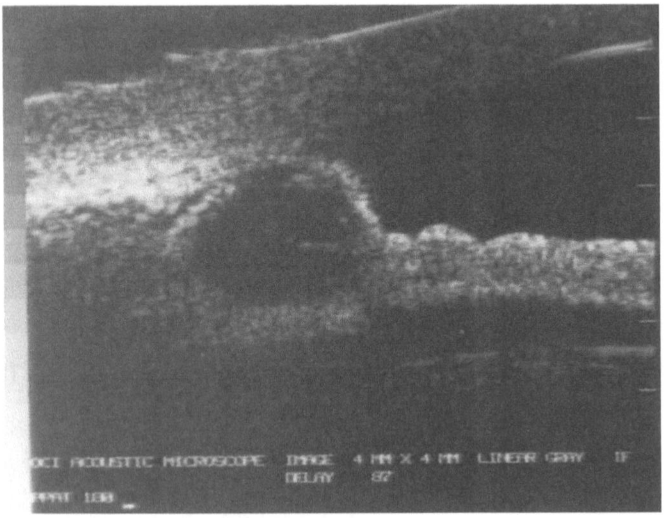

FIGURE 6.25. Ultrasound biomicroscopy of an intrairis cyst shows displacement of iris stroma.

Iris cysts can also be found within the stroma of the iris itself. Figure 6.25 shows such a cyst displacing iris stroma. Small cysts are also found occasionally either as an isolated finding on examination for some other clinical indication, or in association with solid lesions of the iris or ciliary body. Figure 6.26 shows a small cyst on the margin of an iris tumor thought to be metastatic.

Not all localized elevations of the iris without involvement of the iris itself are cysts. Figure 6.27a shows the clinical appearance of a localized iris elevation thought to be a cyst on initial clinical examination. Ultrasound biomicroscopy revealed that the mass lesion causing the local elevation is solid (Figure 6.27b). This lesion turned out to be an extension of a ciliary body tumor.

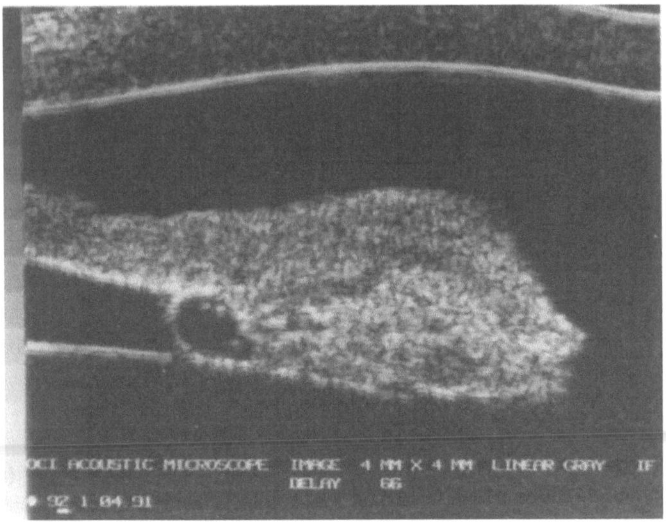

FIGURE 6.26. A small cyst is present on the margin of an iris tumor thought to be metastatic. Published courtesy of *Ophthalmology* (1992;99:1220–1228).

FIGURE 6.27. (**a**) Clinical appearance of localized iris elevation without iris change is typical of a cyst. (**b**) Ultrasound biomicroscopy shows that the lesion under the iris is solid. Published courtesy of *Ophthalmology* (1992;99:1220–1228).

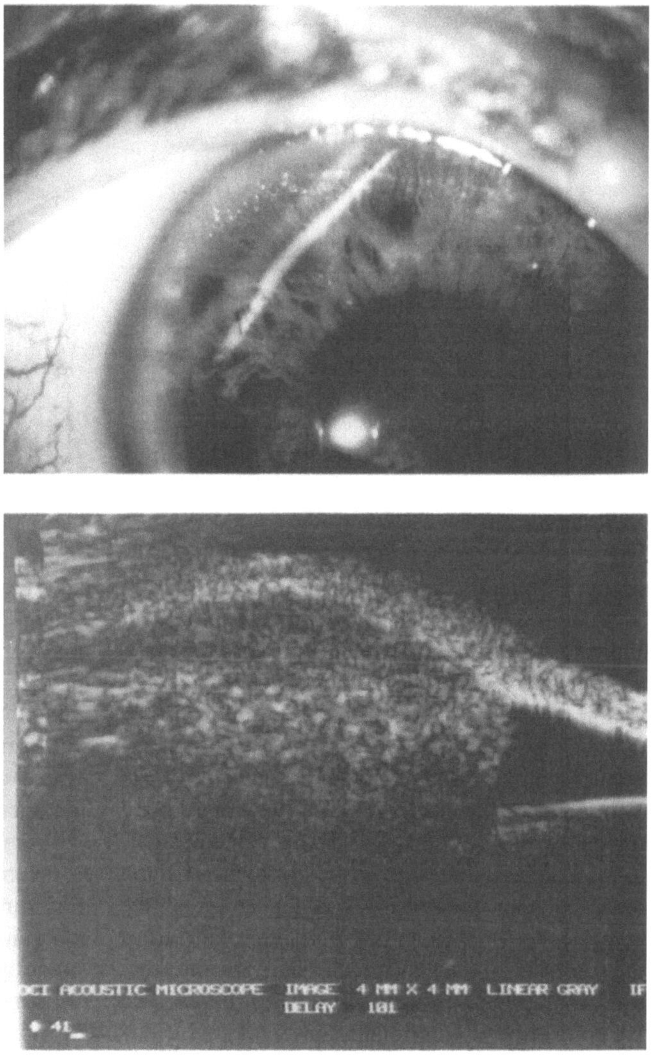

(a)

(b)

An entirely different type of cystic disease that is often multicentric, familial, and a cause of angle closure glaucoma can be found rarely. The ultrasound biomicroscopic appearance of these cysts is quite different from the usual iridociliary cyst. They are thicker walled, much more numerous, and bilateral. Such cysts are discussed in the preceding chapter on glaucoma.

Peripheral Choroidal Tumors

Ultrasound biomicroscopic assessment of choroidal tumors is currently limited to those tumors in a sufficiently anterior position to have some portion imaged. To image a choroidal tumor, the transducer must be placed directly over the tumor base, as penetration is not sufficient to cross the vitreous

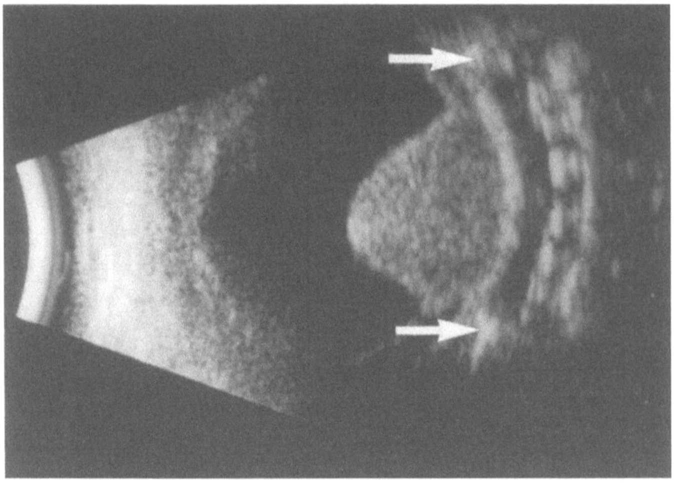

FIGURE 6.28. Conventional B-scan ultrasound shows the margins of an I^{131} plaque below a choroidal melanoma.

cavity. Frequently only part of the anterior margin of a tumor can be imaged, but this capability can add valuable information regarding management of these patients. It is often difficult to differentiate tumors of choroidal origin that come close to, or involve the ciliary body from tumors of ciliary body origin. Ultrasound biomicroscopy aids in this differentiation by clearly defining the ciliary body region. If plaque therapy is being contemplated, ultrasound biomicroscopy adds helpful information regarding the characteristics and position of the anterior margin. The ability to image some part of the substance of the tumor adds diagnostic information. Extrascleral extension of anterior tumors can be differentiated from other causes of pigmented lesions of the sclera and related to the underlying pathology.

Defining the Anterior Margin of Anterior Choroidal Tumors

Peripheral choroidal tumors are frequently in a position in which radioactive plaque therapy can be considered. These plaques must be applied with a sufficient margin around the base of the tumor to assure adequate dose to the entire tumor substance. The I^{131} plaque used in the COMS study [2] should have at least a 2 mm margin around the tumor edge. We have previously defined a method for using conventional ultrasound to image the position of plaques behind tumors [9,10]. Figure 6.28 shows a conventional B-scan ultrasound image of a choroidal tumor with such a plaque in place. This method is helpful for posterior tumors, but can't be used to image the anterior plaque margin with anteriorly placed tumors. Another consideration when plaquing anterior tumors is that due to anatomical considerations, there is a limit as to how anteriorly a plaque can be placed, and still be covered with conjunctiva and not overlap the cornea.

There are basically three methods currently used to determine the position of anterior tumor margins: direct visualization, conventional ultrasound, and transillumination. Direct visualization with indirect ophthalmoscopy can be difficult with anterior tumors, especially larger lesions. Conventional ultrasound in a water bath can image the tumor but does not show details of the anterior ciliary body region clearly. Transillumination can be helpful in showing the relationship of pigmented tumors to the ciliary band, but can give a false impression depending on the shape of the margin, and the presence of hemorrhage. Ultrasound biomicroscopy can produce a clear image of anterior choroidal tumor margins, and the relationship of these margins to anterior segment structures. The position of the anterior margin can be quantitated with reference to the scleral spur. Figure 6.29a shows the clinical appearance of an anterior melanoma. Ultrasound biomicroscopy (Figure 6.29b) shows that this tumor involves the majority of the ciliary body, and has an anterior extent almost to the scleral spur. Histology following enucleation (Figure 6.29c) confirms that the tumor involves the

FIGURE 6.29. (**a**) Clinical appearance of an anteriorly situated melanoma. (**b**) Ultrasound biomicroscopy shows that the tumor involves the majority of the ciliary body, and extends anteriorly almost to the scleral spur. (**c**) Histology of the enucleated specimen shows the extent of ciliary body involvement.

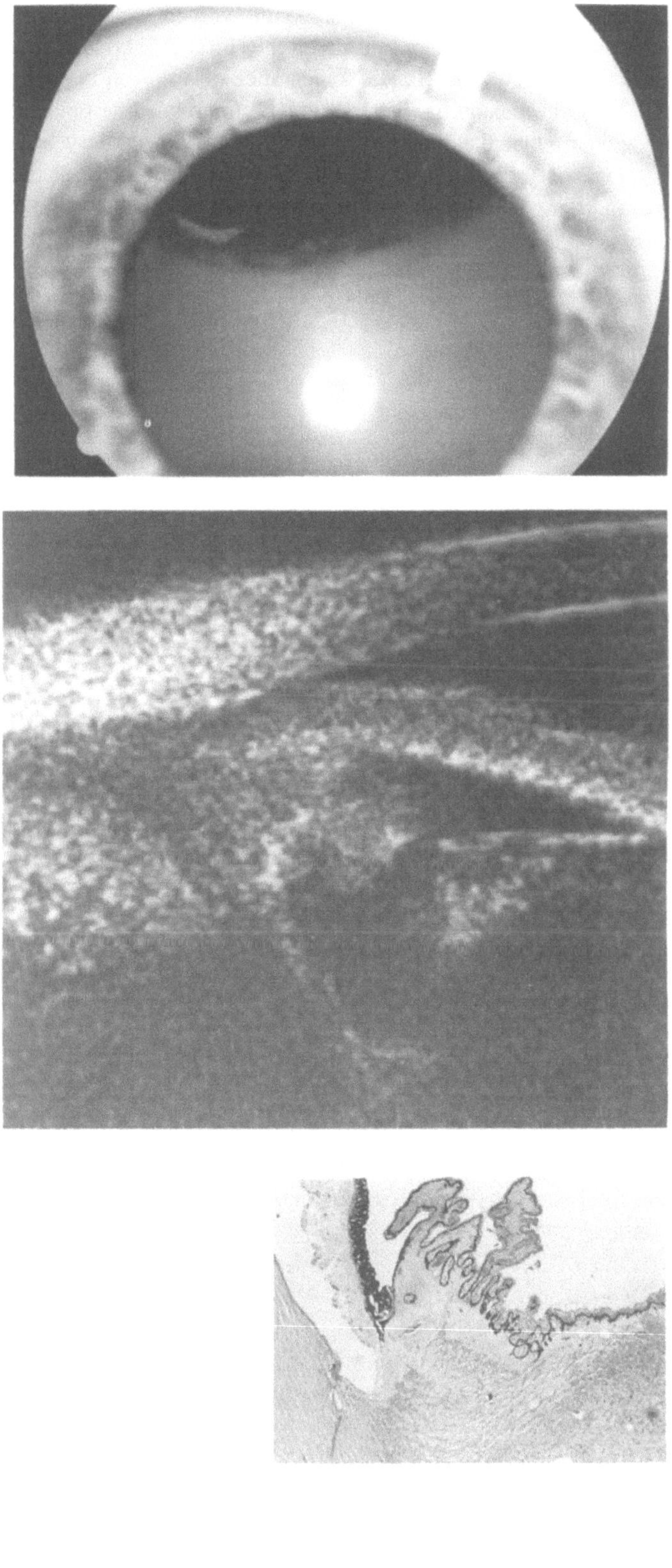

(a) (b) (c)

majority of the ciliary body, with some uninvolved ciliary processes and ciliary muscle on the surface. Figure 6.30a shows the clinical appearance of another anterior melanoma. Ultrasound biomicroscopy reveals that the tumor extends beneath the posterior ciliary body (Figure 6.30b), with the anterior margin of the tumor approximately 1.3 mm posterior to the scleral spur. The posterior ciliary body is imaged as a more weakly reflective region on the anterior margin of the tumor. Pathology of the enucleated specimen reveals that the posterior ciliary body has been stripped off by the leading edge of the melanoma (Figure 6.30c), an appearance that is similar to that seen with ultrasound

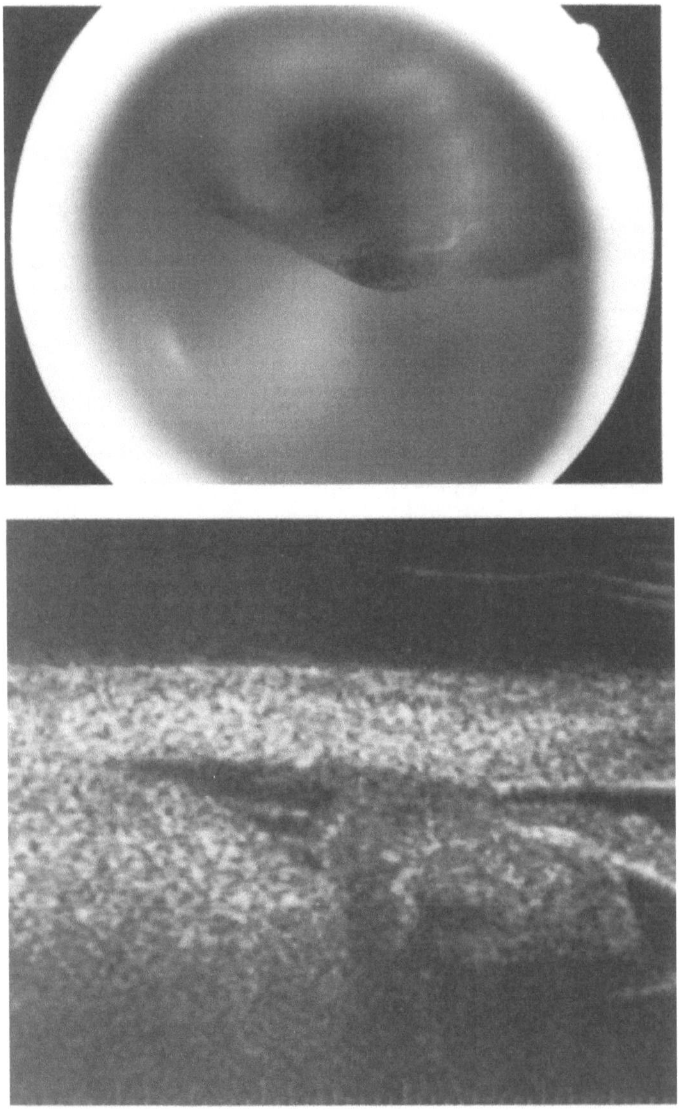

(a)

(b)

FIGURE 6.30. **(a)** Clinical appearance of an anteriorly situated melanoma. **(b)** Ultrasound biomicroscopy shows the anterior margin of the tumor extends 1.3 mm from the scleral spur, stripping off the posterior ciliary body. **(c)** Histology shows the stripping off of the posterior ciliary body by the anterior tumor margin.

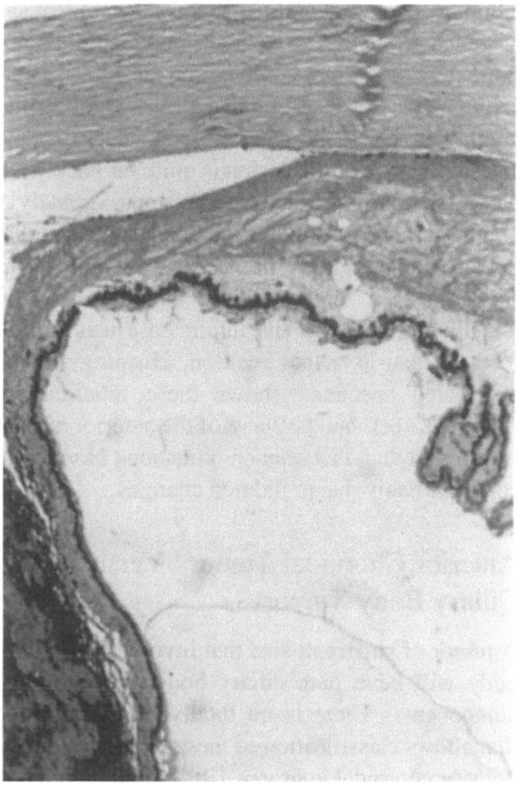

(c)

biomicroscopy. Figure 6.31a shows the clinical appearance of the eye of a patient in which the anterior extent of a tumor could not be visualized clinically, partly because of difficulty in dilating the pupil. Ultrasound biomicroscopy reveals that the anterior margin of this lesion is quite far back from the ciliary body (Figure 6.31b), approximately 5 mm from the scleral spur. Of interest is the fact that the anterior margin of this tumor extends forward from the base. This produced an impression on transillumination that the tumor base was further forward than its actual position. Histology of the enucleated specimen shows these relationships (Figure 6.31c), but the curve of the anterior margin is different than that seen on ultrasound biomicroscopy, probably due to fixation changes.

Anterior Choroidal Tumors Versus Ciliary Body Tumors

A tumor of sufficient size that involves the ciliary body will have both ciliary body and choroidal components. There is no totally clear definition that allows classification of these tumors as ciliary body or choroidal in origin. Ultrasound biomicroscopy aids clarification of the extent of ciliary body involvement, as shown in Figures 6.29 to 6.31. If the tumor involves most of the ciliary body, as illustrated in Figure 6.29, then ciliary body origin can be implied, but not proven. If only part of the posterior ciliary body is involved, as illustrated in Figure 6.30, then the origin is more likely choroidal.

Acoustic Characteristics of Anterior Choroidal Tumors

Ultrasound biomicroscopy can provide some information on the internal acoustic characteristics of anterior choroidal tumors. This could be helpful in differential diagnoses in a way similar to the use of internal acoustic characteristics in differential diagnoses of ocular tumors by conventional ultrasound. The acoustic appearance of the part of choroidal melanomas accessible by ultrasound biomicroscopy is usually that of a medium, uniform reflectivity. The anterior margin frequently shows an area of elevation of adjoining retinal/pars plana region with what appears to be fluid at the edge, as shown in Figures 6.30 and 6.31.

FIGURE 6.31. **(a)** The anteriorly located melanoma in this eye was difficult to visualize. **(b)** Ultrasound biomicroscopy shows the anterior margin of this tumor posterior to the ciliary body with forward curvature from the base. **(c)** Histology shows the relationship of the tumor to the ciliary body. The curvature of the anterior margin is decreased postmortem.

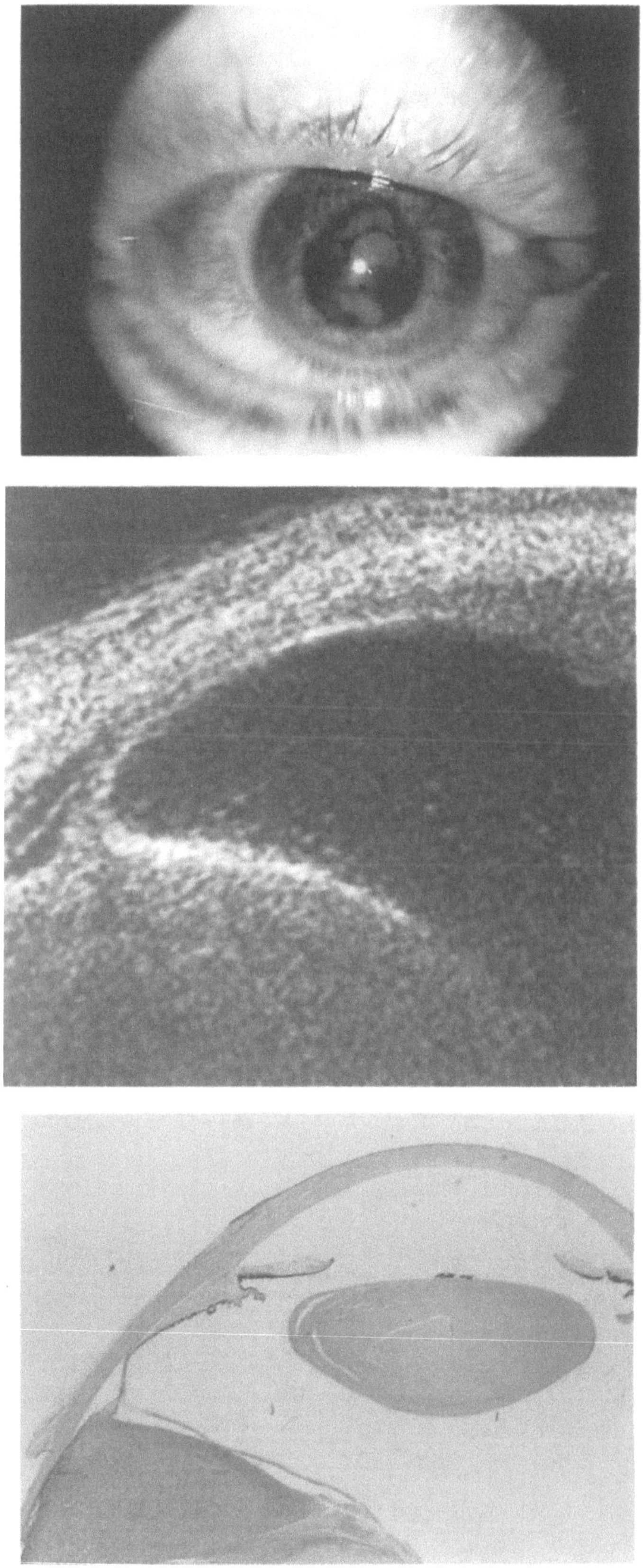

(a)

(b)

(c)

Extrascleral Extension

Figure 6.32a shows the clinical appearance of a pigmented lesion noted on the scleral surface. A small peripheral choroidal lesion 1.5 mm in height could be imaged both clinically and by conventional ultrasound. Because the surface lesion was below the resolution of conventional ultrasound, the two lesions could not be imaged simultaneously, and it was unclear as to whether they were related. Ultrasound biomicroscopy demonstrated that the lesion on the scleral surface (250 μm in height) directly overlay the choroidal tumor (Figure 6.32b). A connecting sonolucent line was noted traversing the sclera (Figure 6.32c), most likely representing the emissary path of tumor cells to the scleral surface.

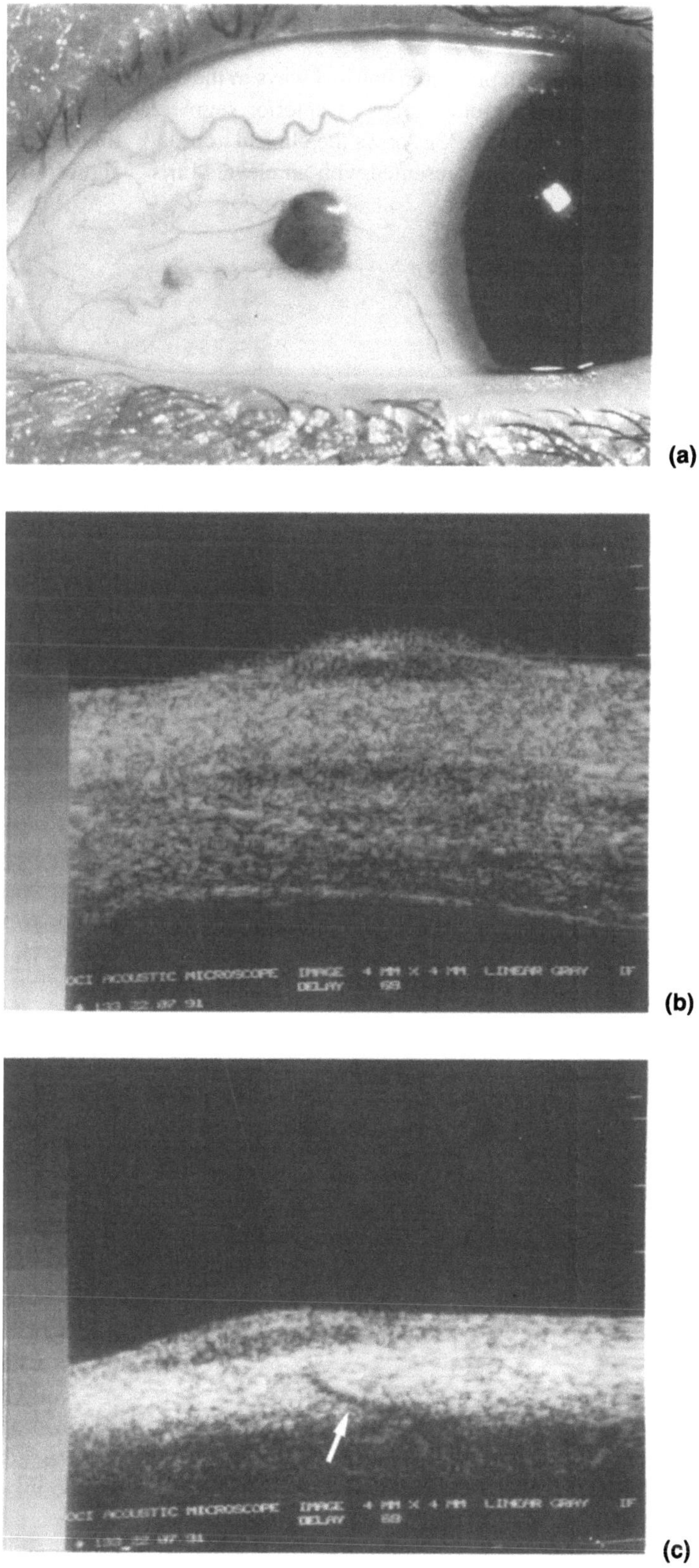

FIGURE 6.32. (**a**) Clinical appearance of a patient with a pigmented scleral nodule. (**b**) Ultrasound biomicroscopy reveals that this nodule directly overlies a choroidal tumor. (**c**) An emissary pathway through the sclera (arrow) is imaged. Published courtesy of *Ophthalmology* (1992;99:1220–1228).

Lymphoma and Leukemia

Lymphomas can present in unusual ways in the eye and can simulate other types of anterior segment pathology. Figure 6.33a shows the clinical appearance of an eye that presented with an elevated iris and kerato-precipitates. Ultrasound biomicroscopy showed that the iris was markedly thickened by a diffuse infiltrate (Figure 6.33b), and the clumps of tumor cells on the back of the cornea could also be imaged (Figure 6.33c). Clinical examination showed a testicular primary.

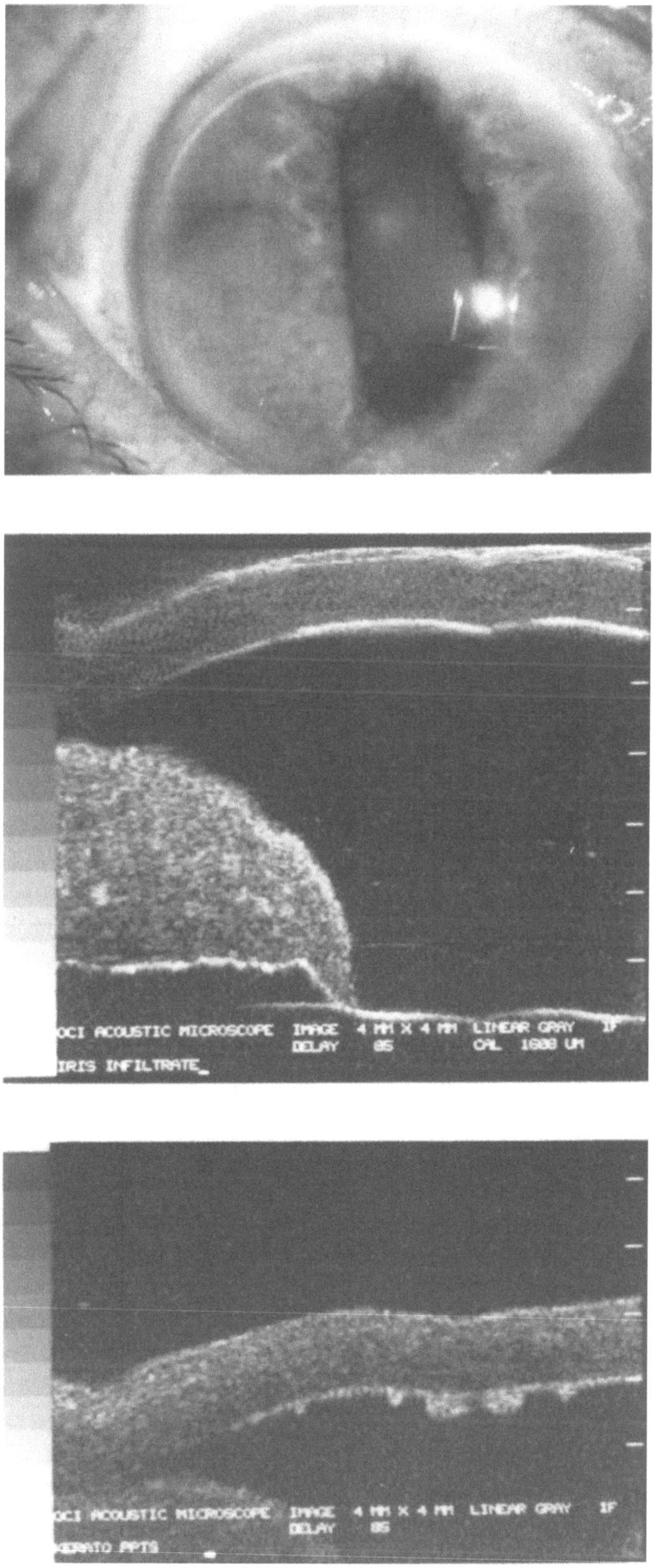

(a) (b) (c)

FIGURE 6.33. **(a)** Clinical appearance of a patient presenting with an elevated iris and kerato-precipitates. **(b)** Ultrasound biomicroscopy reveals massive thickening of the iris with a low-reflective infiltrate. Published courtesy of *Ophthalmology* (1991;98:287–295). **(c)** Ultrasound biomicroscopy images clumps of tumor cells on the posterior corneal surface.

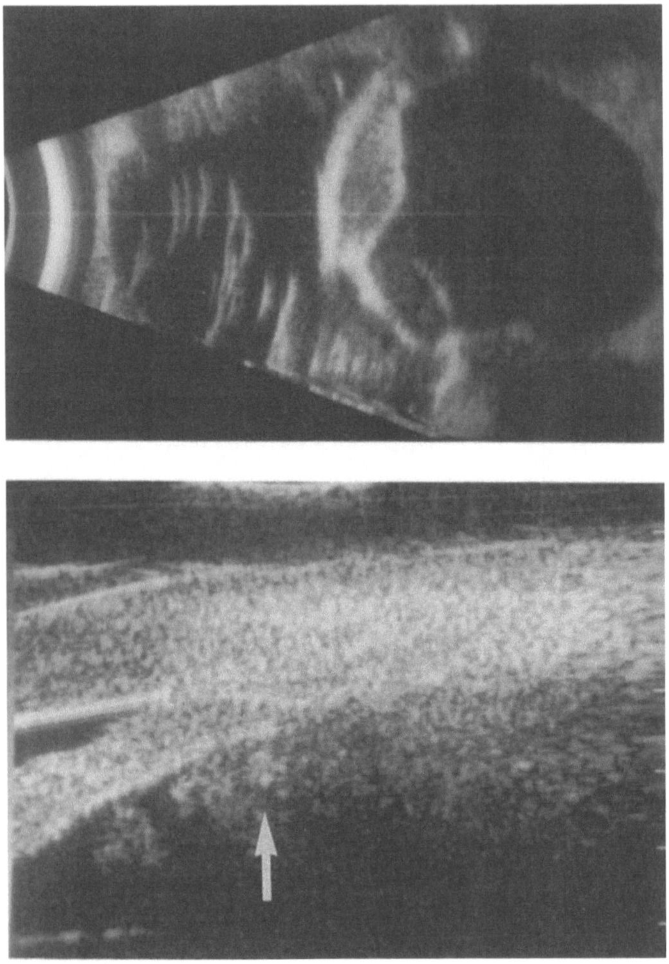

(a)

(b)

FIGURE 6.34. Conventional ultrasound of a patient with lymphoma shows anterior choroidal separation by a low-reflective infiltrate. (**b**) Ultrasound biomicroscopy reveals the infiltrate above the ciliary body, with anterior positioning of the ciliary processes (arrow) closing the peripheral angle.

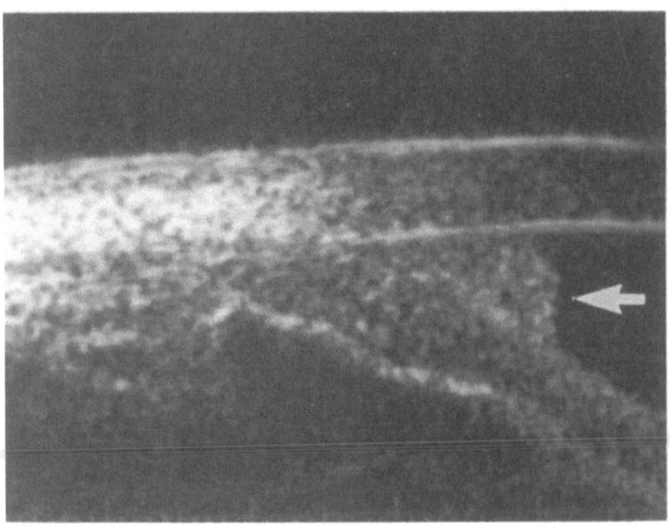

FIGURE 6.35. Ultrasound biomicroscopy of the anterior chamber in a patient with leukemia shows a leukemic hypopyon (arrow) above a slightly thickened iris.

An unusual case of lymphoma presented with glaucoma secondary to shallowing of the anterior chamber. Conventional ultrasound revealed anterior choroidal detachment and the presence of a uniform low-reflective solid infiltrate in the suprachoroidal space (Figure 6.34a). Ultrasound biomicroscopy showed that the infiltrate extended above the ciliary body and had caused anterior rotation of the ciliary processes and angle closure (Figure 6.34b) in a manner similar to that caused by anterior cilio-choroidal effusions. Biopsy confirmed the presence of lymphoma cells in the suprachoroidal space in this patient with a previous history of lymphoma in remission. Radiotherapy improved the glaucoma, and produced resolution of the choroidal infiltrates.

Leukemia can produce iris infiltration and anterior chamber deposits. Figure 6.35 shows an example in which leukemic cells formed a hypopyon in the base of the anterior chamber. Ultrasound biomicroscopy images the hypopyon and the underlying contracted iris, which is also likely involved.

Summary

Ultrasound biomicroscopy is a new method of imaging anterior segment tumors that can add information to that gained by clinical observation. Morphological and internal reflectivity patterns aid differential diagnoses. Ultrasound biomicroscopy is diagnostic in differentiating cysts from solid tumors. Where observation is elected greater precision in detecting tumor change is provided. Where surgical removal or radiotherapy is indicated, an improved ability to determine tumor borders can aid treatment planning.

References

1. Pavlin CJ, McWhae JA, McGowan HD, Foster FS: Ultrasound biomicroscopy of anterior segment tumors. *Ophthalmology* 1992;99:1222–1228.
2. The Collaborative Ocular Melanoma Study Group. Accuracy of diagnosis of choroidal melanomas in the Collaborative Ocular Melanoma Study. COMS report no. 1. *Arch Ophthalmol* 1990;108:1268–1273.
3. Verbeek AM, Mitropoulos P. Diagnostic ultrasound: An aid in the differentiation of anterior segment lesions of the eye. *Int Ophthalmol* 1991; 15:205–212.
4. Dart JK, Marsh RJ, Garner A, Cooling RJ. Fluorescein angiography of anterior uveal melanocytic tumours. *Br J Ophthalmol* 1988;72:326–337.
5. Coleman DJ, Lizzi FL, Jack RL. *Ultrasonography of the Eye and Orbit*. 1977, pp. 173–181. Lea & Febiger, Philadelphia.
6. Shields JA, Sanborn GE, Augsburger JJ. The differential diagnosis of malignant melanoma of the iris. A clinical study of 200 patients. *Ophthalmology* 1983;90:716–720.
7. Jakobiec FA, Silbert G. Are most iris 'melanomas' really nevi? A clinicopathological study of 189 lesions. *Arch Ophthalmol* 1981;99:2117–2132.
8. Shields JA, Kline MW, Augsburger JJ. Primary iris cysts: A review of the literature and report of 62 cases. *Br J Ophthalmol* 1984;68:152–166.
9. Pavlin CJ, Japp B, Payne D, Drysdale AM, Gallie BL. Intraoperative use of ultrasound in the management of choroidal melanomas. In: *Ophthalmic Echography*. Oissoinig KC, ed. 1987, pp. 391–399. Martinus Nijhoff/Dr. W.Junk Publishing, Dordrecht, The Netherlands.
10. Pavlin CJ, Japp B, Simpson ER, McGowan HD, Fitzpatrick PJ. Ultrasound determination of the relationship of radioactive plaques to the base of choroidal melanomas. *Ophthalmology* April 1989;96: 538–542.

7
Trauma

Penetrating or blunt trauma can frequently result in anterior segment abnormalities that are difficult to assess owing to corneal opacity, inflammation, hemorrhage, or other disruption of intraocular tissue resulting in poor visualization. Ultrasound biomicroscopy can be helpful in assessing the anterior segment in these circumstances. The ultrasound biomicroscopic appearance of some typical findings associated with trauma are presented here.

Angle Recession

Angle recession is caused by blunt trauma producing a pressure wave that causes a tear into the ciliary body [1]. It is not infrequently accompanied by late onset glaucoma from concomitant damage to the trabecular meshwork. Angle recession has a typical appearance on ultrasound biomicroscopy [2]. The tear into the ciliary body can be imaged, extending from the angle region. Examples of angle recession are shown in Figure 7.1. As is noted in examination of pathological specimens, the tear is into the ciliary body itself, and does not produce disinsertion of the ciliary body from the scleral spur (Figure 7.1a). The superficial aspect of the tear can have a high reflectivity most likely representing secondary condensation of the ciliary body tissue on this surface (Figure 7.1b). Angle recession can be accompanied by other signs of trauma such as iris tears.

Iridodialysis

In traumatic iridodialysis the iris tends to tear at its thinnest area near the root. The ultrasound biomicroscopic appearance of a traumatic iridodialysis is shown in Figure 7.2. It should be noted that there is little in the way of residual iris tissue remaining attached near the scleral spur. This differs from the ultrasound biomicroscopic appearance of an iridectomy, which is generally more medial in location and shows a small residual portion of the iris root remaining peripherally.

Cyclodialysis

Cyclodialysis refers to the disinsertion of the ciliary body from the scleral spur. This can occur secondary to blunt trauma and surgical trauma [3,4], and generally results in hypotony. The pressure lowering effect of cyclodialysis has been used in the past as a surgical procedure for glaucoma.

The ultrasound biomicroscopic appearance of traumatic cyclodialysis is typical and diagnostic. Figure 7.3 shows a case in which the ciliary body has been disinserted from the scleral spur following blunt trauma. Clinically the pupil is irregular, being displaced toward the site of the cyclodialysis (Figure 7.3a). This sign is not always present. On ultrasound biomicroscopy the anterior ciliary body and iris root are both displaced posteriorly by approximately 2 mm accounting for the displacement of the pupil (Figure 7.3b). This ultrasound biomicroscopic appearance is quite different from angle recession. There is no residual uveal tissue attached to the scleral spur. A space can be seen above the ciliary body, separating it from the overlying sclera.

Clinically this condition can be difficult to diagnose because of the inability to see past the peripheral iris on gonioscopy. As noted in the examples

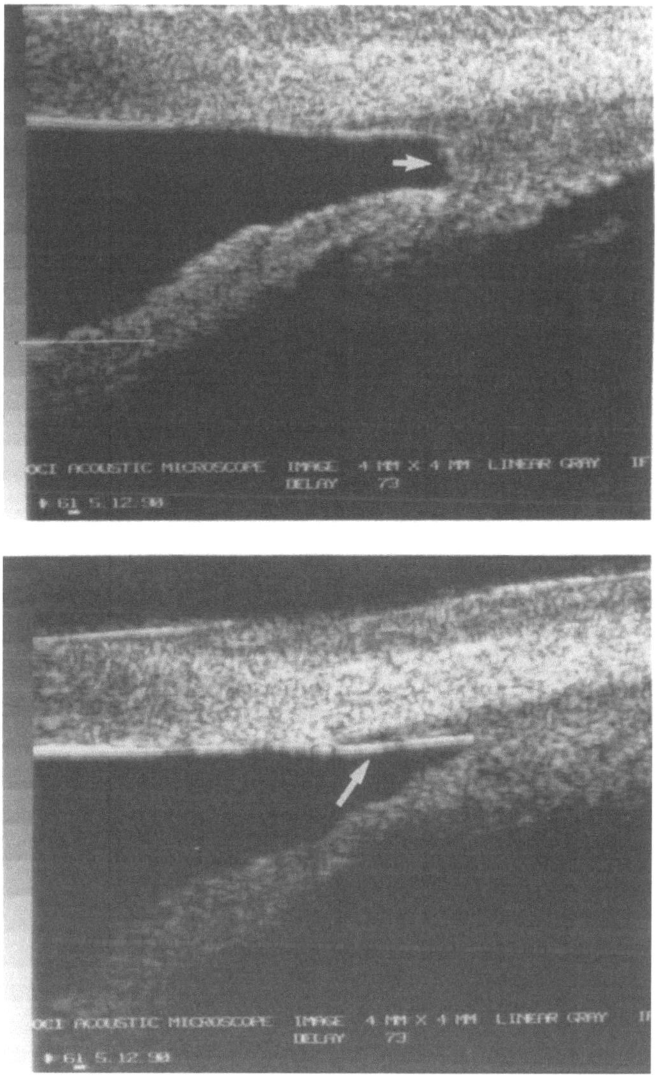

(a)

(b)

FIGURE 7.1. Ultrasound biomicroscopic appearance of angle recession. **(a)** The angle shows a tear into the ciliary body (arrow). The ciliary body remains attached at the scleral spur. Published courtesy of *Ophthalmology* (1991;98: 287–295). **(b)** The inner surface of a ciliary body tear shows a high reflectivity (arrow), most likely representing condensation of ciliary body tissue.

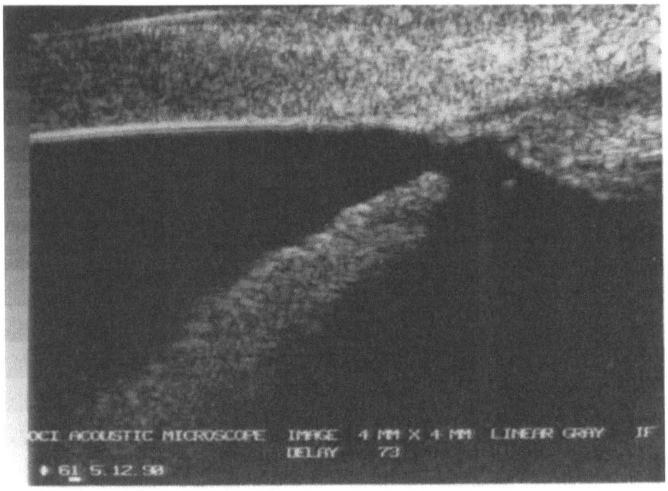

FIGURE 7.2. Ultrasound biomicroscopic appearance of an iridodialysis. The iris is disinserted at the iris root.

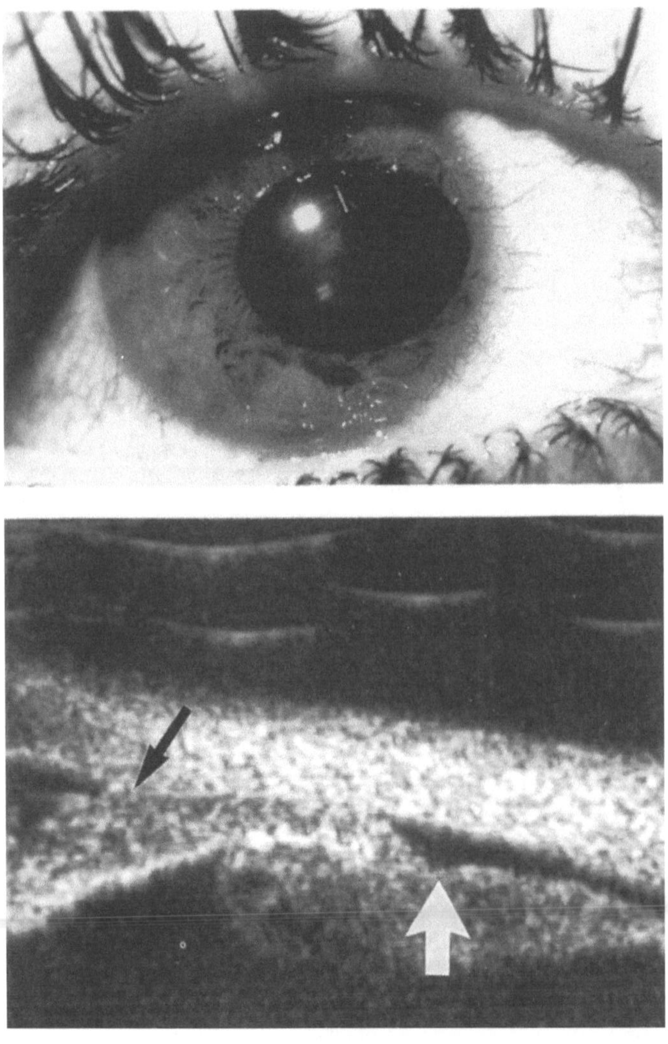

(a)

(b)

FIGURE 7.3. A case of cyclodialysis following blunt trauma. **(a)** Clinical appearance shows displacement of the pupil toward the site of cyclodialysis. **(b)** Ultrasound biomicroscopy shows that the ciliary body and iris root (white arrow) are disinserted from the scleral spur (black arrow) and moved 2 mm posteriorly. The peripheral iris is lying against the scleral spur.

given here, the peripheral iris is lying against the scleral spur, which prevents the gap from being visualized. Methods such as inflating the anterior chamber with fluid at surgery or in the examination room may be required to detect the presence of cyclodialysis and determine its extent. Ultrasound biomicroscopy provides a reliable method of defining the extent of cyclodialysis without entering the anterior chamber.

Traumatic cyclodialysis can be accompanied by shallowing of the anterior chamber and angle closure in the presence of hypotony. Clinical appearance of a case of traumatic iridodialysis secondary to blunt trauma from a hockey stick is shown in Figure 7.4a. The patient presented 3 weeks following injury with shallowing of the anterior chamber and hypotony. In this case the pupil is not displaced. Figure 7.4b shows the typical ultrasound biomicroscopic appearance of disinsertion of the ciliary body from the scleral spur with posterior displacement of the ciliary body and iris, this time by only 0.5 mm. The peripheral iris is lying against the scleral spur, preventing visualization of the cleft by gonioscopy. In this case the cyclodialysis was superior, but the choroidal effusion extended 360°. Figure 7.4c shows the ultrasound biomicroscopic appearance of a region of the eye that has choroidal effusion, but no cyclodialysis. The shallowing of the anterior chamber was produced by the supraciliary effusion rotating the ciliary processes forward, which directly closed the angle and moved the lens forward. The anterior bowing of the iris illustrated in Figure 7.4d indicates pupil block secondary to the forward lens position. It is interesting that pupil block with complete angle closure coexisted with hypotony, most likely secondary to decreased aqueous production. In this case intensive cycloplegia moved the ciliary processes back, deepening the anterior chamber, breaking the pupil

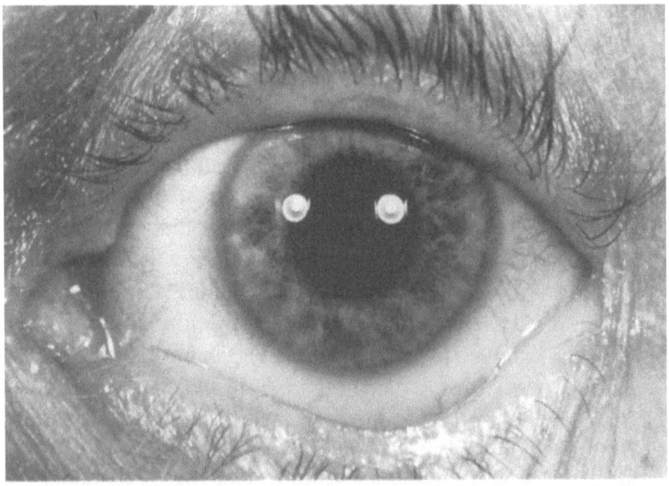

(a)

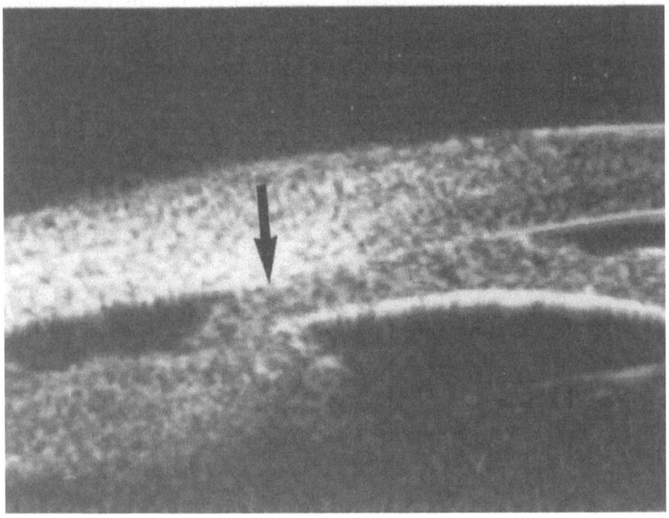

(b)

FIGURE 7.4. Cyclodialysis following blunt trauma with anterior chamber shallowing. **(a)** Clinical appearance of patient with blunt trauma and a shallow chamber. The pupil is not obviously displaced. **(b)** Ultrasound biomicroscopy shows disinsertion of the ciliary body superiorly with displacement of the iris root 0.5 mm posterior to the scleral spur (arrow). Supraciliary fluid is present. **(c)** Ultrasound biomicroscopy in a different region of the angle shows supraciliary fluid (arrow), which has produced chamber shallowing. **(d)** Anterior iris bowing indicates an element of pupil block (arrow) in the presence of hypotony.

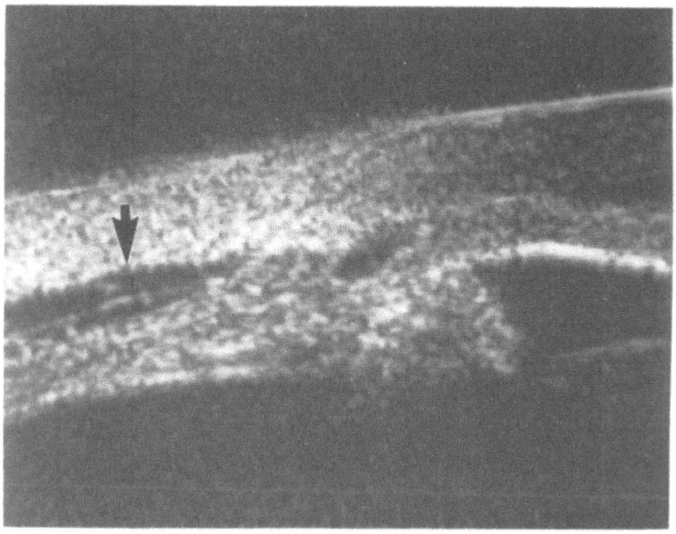

(c)

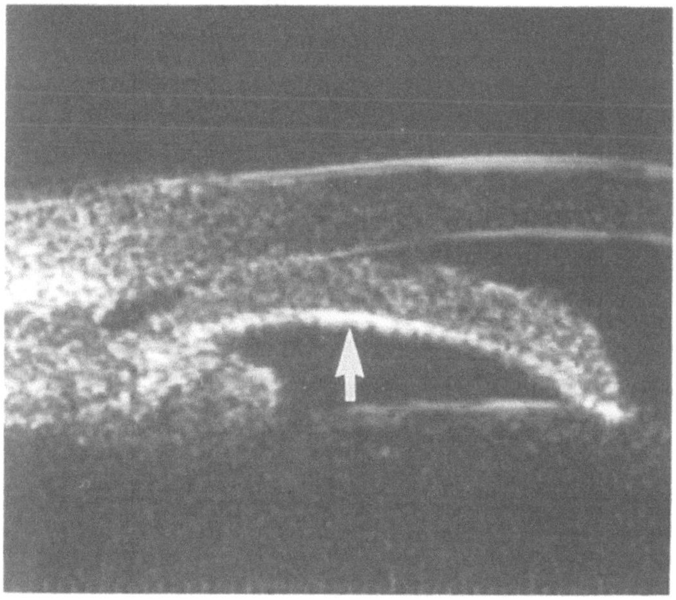

(d)

block, and opening the angle. Figure 7.5a shows the deeper anterior chamber in the region of cyclodialysis. Figure 7.5b shows that the iris has fallen away from the scleral spur in one area. This region could be detected by gonioscopy at this stage, but the full extent of the cyclodialysis could not be ascertained. Figure 7.5c shows persistent supra-choroidal effusion in the region away from the cyclodialysis, but the angle is now open.

FIGURE 7.5. Cyclodialysis following treatment with cycloplegics (same case as in Figure 7.4). (**a**) Ultrasound biomicroscopy of cyclodialysis patient following cycloplegia. The ciliary body has moved back and the chamber has deepened. Gonioscopy would still not allow detection of the iridodialysis site because of the position of the iris against the scleral spur (arrow). (**b**) Iris has fallen away from the scleral spur in one region revealing a continuous opening (arrow). (**c**) In region of the angle away from the cyclodialysis, supraciliary fluid is still present (arrow). The pupil block has broken and the angle is open.

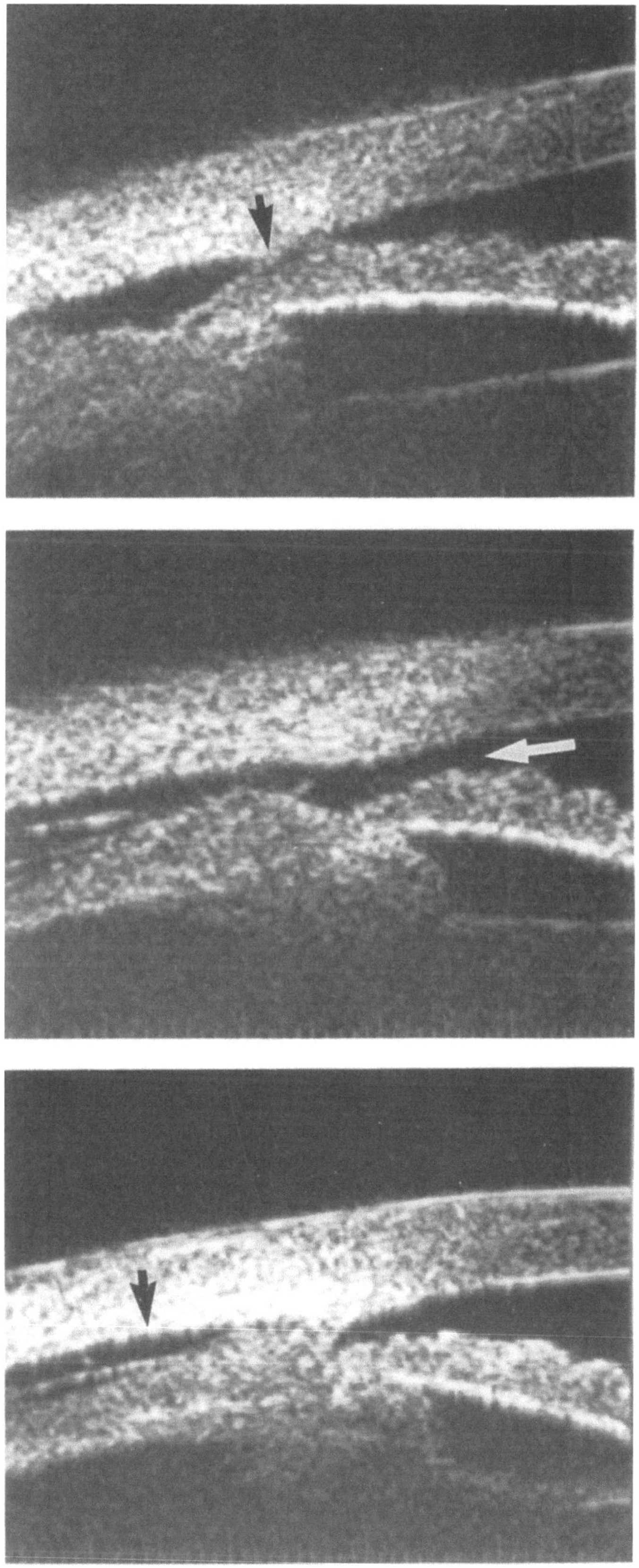

Hyphema

Figure 7.6 shows the appearance of liquid blood in the anterior chamber. The red cells produce scattering of the ultrasound beam. Some layering of the blood can be noted. The blood cells can be noted to be mobile during the examination.

Vitreous Hemorrhage

Hemorrhage into the anterior vitreous can be imaged by ultrasound biomicroscopy. Figure 7.7 shows an area of vitreous hemorrhage in the region just below the posterior ciliary body and pars plana. The blood has the appearance of multiple strands in the anterior vitreous. The vitreous blood in this region is minimally mobile during examination.

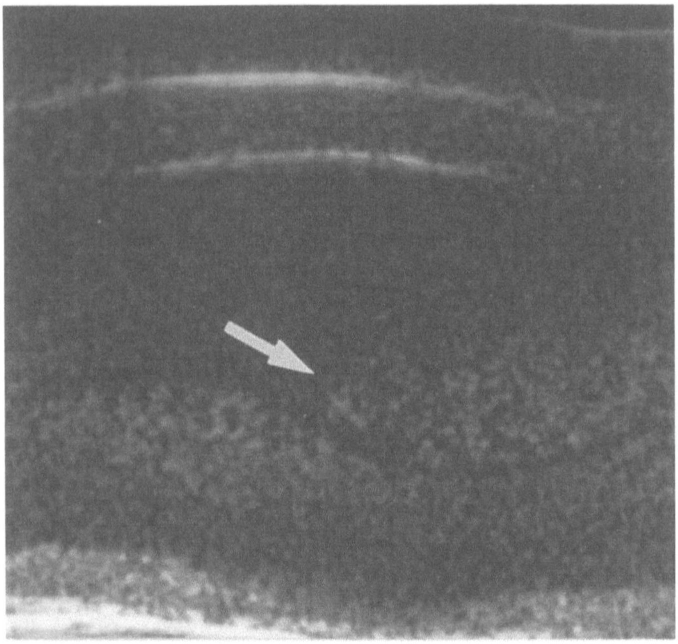

FIGURE 7.6. Ultrasound biomicroscopic appearance of blood in the anterior chamber (arrow). The red blood cells produce low-reflective scattering, some layering, and are mobile with eye movement.

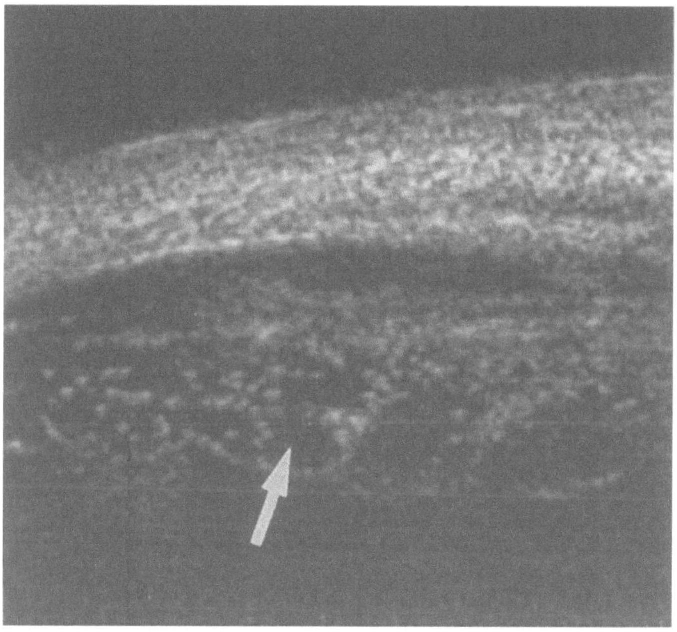

Figure 7.7. Ultrasound biomicroscopic appearance of bleeding into the vitreous below the pars plana region (arrow). The blood has the appearance of strands in the anterior vitreous.

Corneal Blood Staining

Repetitive bleeding accompanied by high intraocular pressure can result in corneal blood staining. This can obscure visualization of anterior chamber structures. A clinical photograph of a patient's eye with corneal blood staining following recurrent hyphema after blunt trauma is shown in Figure 7.8a. In this case no anterior chamber structures were visible. This case provides a good example of the ability of ultrasound biomicroscopy to determine details of anterior segment pathology behind an opaque cornea. This patient had undergone filtering surgery for intractable glaucoma. Ultrasound biomicroscopic examination revealed total occlusion of the pupil (Figure 7.8b). The iris appeared continuous through the center of this eye with only slight irregularity in the position the pupil should have been. The patient had had filtering surgery with iridectomy accounting for the lack of pupil block glaucoma. The patient had regions of angle closure secondary to synechia. Details of anterior chamber pathology can be a helpful guide to the operating surgeon if further surgery such as corneal transplantation is performed in the future.

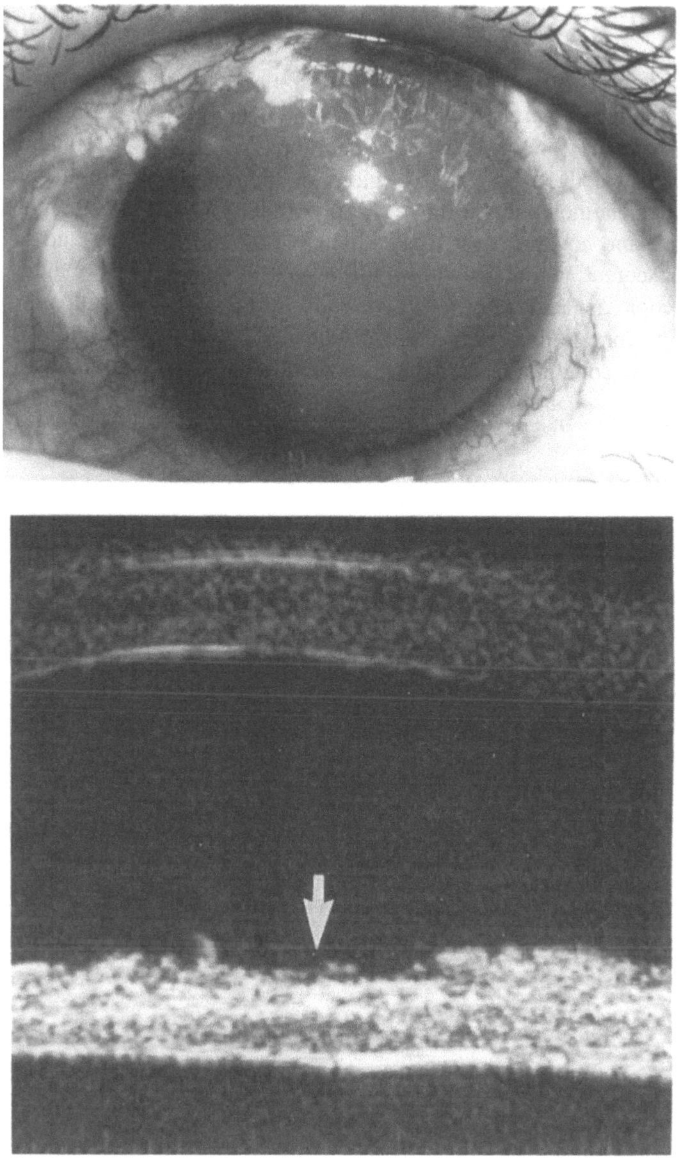

(a)

(b)

FIGURE 7.8. Corneal blood staining following posttraumatic hyphema. **(a)** Clinical photograph of a patient with corneal blood staining. **(b)** Ultrasound biomicroscopy reveals total occlusion of the pupil. No pupil space is detected, with only an area of irregularity where the pupil should be (arrow).

Foreign Bodies

Foreign bodies are generally highly reflective, although this can vary depending on the material of which the foreign body is made. Foreign bodies can be lodged in various regions of the anterior segment including the angle. If they are longstanding and covered with tissue, their nature can be obscured. Figure 7.9 shows ultrasound biomicroscopic appearance of a foreign body in the angle. The foreign body was covered with tissue and its nature could not be confirmed on gonioscopy. The material is highly reflective and produces complete shadowing of all structures behind it. These characteristics differentiate a foreign body from a peripheral iris tumor, or synechiae in this region. Small foreign bodies can be buried in the lens, iris, posterior chamber, and ciliary body. Ultrasound biomicroscopy provides an excellent method of diagnosing and localizing these bodies prior to surgery. Although foreign bodies can be imaged with conventional ultrasound, high-frequency ultrasound provides a cleaner image and better view of surrounding tissue [5].

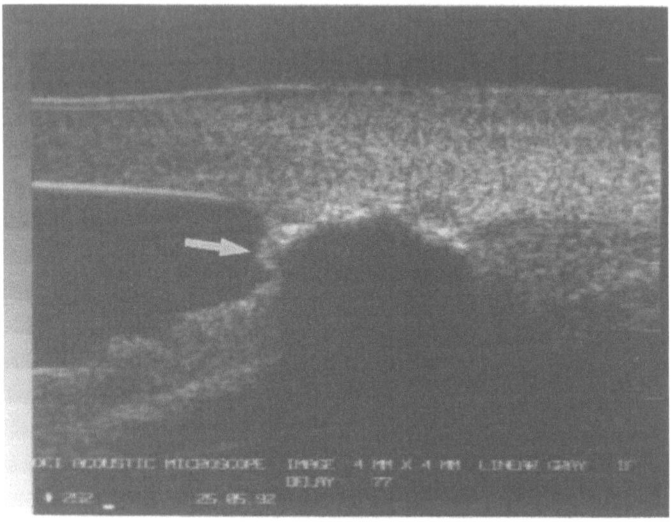

FIGURE 7.9. Ultrasound biomicroscopy of foreign body in the angle (arrow) shows high reflectivity and total shadowing of structures behind it.

Epithelial Downgrowth

Epithelium can be implanted in the anterior chamber secondary to trauma or following anterior segment surgery [6]. Clinical manifestations include cysts, solid tumors, and diffuse epithelial growth. Figure 7.10a shows a large cyst in a surgical case, which completely displaces the iris. A defect at the corneo-scleral junction is present, which likely represents an internal wound gap and the point of invasion of the epithelium. Figure 7.10b shows another view of the cyst, showing complete disruption of the iris and a solid component likely representing epithelial cells.

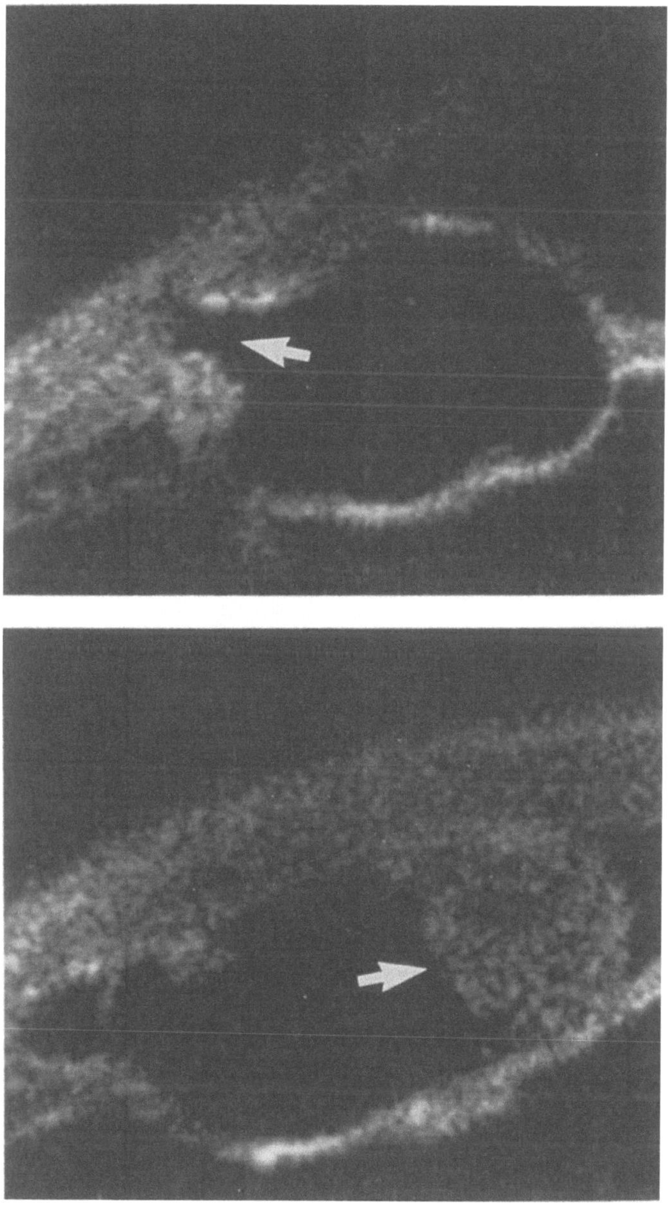

(a)

(b)

FIGURE 7.10. (a) Ultrasound biomicroscopy of epithelial ingrowth shows large cyst with an internal corneo-scleral defect (arrow). (b) Ultrasound biomicroscopic image of the cyst shows iris displacement and a solid component (arrow).

Summary

Ultrasound biomicroscopy is a helpful adjunct in assessing trauma, especially in those cases in which structural changes or opacity obscure relevant pathology. Ultrasound biomicroscopy provides a new method of determining the extent of cyclodialysis prior to therapeutic intervention. The presence of pathology such as angle changes and iris abnormalities behind opaque corneas can be determined prior to surgery. Foreign bodies have a typical appearance on ultrasound biomicroscopy, and can be imaged in the angle and behind the iris.

References

1. Pilger IS, Khwarg SG. Angle recession glaucoma: review and two case reports. *Ann Ophthalmol* 1985;17:197–199.
2. Pavlin CJ, Harasiewicz K, Foster FS. Ultrasound biomicroscopy of anterior segment structures in normal and glaucomatous eyes. *Am J Ophthalmol* 1992; 113:381–389.
3. Slusher MM. Pseudophakic choroidal detachment with cyclodialysis cleft. *Ophthal Surg* 1987;18:191–194.
4. Ormerod LD, Baerveldt G, Sunalp MA, Riekhof FT. Management of the hypotonous cyclo-dialysis cleft. *Ophthalmology* 1991;98:1384–1393.
5. Nouby-Mahmoud G, Silverman RH, Coleman DJ. Using high-frequency ultrasound to characterize intraocular foreign bodies. *Ophthal Surg* 1993;24:94–99.
6. Weiner MJ, Trentacoste J, Pon DM, Albert DM. Epithelial downgrowth: A 30 year clinico-pathological review. *Br J Ophthalmol* 1989;73:6–11.

8
Corneal Disease

Corneal disease can generally be assessed well by direct slit lamp observation. Most pathology occurring in a relatively clear cornea can be observed directly and the depth of the corneal changes determined. Exceptions occur when corneal opacity increases, or the cornea is covered, as with a conjunctival flap. In these circumstances, ultrasound biomicroscopy allows assessment of internal corneal changes, assessment of corneal dimensions, and assessment of underlying changes in the anterior chamber. Internal reflectivity patterns provide a different type of information than that obtained by direct observation. Quantitative assessment of corneal thickness is improved compared to current ultrasound pachymeters, which operate in the 20 MHz range.

Because penetration of corneal thickness is usually not difficult, higher frequency transducers can be used. The corneal stroma and epithelium can be imaged and measured separately.

Corneal Edema

Corneal edema can occur from many causes, most involving some form of endothelial pathology. Ultrasound biomicroscopy provides a new highly accurate method of assessing corneal thickness changes. Figure 8.1 shows the ultrasound biomicroscopic appearance of a normal cornea. As outlined in the section on normal cornea, the interface between fluid and normal corneal epithelium shows a smooth high reflectivity. Another highly reflective line is imaged below this from Bowman's membrane. The stroma shows a low-medium reflectivity, and the endothelial surface is imaged as a highly reflective line. Figure 8.2 shows an ultrasound biomicroscopic appearance of a thickened edematous cornea. In corneal edema, the epithelial surface echo is more irregular, and the epithelium shows some internal reflectivity that is not apparent in normal cornea. The distance from the surface echo to the echo from Bowman's membrane is increased in keeping with epithelial thickening. The stromal reflectivity is generally increased in corneal edema. This is most likely due to the separation of the corneal lamellae by edema fluid. In bullous keratopathy, bullae can be imaged as a separation of the epithelium from Bowman's membrane (Figure 8.3).

The thickness of the corneal stroma can be measured independently of epithelial thickness, by measuring the distance from the Bowman's membrane reflection to the reflection from the endothelial surface. This capability may prove valuable in the assessment of graft rejection or other causes of corneal thickening.

Corneal Opacification and Underlying Changes

There are a multitude of causes of corneal opacification. Opacification can result from corneal dystrophies, trauma, or inflammatory disease. Ultrasound biomicroscopy provides some information on the scarring process, allows quantitative assessment of corneal thinning, and provides information on underlying anterior segment changes. Generally the region of a corneal scar shows a higher reflec-

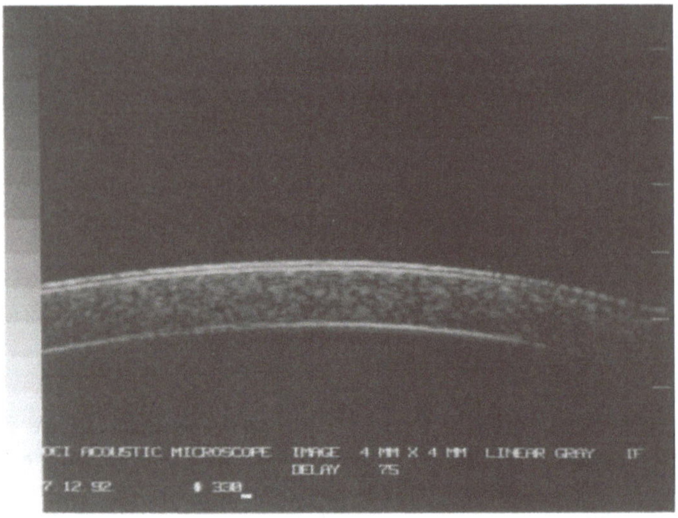

FIGURE 8.1. Ultrasound biomicroscopic image of normal cornea. The two smooth highly reflective surface echoes are from the epithelial surface and Bowman's membrane. The stroma shows a low regular reflectivity. The descemet's membrane/endothelial surface is imaged as a smooth highly reflective line.

tivity than the surrounding normal cornea, probably due to the disruption of the very regular corneal lamellae present in normal corneal structure. Figure 8.4 shows a scarred cornea with high stromal reflectivity. If calcification is present, the reflectivity increases to very high levels and shadowing of structures posterior to the calcification is seen. This is due to the almost total reflection and absorption of the sound waves by the calcium. Figure 8.5 shows a thickened cornea with areas of superficial calcification with total shadowing of corneal structure behind it.

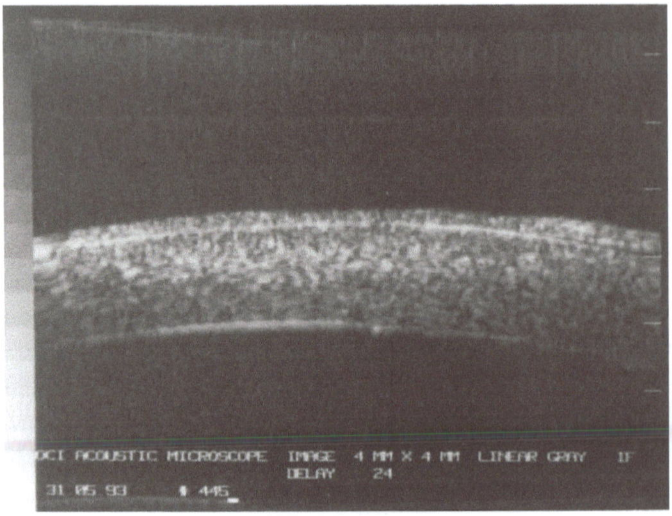

FIGURE 8.2. Ultrasound biomicroscopic image of an edematous cornea. The epithelium is thickened and irregular. The stroma is thickened and shows increased reflectivity.

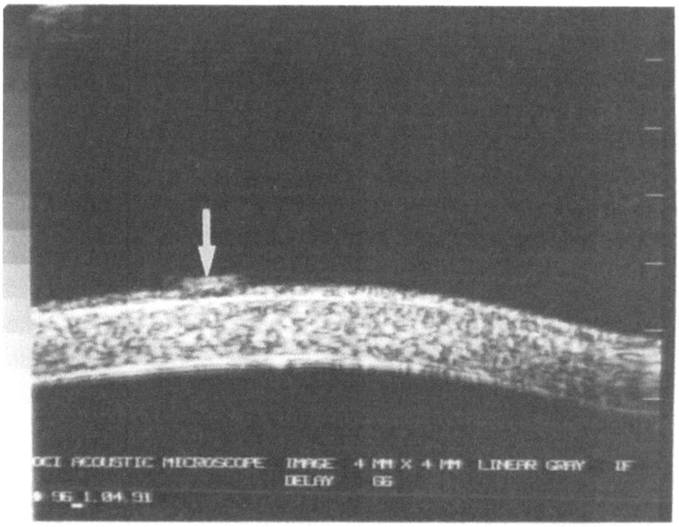

FIGURE 8.3. An epithelial bullae (arrow) in an edematous cornea is imaged on the corneal surface.

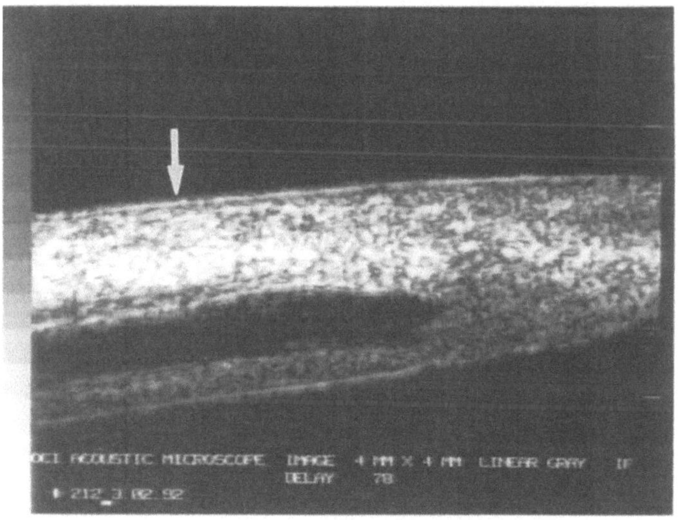

FIGURE 8.4. Scarred cornea secondary to inflammation shows increased stromal reflectivity.

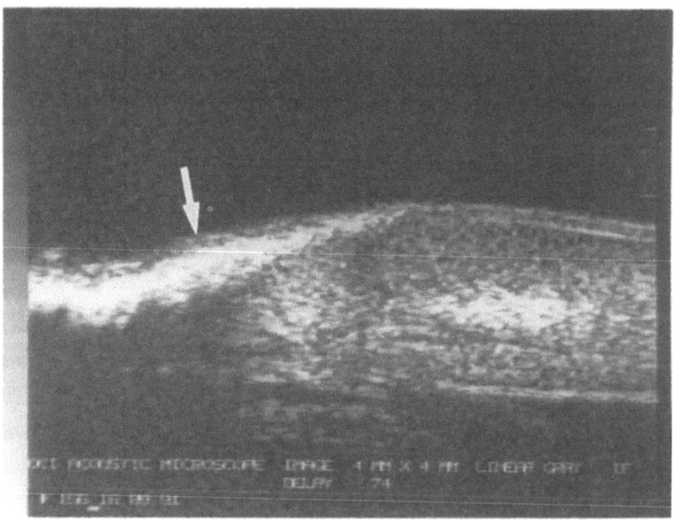

FIGURE 8.5. Scarred thickened cornea with an area of calcification (arrow) producing complete shadowing of structures behind it.

Underlying changes can be detected by ultrasound biomicroscopy. Figure 8.6 shows the appearance of an adherent leukoma. The iris strands can be seen extending up to the overlying cornea. The region of attachment to the cornea is clearly visualized. Figure 8.7 shows underlying iris adhesions and a closed angle in a case with an opaque cornea secondary to trauma. Figure 8.8a shows the clinical appearance of a case of lipid keratopathy. It is apparent that no details of the anterior segment can be discerned behind this virtually complete opacity. The ultrasound image of the cornea shows thickening, increased reflectivity, and irregularity (Figure 8.8b). Beneath this opacity the chamber is shallow and the angle extremely narrow.

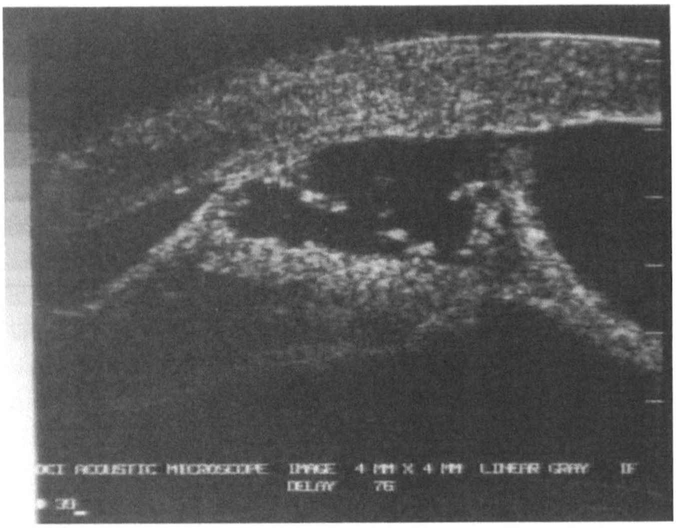

FIGURE 8.6. Adherent leukoma. Strands of iris tissue extend anteriorly and are adherent to the posterior corneal surface.

FIGURE 8.7. Traumatic corneal opacity with angle closure and anterior synechiae (arrow) behind the opacity.

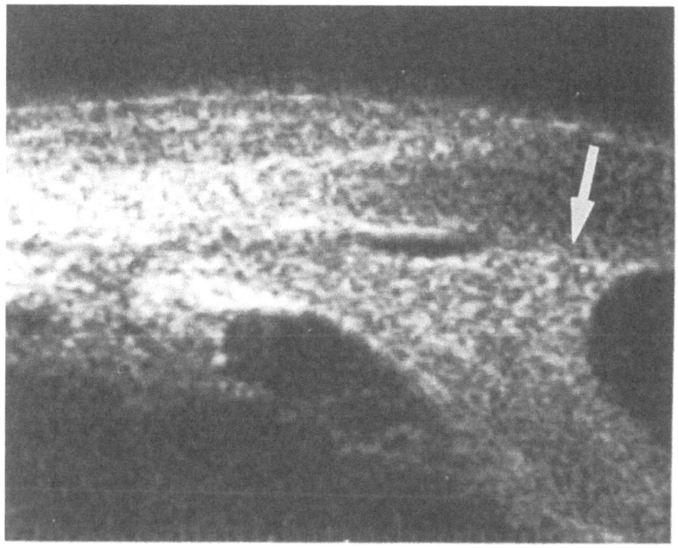

FIGURE 8.8. **(a)** Clinical photograph of a case of lipid keratopathy. No anterior chamber details are visible. **(b)** Ultrasound biomicroscopy reveals a thickened cornea with a shallow underlying anterior chamber. The iris (arrow) is touching the posterior cornea.

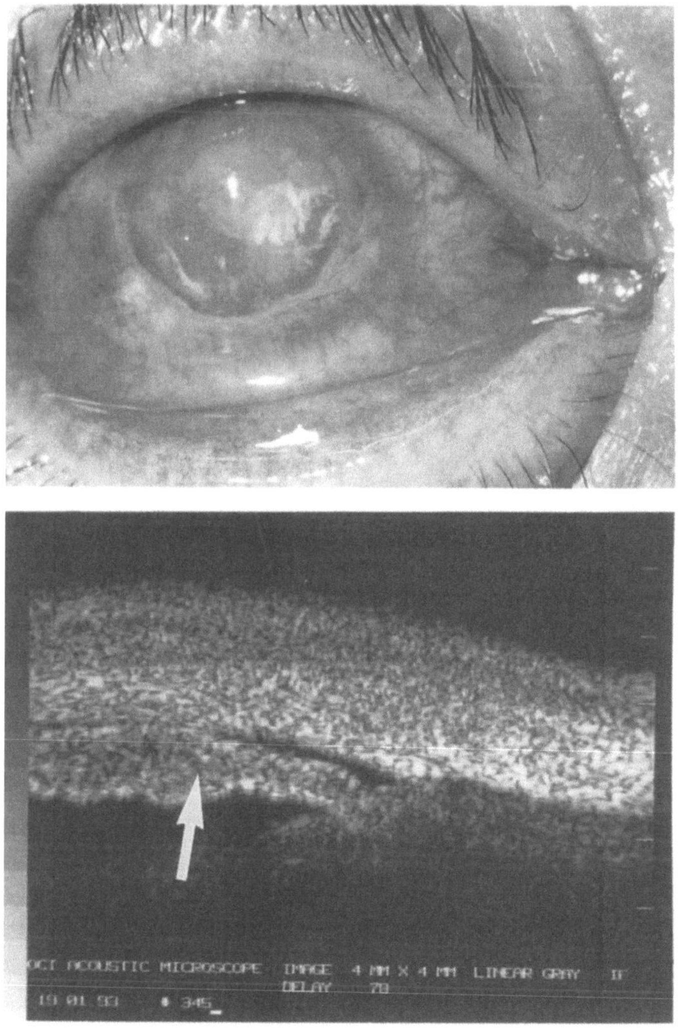

(a)

(b)

Conjunctival Flaps

After a conjunctival flap is applied, it is difficult to assess the underlying cornea and the anterior chamber. Ultrasound biomicroscopy allows a method of assessing these structures through the conjunctival flap. The corneal tissue can be differentiated from the conjunctival tissue and the corneal thickness noted. In addition, the state of the underlying iris and angle structures can be assessed. Figure 8.9 shows a conjunctival flap in position. The cornea beneath the flap shows relatively normal thickness.

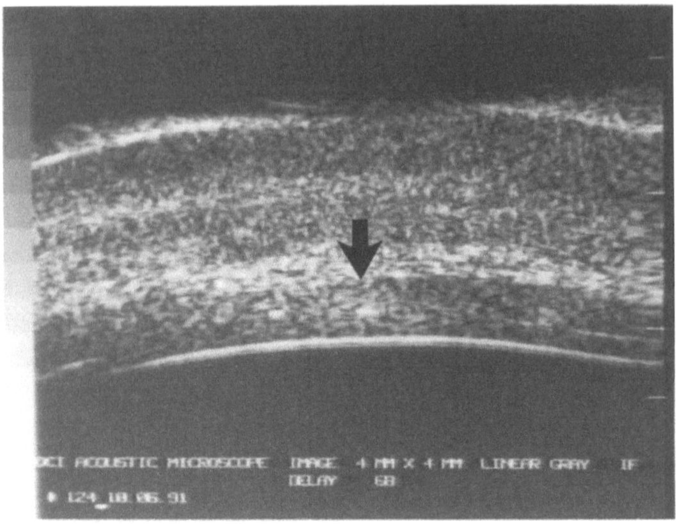

FIGURE 8.9. Conjunctival flap. The cornea (arrow) can be differentiated beneath the conjunctival tissue and is of relatively normal thickness.

Corneal Grafts

Ultrasound biomicroscopy provides a new method of assessing corneal grafts. As noted above, edema and thickening of corneal stroma and epithelium can be assessed independently and with a new level of accuracy. In addition, aberrations at the graft-host junction can be assessed. This area is often difficult to visualize at the slit lamp because of the scarring present due to healing at the suture line and the frequent opacity of the residual host cornea. Gonioscopy often fails to provide a clear view of the region immediately underlying the peripheral cornea. The problem is compounded if there is any opacity of the graft itself. Ultrasound biomicroscopy provides a method of visualizing this area in depth. The graft-host junction is usually identifiable by a change in reflectivity from the more weakly reflective graft and the more highly reflective pathological host cornea. Figure 8.10 shows an image of a graft-host junction with an irregular internal apposition of Descemet's membrane. Aberrations such as a step or irregularity between the host cornea and the graft are easily discernible. Figure 8.11a shows an opaque graft. A step between the graft and the host cornea is noted on ultrasound biomicroscopy (Figure 8.11b). Any posterior wound gaping can also be imaged. These capabilities provide a method of determining the accuracy of graft placement. Underlying abnormalities such as angle closure and iris adhesion to the graft-host junction can also be visualized. Figure 8.11c shows a closed angle with adhesion of the iris margin to the graft-host junction.

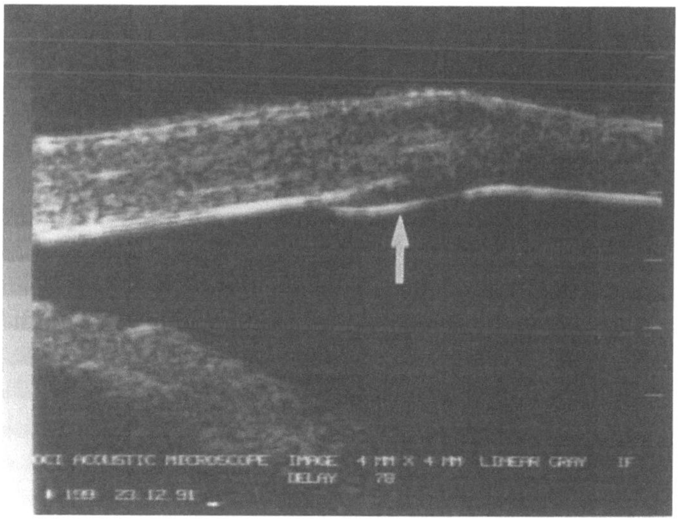

FIGURE 8.10. Graft-host junction is discernible by the irregularity and change in thickness at the suture line.

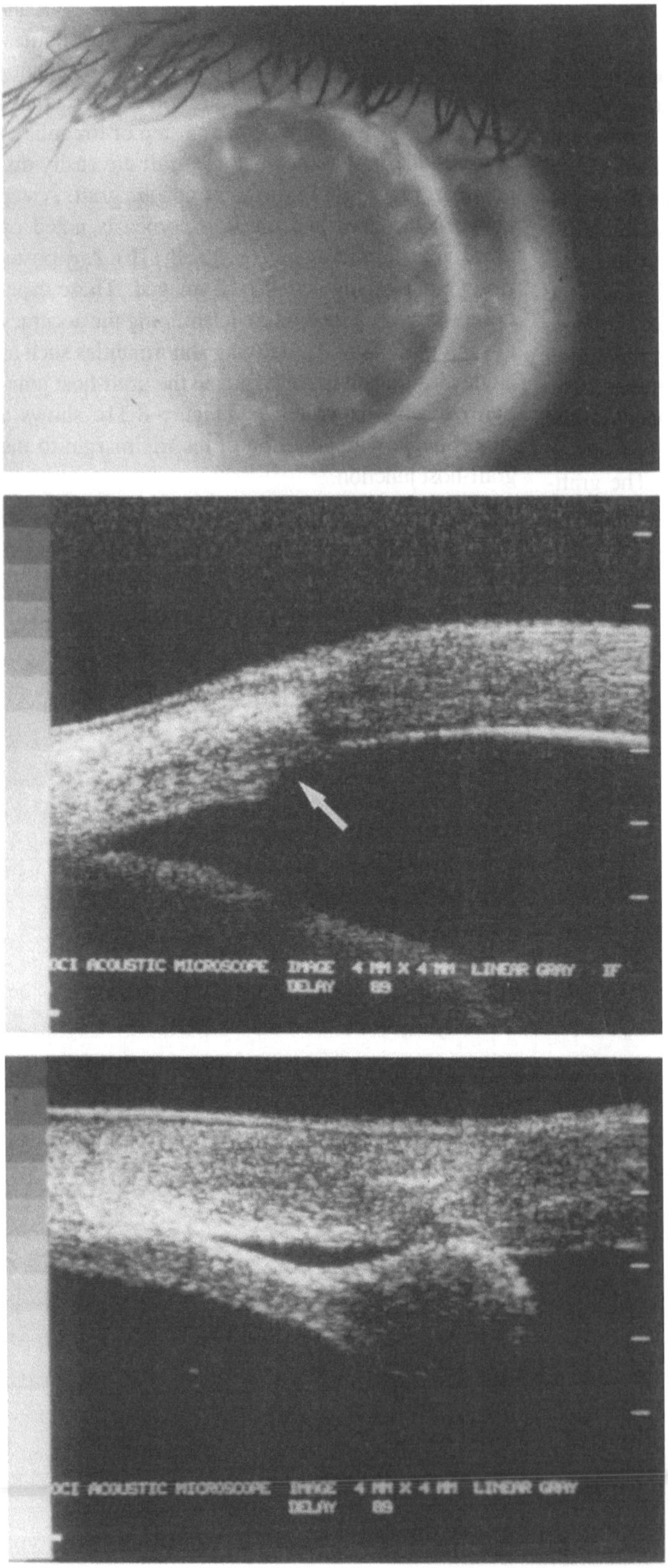

FIGURE 8.11. (**a**) Clinical photograph of an opaque corneal graft. (**b**) Graft-host junction shows a step on the graft side. (**c**) Iris below the graft has closed the angle and is adherent to the graft-host junction. Published courtesy of *Ophthalmology* (1991;98:287–295).

Corneal Dystrophies

Ultrasound biomicroscopy can image changes that occur in the weakly reflective regular corneal lamellae. Figure 8.12a shows a cornea with granular dystrophy. The granules of hyaline material are clearly imaged on ultrasound biomicroscopy (Figure 8.12b). The granules show increased reflectivity and are located mostly in the superficial stroma. This patient underwent an excimer laser superficial keratectomy in an attempt to decrease the opacities in the superficial cornea. Figure 8.12c shows the same cornea posttreatment. On ultrasound biomicroscopy the cornea shows some flattening. The loss of Bowman's membrane is apparent and the residual granules now come very close to the corneal surface (Figure 8.12d). The following section elaborates on changes seen with excimer laser photoablation.

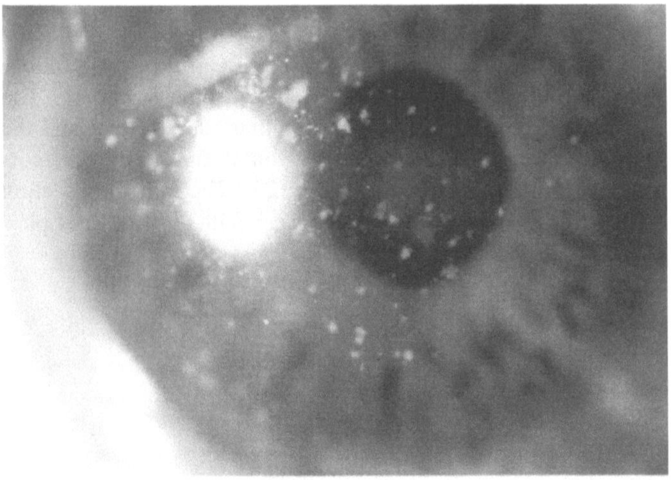

(a)

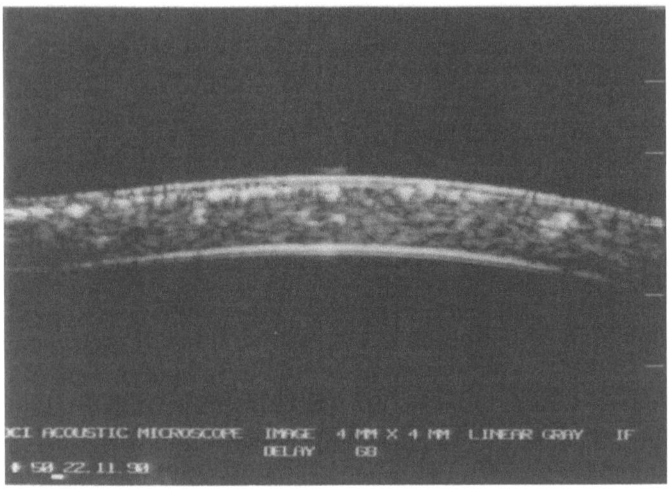

(b)

FIGURE 8.12. **(a)** Clinical appearance of a granular dystrophy. **(b)** On ultrasound biomicroscopy, the highly reflective hyaline bodies are outlined against the stroma in the superficial cornea. **(c)** Clinical appearance of granular dystrophy postexcimer laser therapeutic keratectomy. **(d)** Ultrasound biomicroscopy shows loss of Bowman's membrane. Some residual granules extend close to the surface. Reprinted with permission from reference [5].

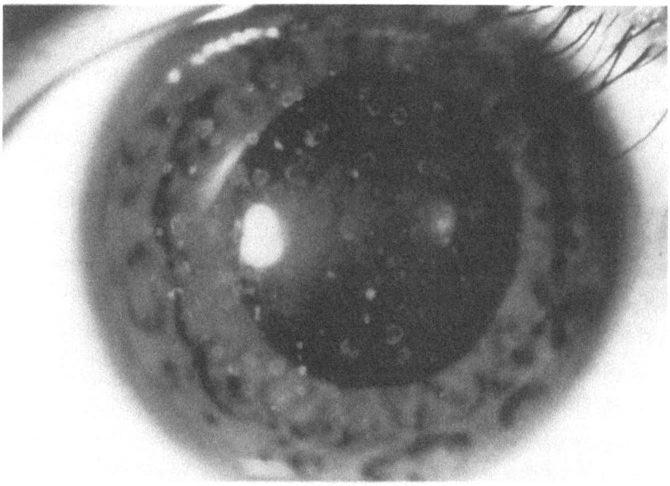

(c)

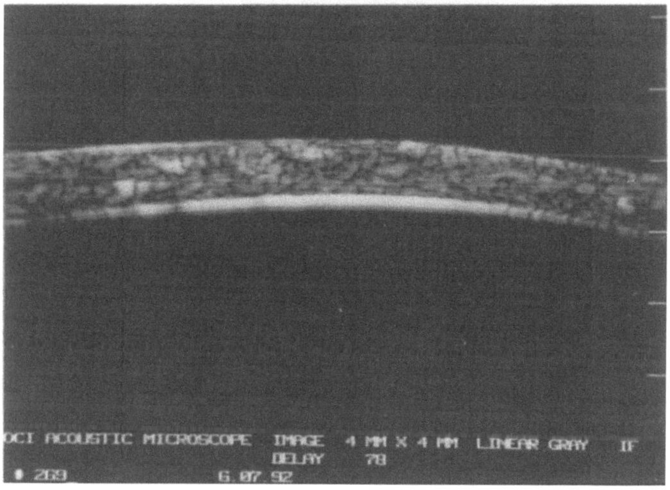
OCI ACOUSTIC MICROSCOPE IMAGE 4 MM X 4 MM LINEAR GRAY IF
DELAY 78
269 6.07.92

(d)

Refractive Surgery

Excimer laser photokeratectomy is used for correction of refractive errors and as a therapeutic method in superficial corneal disease [1–4]. Ultrasound biomicroscopy of the site of laser photoablation reveals the change in surface configuration that takes place [5]. The anterior corneal curvature shows flattening. The usual double-layered superficial appearance of the highly reflective epithelial surface and Bowman's membrane found in normal eyes is replaced by a less clear division between the surface epithelium and underlying stroma (Figure 8.13). This is most likely due to loss of Bowman's membrane, with the resulting stromal-epithelial interface being less of a specular reflector. Figure 8.14a shows clinical appearance of a patient who had undergone laser photokeratectomy for a small refractive error. The amount of corneal haze is minimal. Ultrasound biomicroscopy was done at a high frequency of 75 MHz. Figure 8.14b shows the ultrasound biomicroscopic appearance of the border between the unaffected cornea and the affected cornea. The double line of reflectivity gives way to the single line of reflectivity of the treated portion.

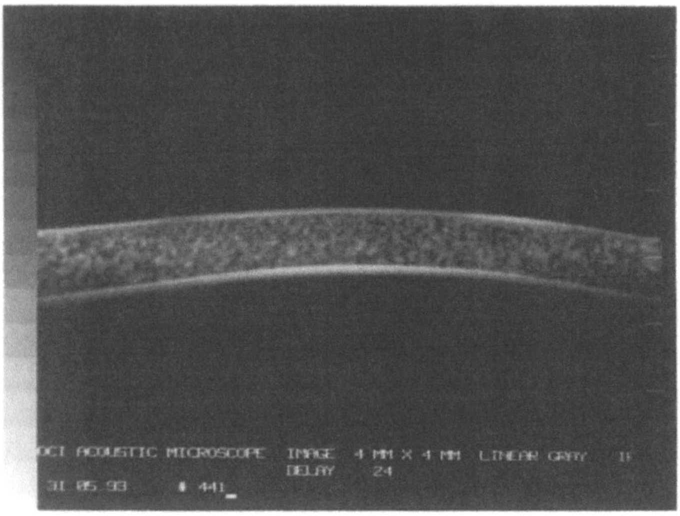

FIGURE 8.13. Excimer laser treated cornea shows only a single reflection from the epithelial surface. The echo from Bowman's membrane is absent. Reprinted with permission from reference [5].

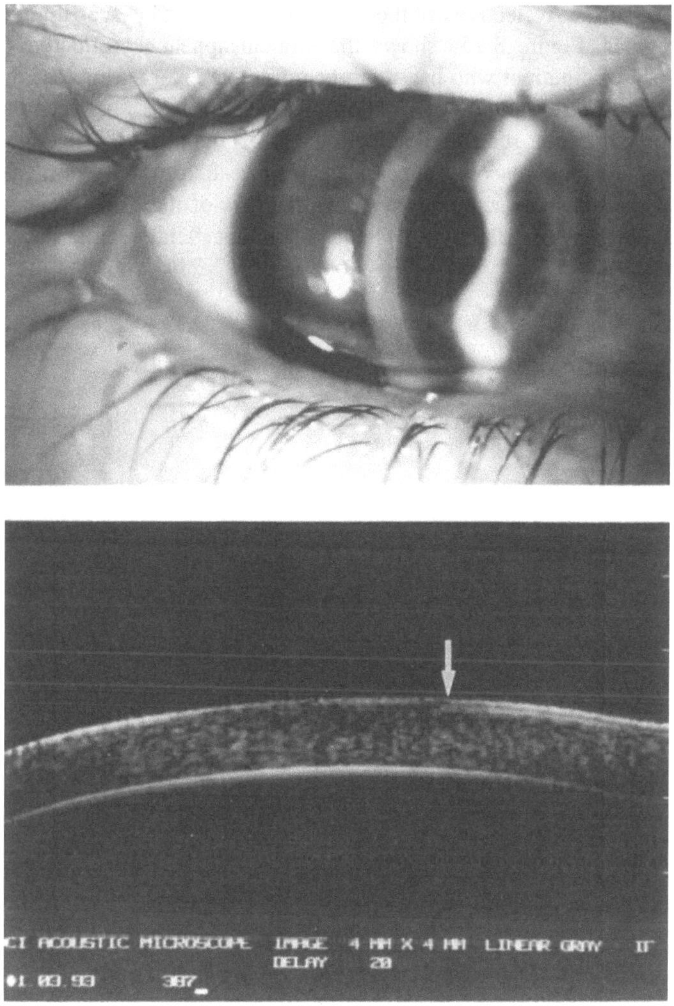

(a)

(b)

FIGURE 8.14. **(a)** Clinical photograph postexcimer shows minimal scarring. **(b)** Ultrasound biomicroscopy of the treatment junction (arrow) shows transition from the double line of the unaffected cornea to the single line of the treated cornea. Reprinted with permission from reference [5].

The surface reflectivity of the stroma is smooth and regular. Figure 8.15a shows the clinical appearance of a patient who had a larger refractive error and a greater amount of ablation. The patient had some irregular scarring noted clinically. The ultrasound biomicroscopic appearance (Figure 8.15b) of the transition zone again shows the loss of the double line of reflectivity. The areas of superficial scarring in the treated zone show up as more highly reflective areas on ultrasound biomicroscopy. In this case the stromal scarring allows differentiation between the stromal surface and epithelial surface.

As corneal imaging techniques evolve, the ability to measure corneal epithelial thickness and cor neal topography may further aid assessment of excimer laser patients [6,7].

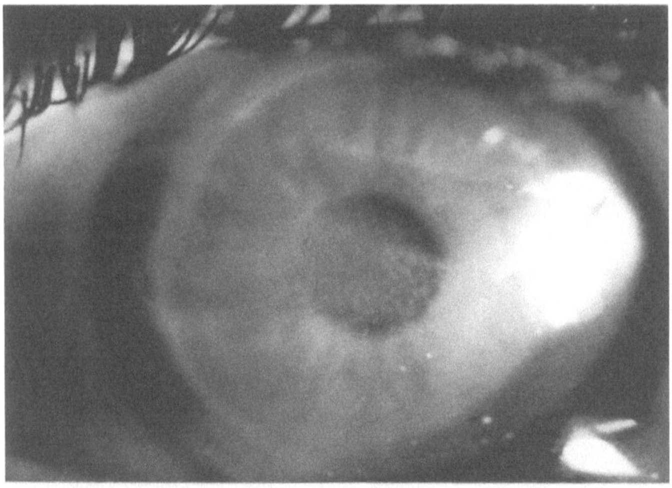
(a)

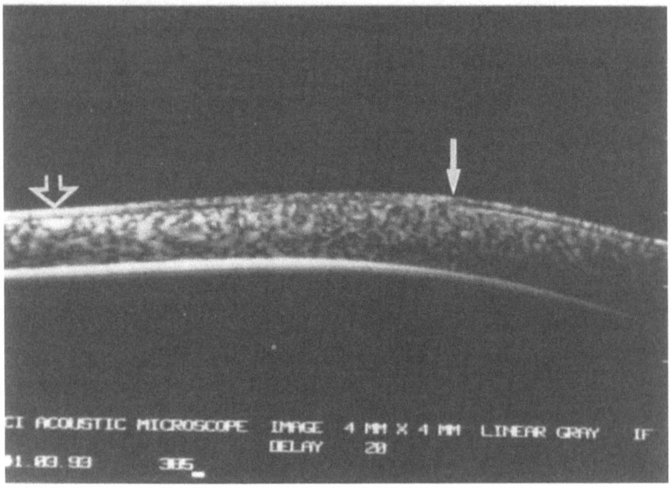

(b)

FIGURE 8.15. **(a)** Clinical photograph of highly myopic excimer patient shows some superficial scarring. **(b)** Ultrasound biomicroscopy shows the treatment junction (closed arrow). The superficial corneal scarring is imaged as highly reflective areas (open arrow) that outline the superficial stroma. The cornea is thinned in the treatment region. Reprinted with permission from reference [5].

Summary

Higher frequency transducers in the range of 75 MHz and up can be used to assess the cornea. This provides improved resolution and more accurate measurement. Ultrasound biomicroscopy provides a new way of assessing corneal edema that allows objective differentiation and measurement of the corneal stroma and epithelium. Ultrasound biomicroscopy provides a new method of assessing the accuracy of graft placement, and imaging underlying changes presurgery in eyes with corneal opacification. This imaging method also holds promise as a method of monitoring the results of various types of refractive surgery.

References

1. Trokel SL, Srinivasan R, Braren B. Excimer laser surgery of the cornea. *Am J Ophthalmol* 1983; 96:710.
2. Marshall J, Trokel S, Rothery S, Krueger R. Photoablative reprofiling of the cornea using excimer laser photo-refractive keratectomy. *Lasers Ophthalmol* 1986;1:21–48.
3. Seiler T, Kahle G, Kriegerowski M. Excimer laser myopic keratomileusis in sighted and blind myopic eyes. *Refract Corneal Surg* 1990;6:165–73.
4. Seiler T, Wollensak J. Myopic photorefractive keratectomy with the excimer laser. One year follow-up. *Ophthalmology* 1991;98:1156–1163.
5. Pavlin CJ, Harasiewicz K, Foster FS. Ultrasound biomicroscopic assessment of the cornea following excimer laser photokeratectomy. *J Cat Refract Surg* 1994;20(Supp.):206–211.
6. Reinstein DZ, Silverman RH, Coleman DJ. High-frequency ultrasound measurement of the corneal epithelium. *Refrac Corneal Surg* 1993;9:385–387.
7. Reinstein DZ, Silverman RH, Rondean MJ, Coleman DJ. Epithelial and corneal thickness measurements by high-frequency ultrasound digital signal processing. *Ophthalmology* 1994;101:140–146.

9
Scleral Disease

As noted in the chapter on normal ultrasound biomicroscopic findings, the sclera can be clearly defined because of its high internal reflectivity compared to surrounding tissues. This allows differentiation between events taking place above or below the sclera and those taking place within the sclera itself. Ultrasound biomicroscopy thus provides a new way of imaging scleral tissue [1] that adds supportive information to the well-established clinical methods of differentiating anterior scleral disease [2,3]. Although the sclera can be imaged by conventional ultrasound, the resolution is not sufficient to clearly differentiate the sclera from surrounding tissue. Conventional ultrasound has been useful in detecting changes in posterior scleritis [4–7], but has limited application in anterior disease. Examination of the sclera can be performed at any point where the moving transducer can be placed directly over the tissue being examined. Exactly how peripheral this is in the individual patient is dependent on anatomical considerations, including the size of the palpebral fissure, the prominence of the globe, and the site of examination (temporal side greater than nasal). Generally these sites are anterior to the equator. Penetration is not adequate to cross the globe to examine the posterior sclera.

Localized Scleral Staphyloma

Localized scleral staphyloma are uncommon, but can create a problem in differential diagnoses between other causes of a black dot on the surface of the globe [8] such as a conjunctival melanoma or extrascleral extension of a peripheral tumor [9]. Figure 9.1a shows the clinical appearance of a pigmented nodule on the surface of the eye that was noted before cataract surgery. Ultrasound biomicroscopy revealed a ciliary coloboma open to the posterior chamber internally with marked scleral thinning (Figure 9.1b). The coloboma involved the ciliary processes with ciliary processes imaged to each side of the gap in the transverse view (Figure 9.1c). Ultrasound biomicroscopic appearance of another case with a similar clinical presentation is shown in Figure 9.2a. The ciliary body defect is more anterior in this case and extends into the cornea as noted in Figure 9.2b. The transverse view shows two chambers in the colobomatous region (Figure 9.2c). Ultrasound biomicroscopy clearly outlines the structural makeup of these defects and differentiates them from other causes of a pigmented nodule in this region.

Episcleritis

Episcleritis can often be difficult to differentiate from inflammation involving the sclera on clinical grounds alone. Figure 9.3a shows the clinical appearance of a region of localized inflammation. Ultrasound biomicroscopic examination presents the finding of thickened episcleral tissue without apparent involvement of the sclera (Figure 9.3b). A clear margin can be observed between the episcleral thickening and the scleral surface. The sclera appears to be of normal thickness and normal internal reflectivity in this region. A small superficial area of ulceration was evident clinically and on

FIGURE 9.1. (**a**) Clinical appearance of a localized scleral staphyloma near the limbus. (**b**) Ultrasound biomicroscopy shows a ciliary body defect with localized scleral thinning. (**c**) Ultrasound biomicroscopic image in a transverse orientation shows the ciliary processes on either side of the coloboma. Published with permission from *The American Journal of Ophthalmology* (1993; 116:628–635). Copyright by The Ophthalmic Publishing Company.

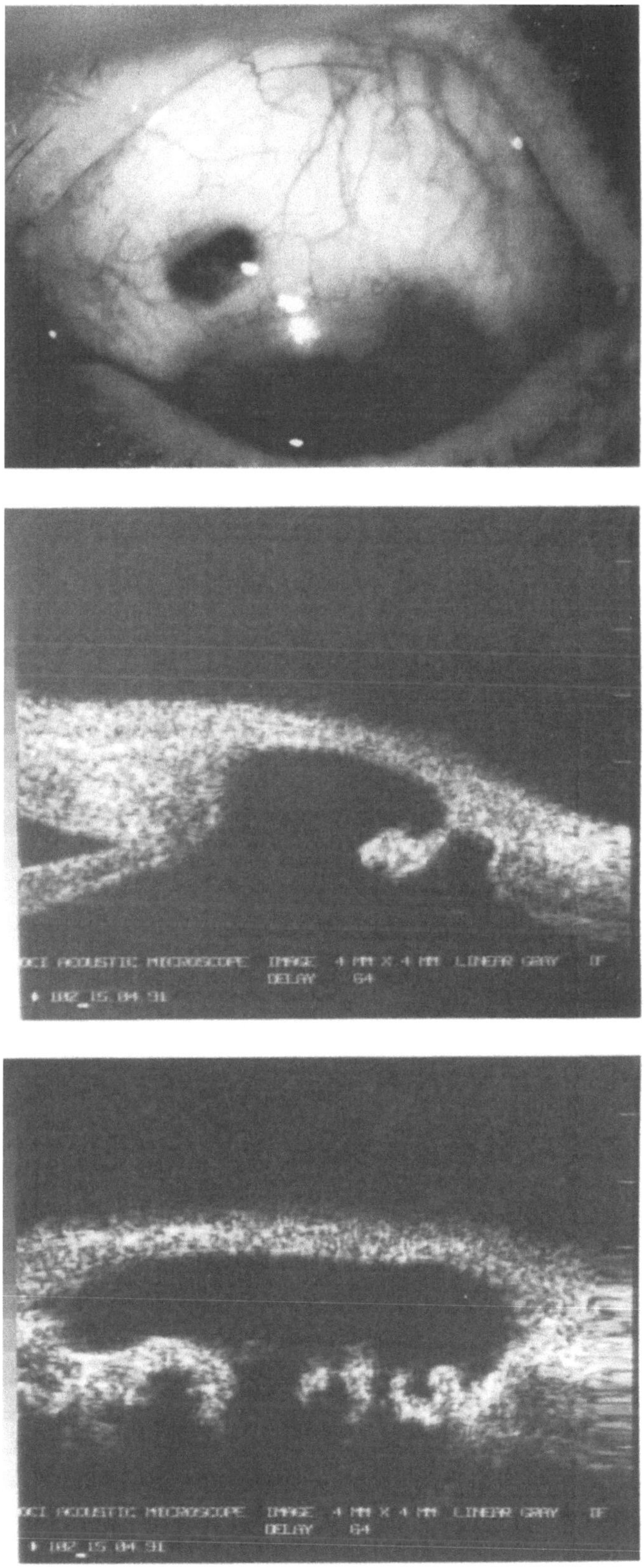

(a)
(b)
(c)

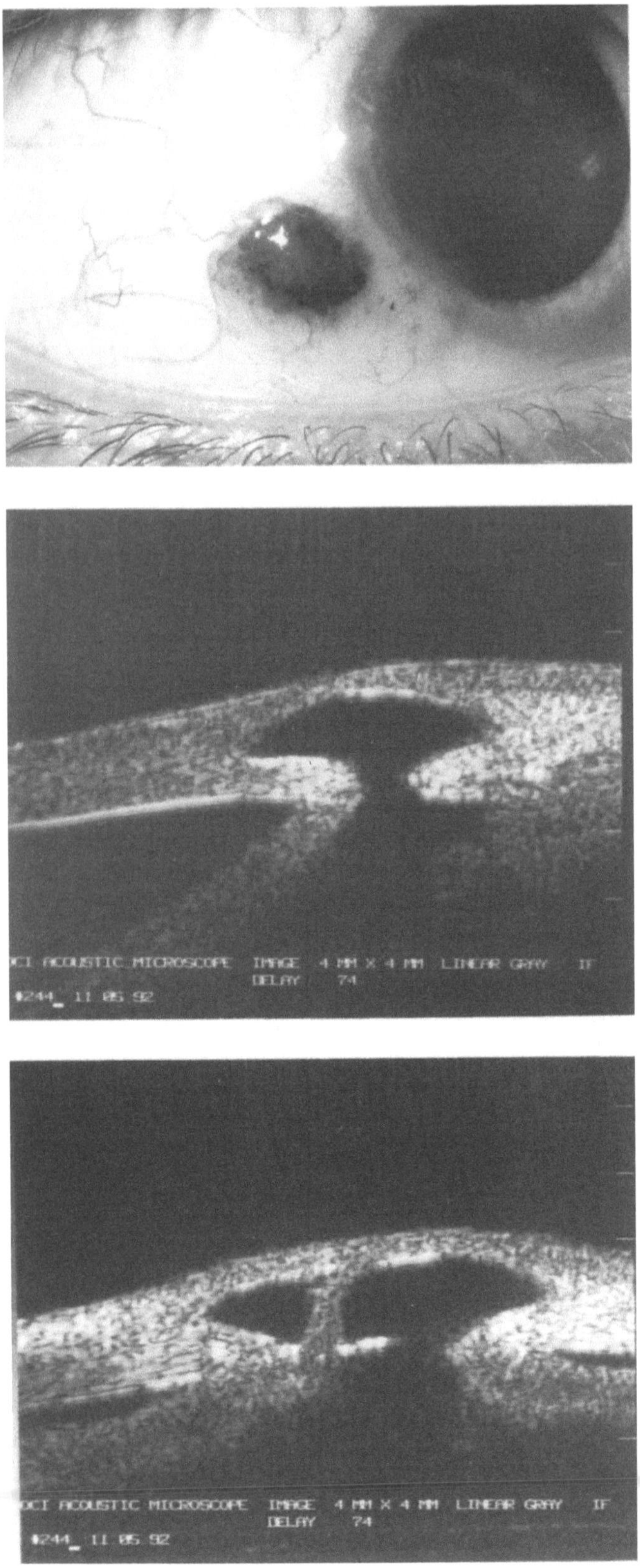

(a)

(b)

(c)

FIGURE 9.2. **(a)** Clinical appearance of a more anterior scleral staphyloma. **(b)** Ultrasound biomicroscopy shows the anterior extension into the cornea. **(c)** Transverse image of this staphyloma shows two separate chambers.

FIGURE 9.3. **(a)** Clinical appearance of localized area of episcleral inflammation. **(b)** Ultrasound biomicroscopy shows thickened episcleral tissue with no involvement of the sclera itself. A small superficial ulceration is noted (arrow). Published with permission from *The American Journal of Ophthalmology* (1993;116:628–635). Copyright by The Ophthalmic Publishing Company.

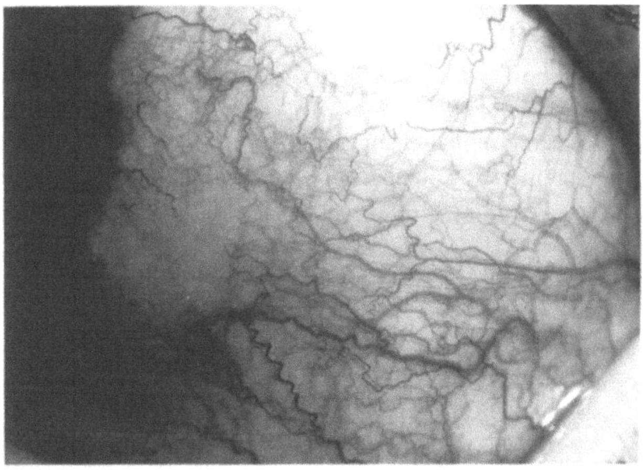

(a)

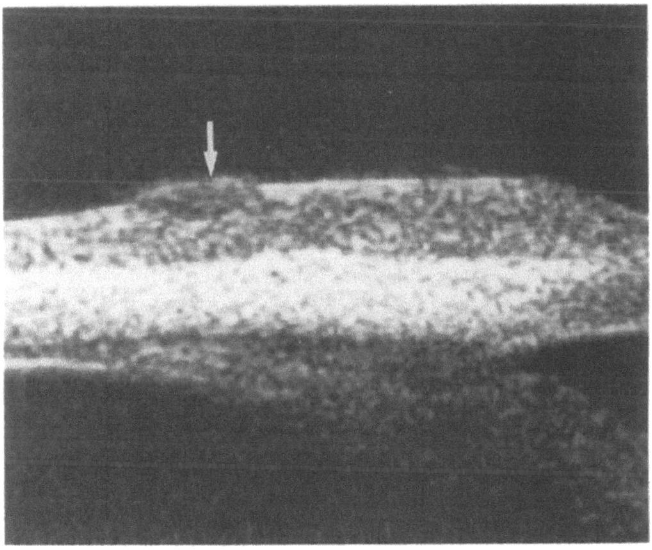

(b)

ultrasound biomicroscopy. It should be noted that inflammatory scleral involvement that is insufficient to show areas of reflectivity change in the sclera itself could be missed.

Underlying retinal changes can be imaged. Figure 9.4 shows a region of shallow retinal separation in a case of episcleritis. Thickening of the episcleral layer is present. The inner scleral surface shows the thin choroidal layer, and below it a shallow retinal separation. It cannot be certain whether this finding is secondary to inflammation or represents a small peripheral retinal separation that can be occasionally seen in normal eyes.

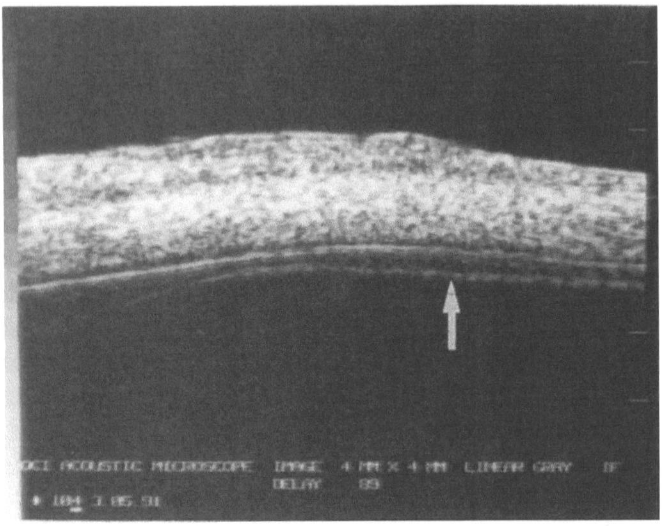

FIGURE 9.4. A case of episcleritis shows thickened episcleral tissue. Below the normal sclera is a thin layer of choroid and a slightly detached retina (arrow).

Diffuse Scleritis

Figure 9.5a shows the clinical appearance of a patient with diffuse scleritis extending over the superior aspect of the right globe. Ultrasound biomicroscopy showed episcleral thickening. The sclera itself had a mottled internal reflectivity with areas of lower reflectivity scattered throughout the involved region (Figure 9.5b). Sclera outside the involved region showed a normal appearance with uniform, high reflectivity of sclera. The diffuse mottling most likely represents scleral infiltration with inflammatory cells and edema of collagen bundles.

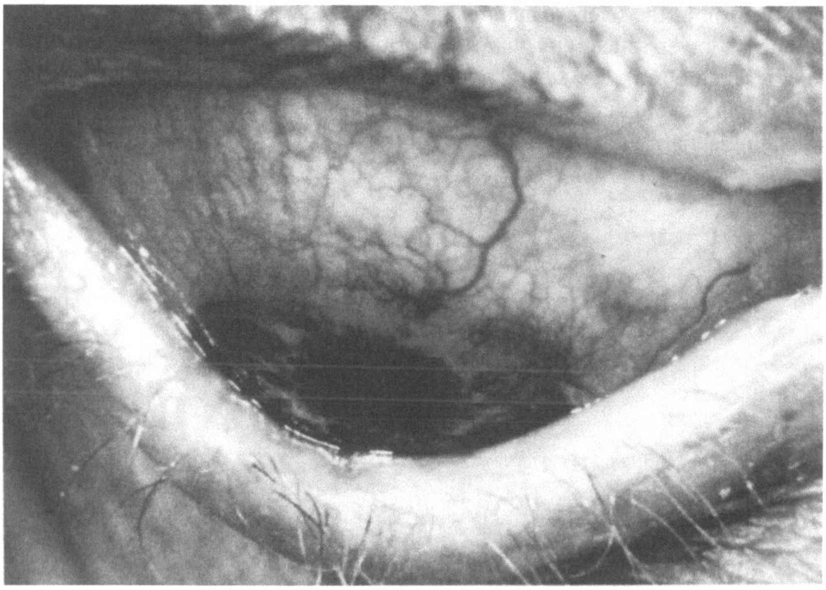

(a)

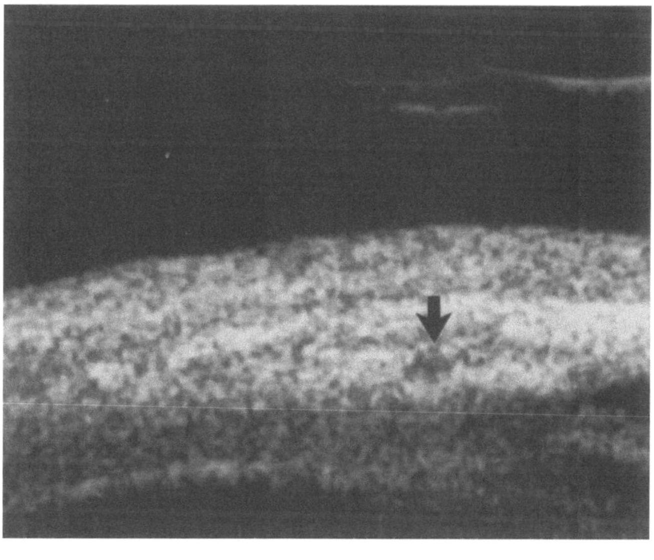

(b)

FIGURE 9.5. **(a)** Clinical appearance of diffuse scleritis extending over the superior globe. **(b)** Ultrasound biomicroscopy shows mottled areas of lower reflectivity in the sclera (arrow). Published with permission from *The American Journal of Ophthalmology* (1993; 116:628–635). Copyright by The Ophthalmic Publishing Company.

Nodular Scleritis

Figure 9.6a shows the clinical appearance of an acute region of scleral inflammation presenting clinically as a localized elevation. Ultrasound biomicroscopy in the region of the acutely inflamed nodule shows thickening of the episcleral layer. This finding is usually present in scleral disease in addition to the involvement of the sclera itself. Involvement of the sclera is manifest as a localized nodule of lower reflectivity than the surrounding sclera (Figure 9.6b). The scleral nodule is differentiated from surrounding sclera by a distinct border extending about two-thirds of the way through the scleral substance. This produces a scooped-out appearance to the sclera, indicating that the process went deep into the scleral tissue, but not all the way through. After resolution of the acute phase there was no obvious scleral thinning on clinical examination. However, scleral thinning was clearly present on ultrasound biomicroscopy (Figure 9.6c). Scleral thinning of intermediate degree without the uveal show typical of marked thinning can be difficult to detect clinically. Ultrasound biomicroscopy can provide an objective guide to thinning, and more clearly define the dividing line between necrotizing and non-necrotizing forms of the disease.

FIGURE 9.6. **(a)** Clinical appearance of acute nodular scleral inflammation in the right eye. **(b)** Ultrasound biomicroscopy shows nodular thickening of the sclera (arrow) with the more weakly reflective nodule extending about two-thirds of the way through the scleral substance. **(c)** Ultrasound biomicroscopy several weeks later shows decrease in size of the nodule with residual scleral thinning (arrow). Published with permission from *The American Journal of Ophthalmology* (1993;116:628–635). Copyright by The Ophthalmic Publishing Company.

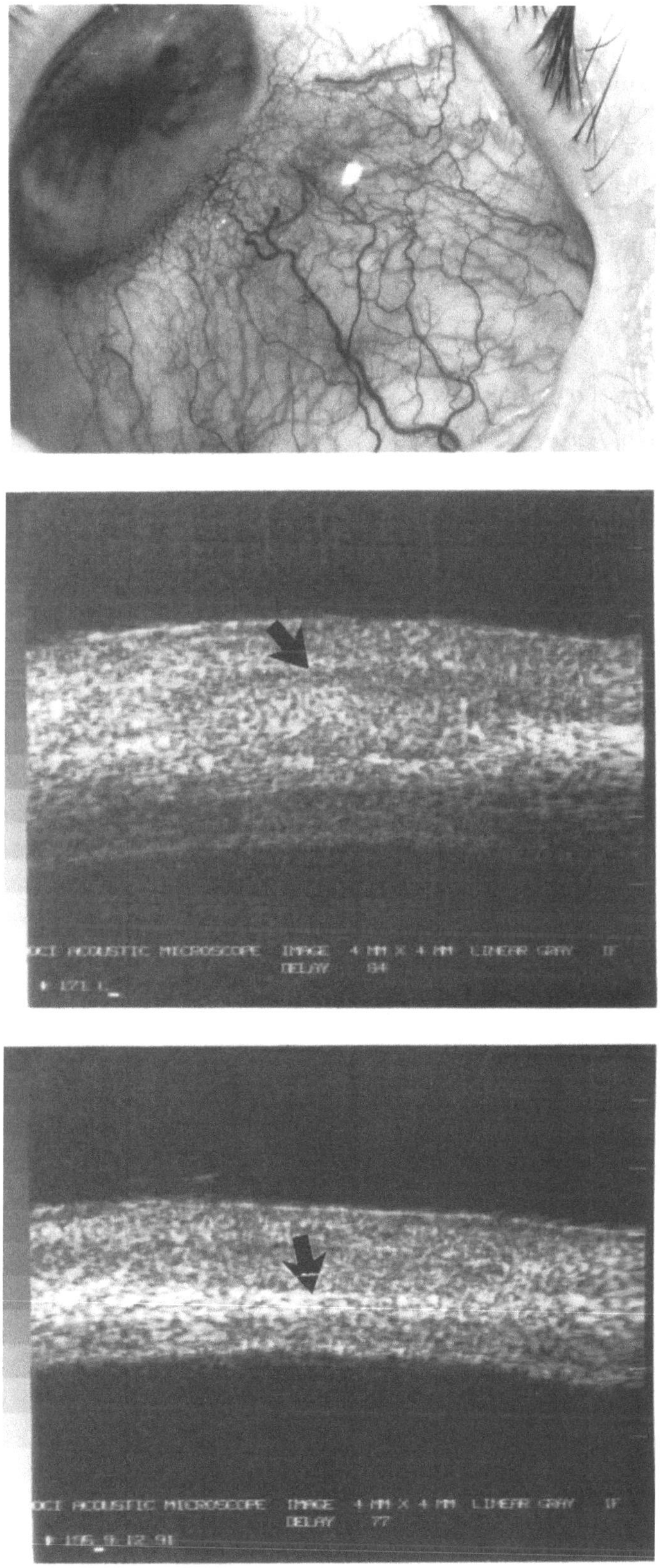

(a)

(b)

(c)

Necrotizing Scleritis

Necrotizing scleritis by definition results in regions of scleral thinning [10–12]. In cases in which the sclera is thinned, ultrasound biomicroscopy allows an objective method of assessing the degree of thinning. Figure 9.7 shows scleral thinning commencing at the limbus and extending peripherally. Figure 9.8a shows the clinical appearance of an area of scleral thinning and Figure 9.8b shows the ultrasound biomicroscopic appearance of this area. In this case the thinned sclera can be well visualized

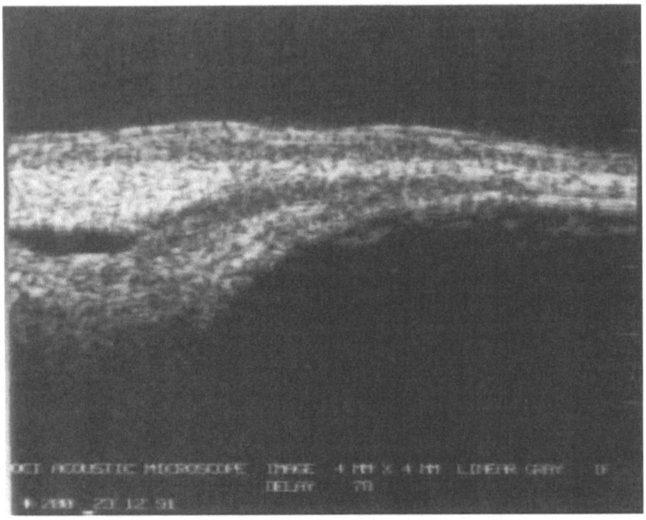

FIGURE 9.7. Area of scleral thinning commencing at the limbus and extending peripherally.

FIGURE 9.8. **(a)** Clinical appearance of old area of scleral thinning. **(b)** Ultrasound biomicroscopic section through the area of scleral thinning. The thinned sclera is still detectable (arrows). Published with permission from *The American Journal of Ophthalmology* (1993; 116:628–635). Copyright by The Ophthalmic Publishing Company.

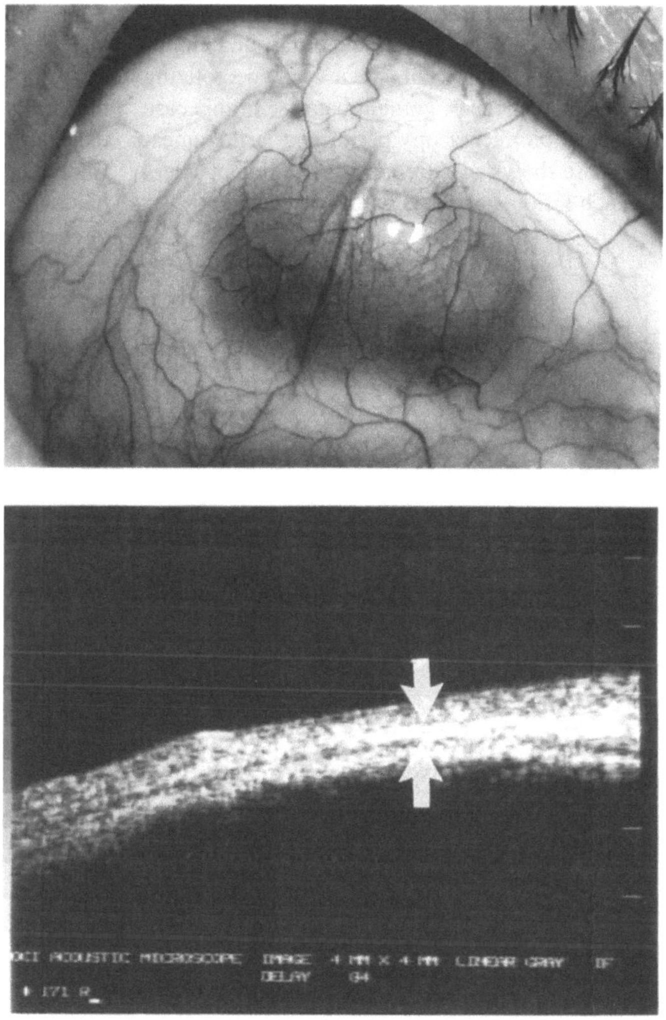

(a)

(b)

and differentiated from surrounding tissue. Figure 9.9a and b shows the clinical and ultrasound biomicroscopic appearance of a case of necrotizing scleritis in Wegener's granulomatosis. In this case ultrasound biomicroscopy performed in the quiescent phase shows an extremely thin region of sclera in which residual sclera is barely detectable.

The ultrasound biomicroscopic appearance of the case in Figure 9.9 showed underlying vitreous fibrils. Figure 9.10 shows another case in which the fibrils are seen in cross section, showing that these are fine linear structures. We have seen this finding quite frequently in necrotizing scleritis and have also noted that it is occasionally a transient phenomena, disappearing in time [13].

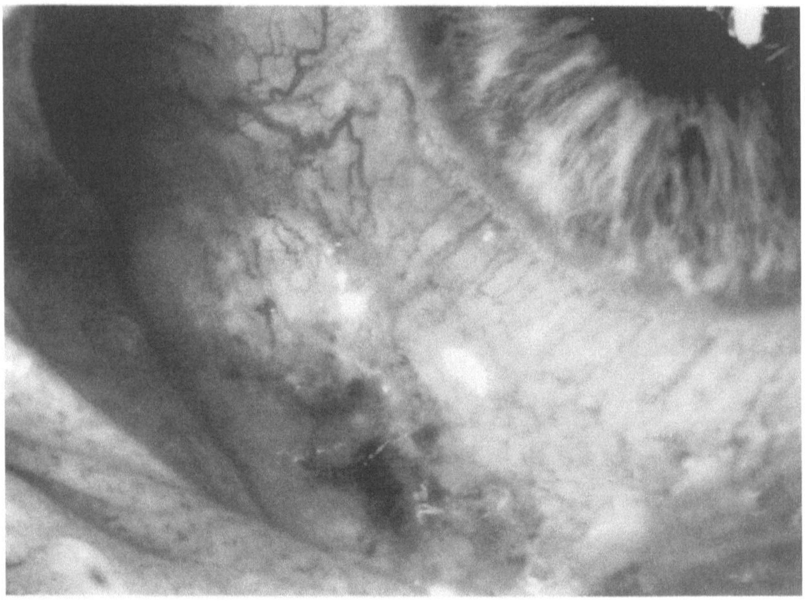

(a)

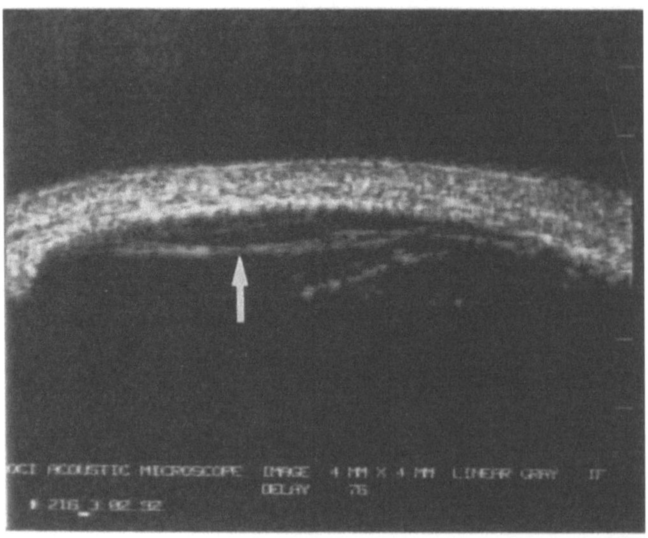

(b)

Figure 9.9. **(a)** Clinical appearance of acute phase of necrotizing scleral disease in a case of Wegener's granulomatosis. **(b)** Ultrasound biomicroscopy shows minimal scleral tissue. Strands are seen in the underlying vitreous (arrow). Published with permission from *The American Journal of Ophthalmology* (1993;116:628–635). Copyright by The Ophthalmic Publishing Company.

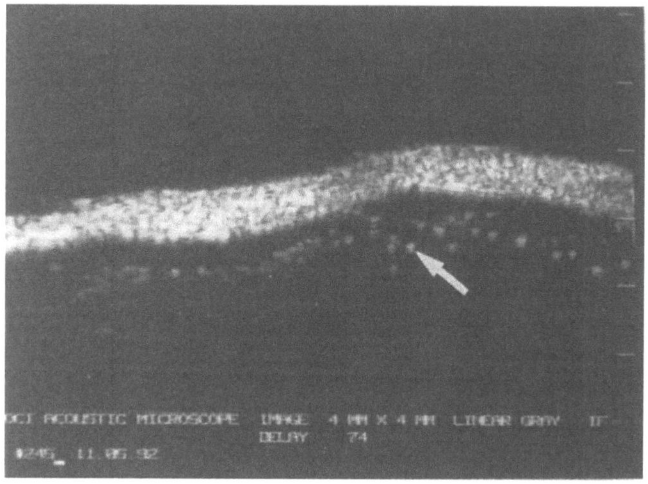

FIGURE 9.10. Transverse section through a region of vitreous fibrils shows that these are fine linear bands (arrow).

Summary

Ultrasound biomicroscopy provides a new tool for examination of the sclera and adjacent tissue. It adds complementary information to well-established clinical criteria for classifying scleral disease. Ultrasound biomicroscopy allows differentiation between changes involving the episclera and those involving the sclera itself. Ultrasound biomicroscopy allows one to follow the natural history of scleral disease including progression to scleral thinning. In cases in which the sclera is thinned, ultrasound biomicroscopy allows an objective measurement of the degree of thinning. A very small layer of residual scleral tissue can be detected. This ability may have value in predicting the stability of this region of the eye, and determining whether reinforcement surgery is required. Underlying changes in the choroidal layers, retinal layers, and underlying vitreous can also be detected.

References

1. Pavlin CJ, Easterbrook M, Hurwitz JJ, Harasiewicz K, Foster FS. Ultrasound biomicroscopy in the assessment of anterior scleral disease. *Am J Ophthalmol* 1993;116:628–635.
2. Watson PG, Hayreh SSH. Scleritis and episcleritis. *Br J Ophthalmol* 1976;60:163.
3. Watson PG, Hazleman BL. *The Sclera and Systemic Disorders*. 1976. WB Saunders, London.
4. Johnson MH, De FG, Zimmerman RA, Savino PJ. Scleral inflammatory disease. *Am J Neuroradiol* 1987;8:861.
5. Calthorpe CM, Watson PG, McCartney AC. Posterior scleritis: A clinical and histological survey. *Eye* 1988;2:267.
6. Wald KJ, Spaide R, Patalano VJ, Sugin S, Yannuzzi LA. Posterior scleritis in children. *Am J Ophthalmol* 1992;113:281.
7. Byrne SF, Green RL. *Ultrasound of the Eye and Orbit*. 1992, pp. 88–90. Mosby Year Book, St. Louis.
8. Duane TD, Jaeger AE. *Biomedical Foundations of Ophthalmology*. Vol. 1. JB Lippincott, Philadelphia.
9. Pavlin CJ, McWhae JA, McGowan HD, Foster FS. Ultrasound biomicroscopy of anterior segment tumors. *Ophthalmology* 1992;99:1222.
10. Young RD, Watson PG. Microscopical studies of necrotising scleritis. II. Collagen degradation in the scleral stroma. *Br J Ophthalmol* 1984;68:781.
11. Young RD, Watson PG. Microscopical studies of necrotising scleritis. I. Cellular aspects. *Br J Ophthalmol* 1984;68:770.
12. Rao NA, Mark GE, Hidayat AA. Necrotizing scleritis. A clinicopathologic study of 41 cases. *Ophthalmology* 1985;92:1542.
13. Tucker S, Pavlin CJ, Hurwitz JJ. Scleral melt following cryotherapy for malignant melanoma of the conjunctiva. *Ophthalmology* 1993;100:572.

10 Intraocular Lenses

Ultrasound biomicroscopy can be helpful in analyzing intraocular lens position and determining the source of the problem if all does not go well. Anterior chamber depth after surgery can be measured with a high degree of accuracy. The margins of the optic can be easily imaged and decentration analyzed. Optics display highly reflective anterior and posterior borders, with frequent presence of reverberation artifacts behind the lens. The high reflectivity of the poly(methyl methacrylate) (PMMA) haptics in one-piece lenses makes the haptic position easy to locate. Proline haptics are not quite as reflective, but can usually be located. Haptic location in relationship to surrounding structures can be determined, and, in the case of posterior chamber lenses, one can usually determine if the haptic is in the capsular bag.

Anterior Chamber Lenses

Anterior chamber lenses are well imaged because of the highly reflective nature of their usual one-piece PMMA construction. The relationship of the anterior chamber lens haptic to the iris and angle structures can be ascertained. Figure 10.1 shows the location of an anterior chamber lens haptic, which is slightly medial to the angle. In situations in which lens removal is being considered, the presence of tissue covering the haptic in the angle region can be imaged. If visualization of the angle is poor, which is frequently the case in these patients because of corneal edema, this information can aid the surgeon considering explantation. Figure 10.2 shows a portion of a peripheral anterior chamber lens haptic buried in tissue in the angle region.

Posterior Chamber Lenses

Figure 10.3 shows the anterior chamber with a posterior chamber intraocular lens in position. The distance from the inner cornea to the lens surface is easily calculated. Figure 10.4 shows the margin of an intraocular lens optic in relationship to the overlying iris. The optic is highly reflective and the anterior and posterior surfaces are clearly imaged. Reverberation artifacts are noted behind the lens.

Determining Haptic Position

Highly reflective posterior chamber lens haptics can generally be located using ultrasound biomicroscopy. The technique involves locating the optic and then using radial views in the approximate orientation of the haptic. When the haptic is located it can be traced to the position that most closely approaches the ocular wall. Residual zonule and

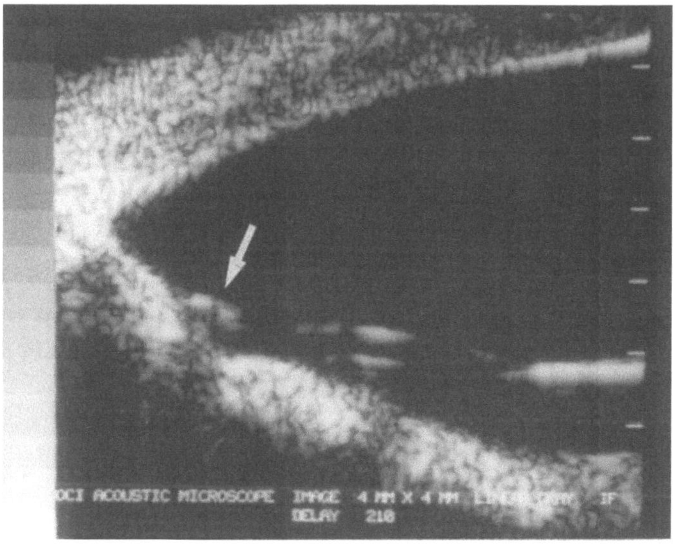

FIGURE 10.1. Ultrasound biomicroscopy shows haptic of anterior chamber lens indenting the iris medial to the angle (arrow).

capsule form an irregularly reflective membrane. Haptics that are in the bag are generally located medial to the ciliary processes and can be seen to be in close relationship to this membrane. It is not always easy to clearly define the actual margin of the capsule extending around the haptic. Figure 10.5 shows a haptic that is in the capsular bag. The haptic is medially located and the capsule can be seen around the haptic margin. Haptics that are not in the capsular bag are usually imaged peripherally in the region of the ciliary sulcus as shown in Figure 10.6.

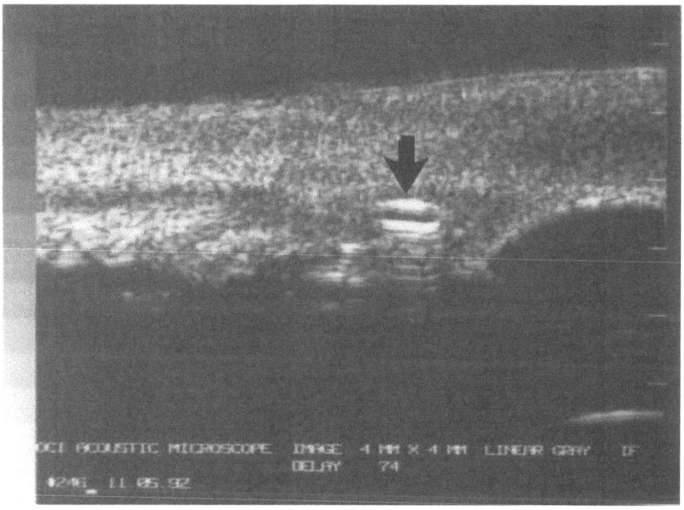

FIGURE 10.2. Ultrasound biomicroscopy shows anterior chamber lens haptic encased in tissue in the angle (arrow).

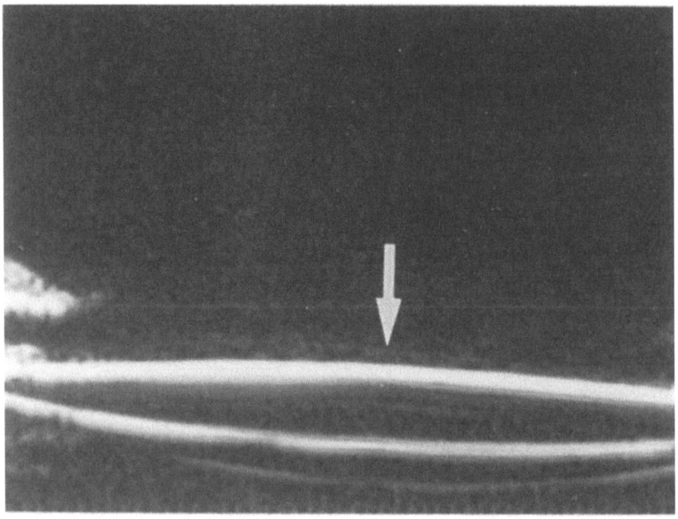

FIGURE 10.3. Anterior chamber with a highly reflective posterior chamber lens in position (arrow).

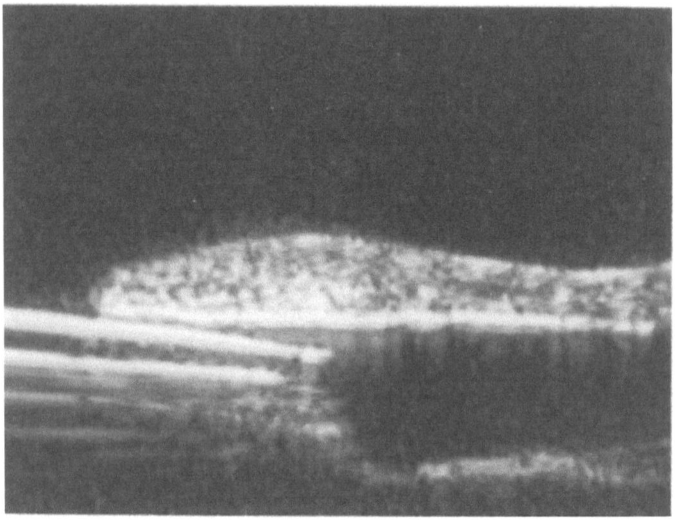

FIGURE 10.4. Iris margin over the edge of a posterior chamber lens. The optic of the lens images with a bright anterior and posterior surface echo with reverberation echoes behind it.

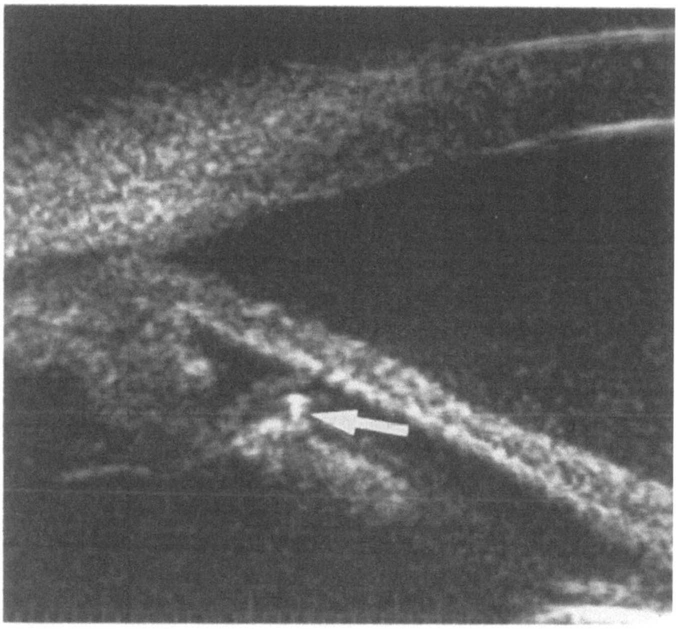

FIGURE 10.5. Posterior chamber lens haptic located in the capsular bag. Location is medial to the ciliary process. The capsule can be noted around the haptic (arrow). Reprinted with permission from reference [11].

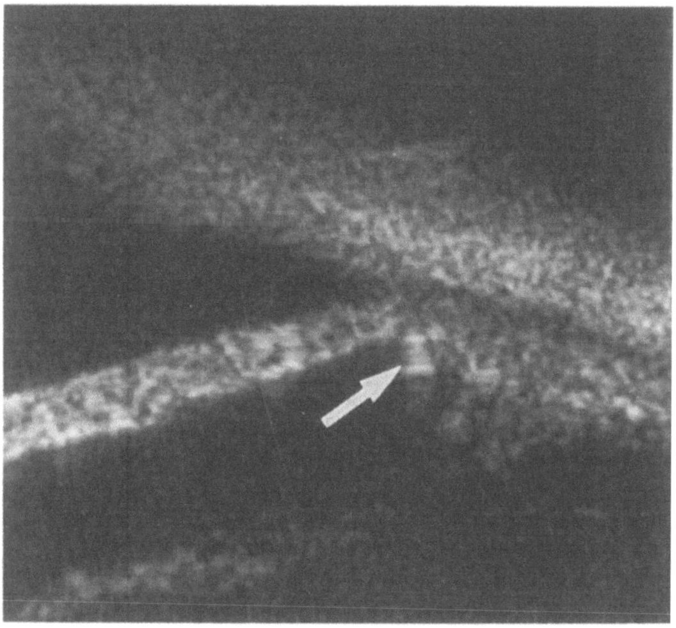

FIGURE 10.6. Posterior chamber lens haptic in the ciliary sulcus (arrow). Reprinted with permission from reference [11].

Intraocular Lens Complications

Transsclerally Sutured Intraocular Lens Haptic Position

We have recently published information on a series of cases with transsclerally sutured posterior chamber lenses [1]. This procedure is used in cases in which adequate capsule for fixation is missing [2–5]. To avoid complications from anterior chamber lenses, the haptic of a posterior chamber lens is fixated by placing a suture through the scleral wall behind the iris. The ciliary sulcus is felt to be the most desirable location for placement of the haptics of these lenses. We examined a series of these cases after surgery. The location of the haptics in these cases was easily accomplished. We traced the haptic to the position most closely approaching the ocular wall and classified the location as in the sulcus, posterior to the ciliary processes, or anterior to the sulcus accompanied by some degree of angle closure. We found that in the majority of cases the loops were not located in the sulcus. The majority were located anterior to the sulcus, pinning the peripheral iris to the trabecular meshwork region. Figure 10.7 shows an example of a haptic located in the ciliary sulcus. Figure 10.8a and b shows haptics located posteriorly, behind

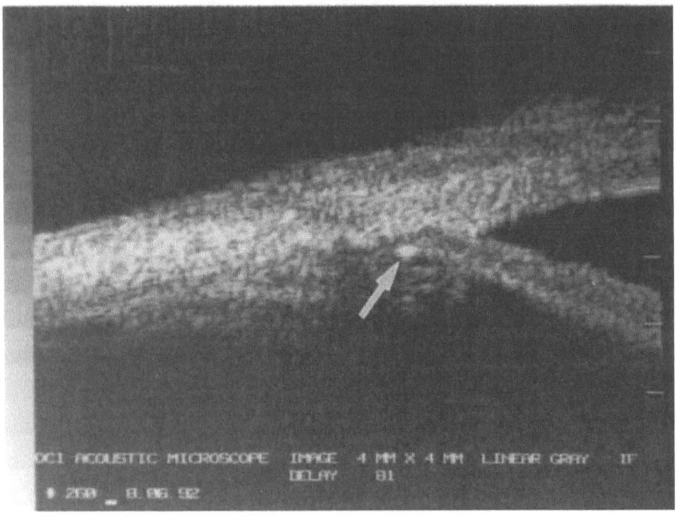

FIGURE 10.7. Haptic of transsclerally sutured posterior chamber lenses in the ciliary sulcus (arrows). Reprinted with permission from reference [1].

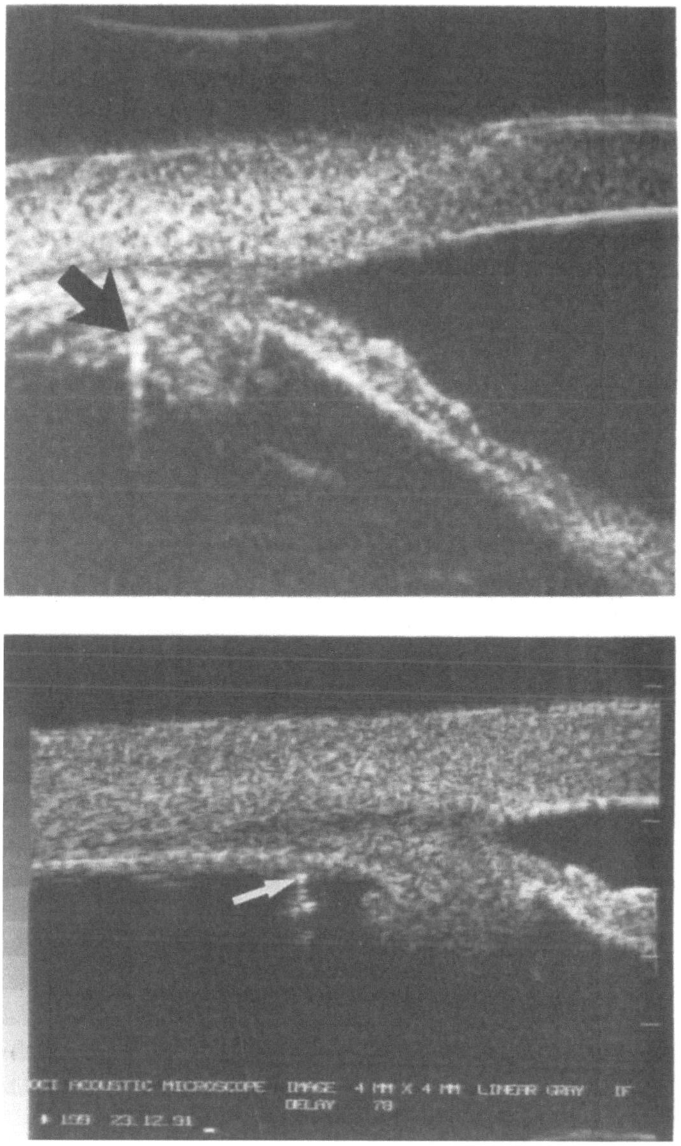

(a)

(b)

FIGURE 10.8. Haptics of transsclerally sutured posterior chamber intraocular lenses located posterior to the ciliary processes (arrows). **(a)** The haptic is just on the posterior margin of the ciliary process. **(b)** The haptic is further back behind the process.

the ciliary body. Figure 10.9a and b shows haptics located anteriorly, pinning the peripheral iris to the inner ocular wall. We have shown that in this essentially blind procedure it is difficult to assure positioning of the haptic in the ciliary sulcus. Duffey et al. [6] determined that a scleral exit point just under 1 mm from the limbus corresponded to the ciliary sulcus in eye bank eyes. This requires that the needle pass through the sclera in a perpendicular fashion. A needle passing along the plane of the iris, however, would pass through the sclera with the inner entry point being more anterior than the outer exit point. This most likely accounts for the fact that a large number of cases in our series showed anterior location of the haptic and pinning of the iris to the trabecular meshwork in spite of exit points that were 1 to 2 mm from the limbus.

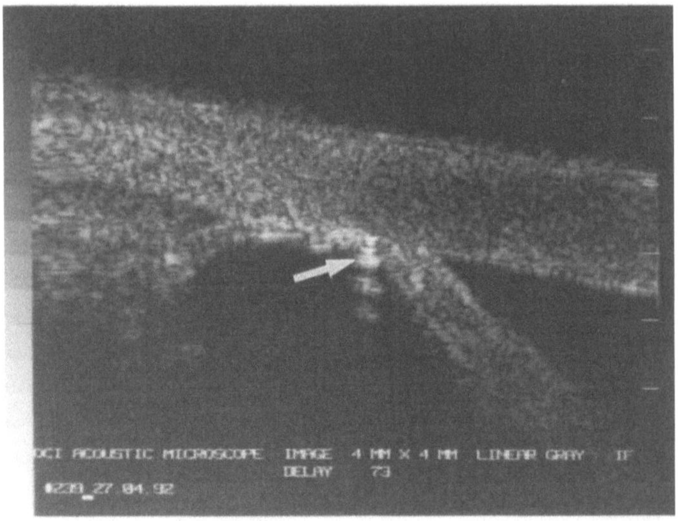

(a)

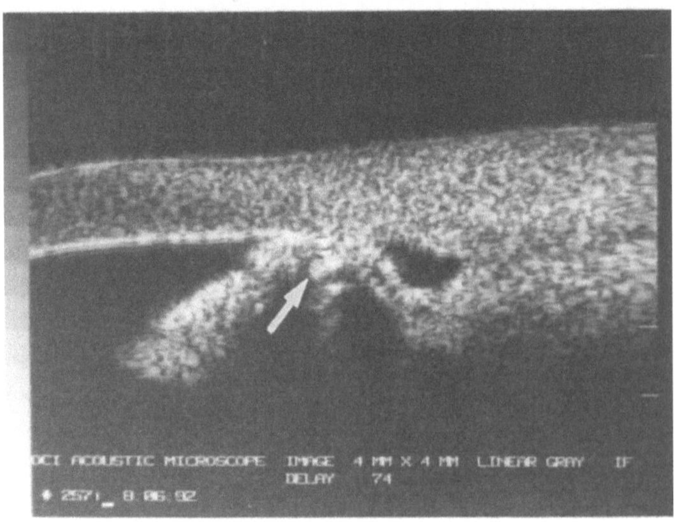

(b)

FIGURE 10.9. Haptics of transsclerally sutured posterior chamber intraocular lens located anteriorly pinning the iris to the inner wall (arrows). **(a)** The haptic is pinning the angle closed. **(b)** More anteriorly placed haptic is pinning the peripheral iris to the inner cornea. Reprinted with permission from reference [1].

Hypotony

Hypotony is an uncommon complication of intraocular lens implantation. Cyclodialysis must be ruled out in these cases. Techniques of ruling out cyclodialysis by ultrasound biomicroscopy are covered in the section on trauma. An unusual case of postoperative hypotony in which there was a dense membrane over the intraocular lens is illustrated in Figure 10.10a. Figure 10.10b shows that this membrane was attached to the margin of the ciliary process and was producing tension and elongation of the process, which may have had a bearing on the production of hypotony in this case. Laser treatment of this membrane relieved tension and allowed the pressure to return to normal.

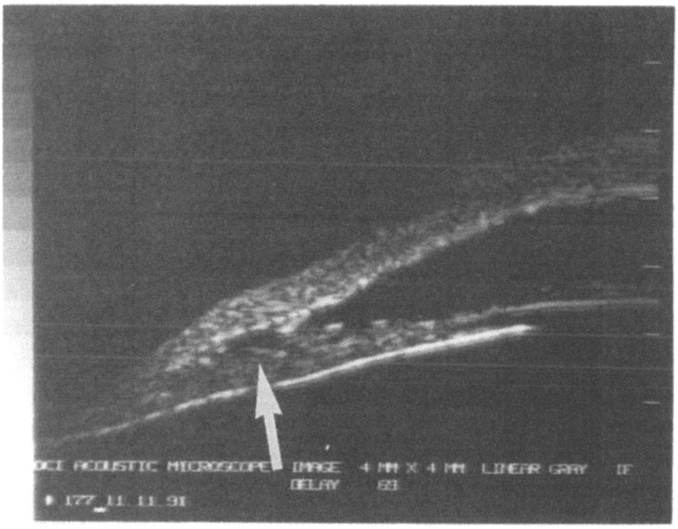

(a)

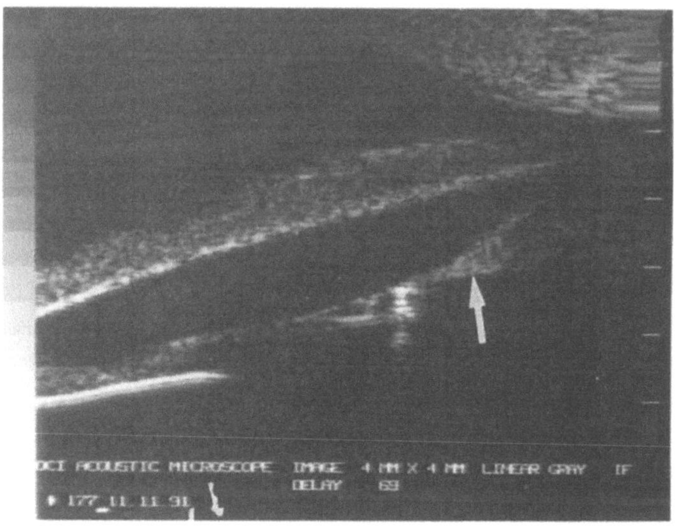

(b)

FIGURE 10.10. (a) Membrane on the surface of a posterior chamber intraocular lens (arrow). (b) Ciliary process attached to this membrane shows elongation due to tension (arrow).

Recurrent Hyphema

Late onset of recurrent hyphema is an uncommon complication associated with posterior chamber lenses. Bleeding from the wound site has to be ruled out [7]. Iris transillumination defects and iris tucking have been noted, implicating haptic-iris touch in the etiology [8–10]. In two cases in which no bleeding site could be determined in the wound, we found remarkably similar findings [11]. The superior loops were sulcus fixated and indenting the peripheral iris (Figure 10.11a and b). Blood could be imaged in the anterior chamber and traced back below the iris in one case (Figure 10.12). Of interest was the fact that both cases had iridecto-

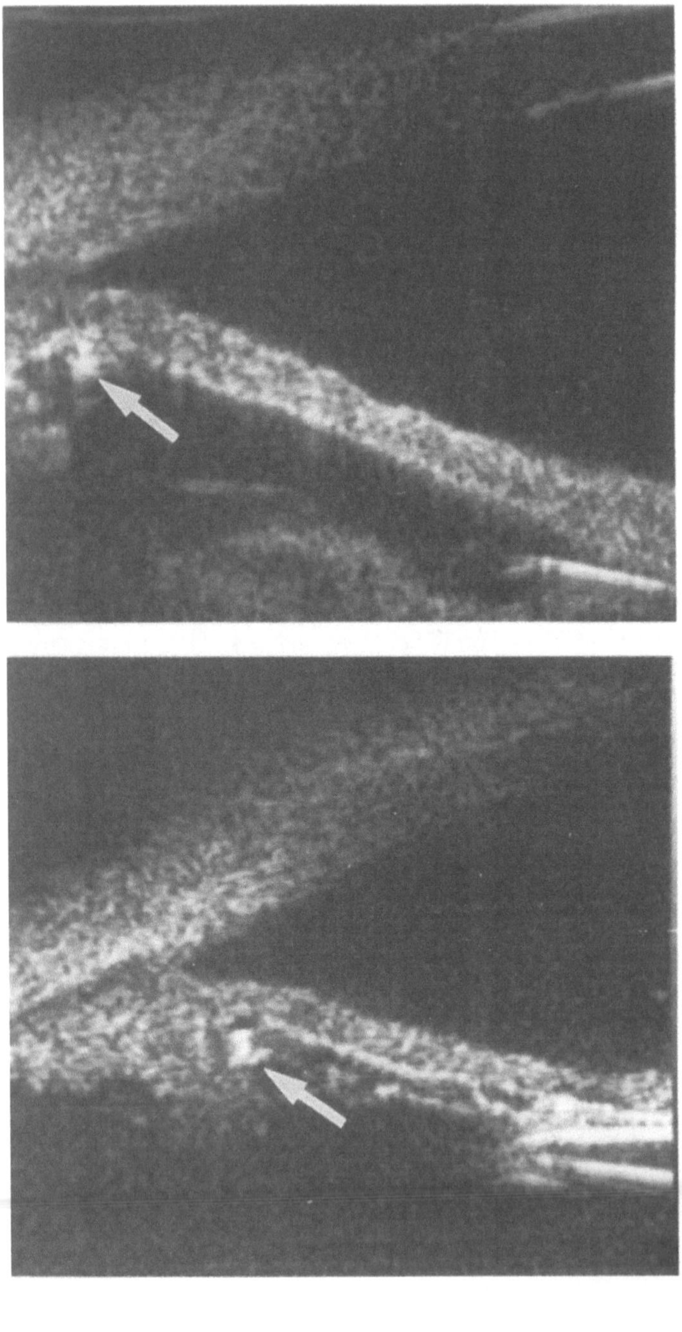

(a)

(b)

FIGURE 10.11. Haptics indenting the peripheral iris in two cases of recurrent hyphema. **(a)** The haptic (arrow) in case one is imaged indenting the peripheral iris. **(b)** The haptic (arrow) in case two is indenting the peripheral iris. There is a small break in the iris epithelium above the haptic. Reprinted with permission from reference [11].

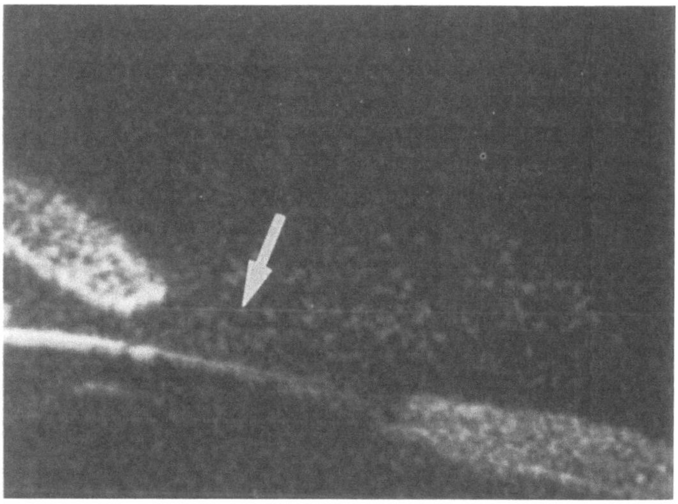

FIGURE 10.12. Blood is imaged in the anterior chamber extending under the iris (arrow). Reprinted with permission from reference [11].

mies close to the haptic position, and in both cases the iridectomies were partial thickness as indicated by residual iris pigment epithelium partially detached and extending under the iridectomy opening (Figure 10.13). Our findings support haptic-iris touch as being the etiology of this syndrome. Small vessels are likely formed at this site and chronically irritated by the presence of the haptic, resulting in recurrent bleeding.

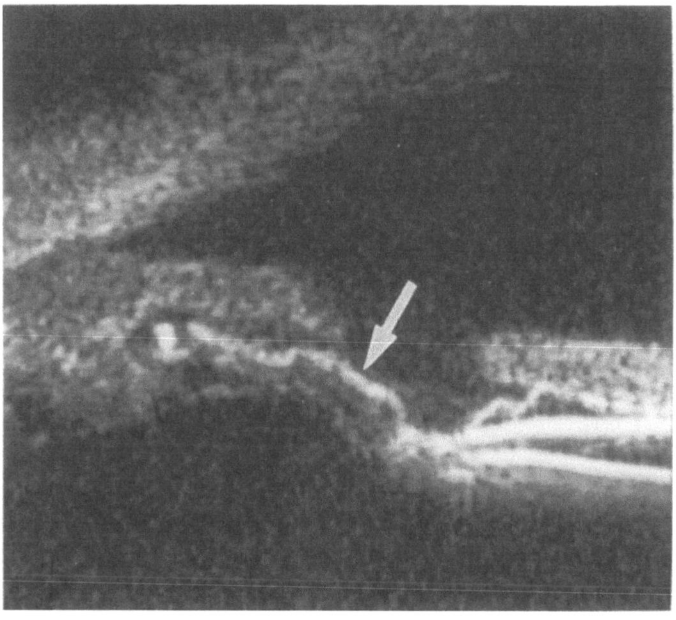

FIGURE 10.13. The iris epithelium is detached under the area of the iridectomy and is imperforate (arrow). Reprinted with permission from Reference [11].

Pupil Block

Iridectomies are not commonly performed with routine extracapsular cataract extraction with posterior lens implantation. An occasional patient will develop pupil block glaucoma. Clinically this presents as an iris bombé. Figure 10.14a shows the bowing forward of the iris in such a case, causing narrowing of the angle. The adhesion of the iris to the lens surface is well visualized in Figure 10.14b. There is a membrane present on the lens surface, most likely of inflammatory origin, which causes this adhesion. Another similar case is shown in Figure 10.15 with a wide iris adhesion to the lens margin.

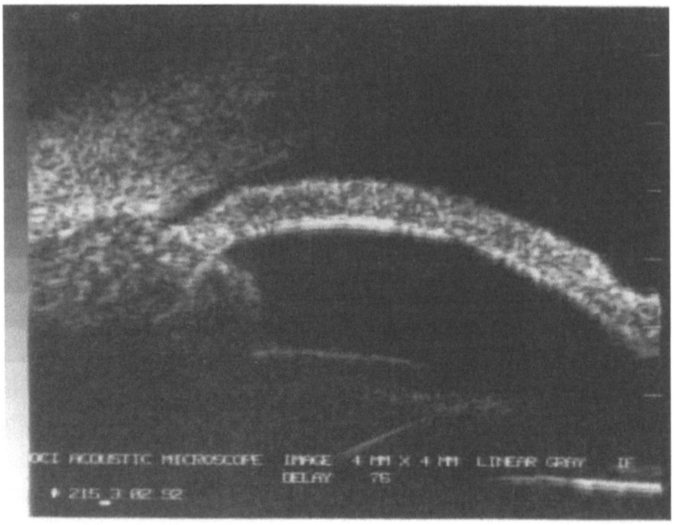

(a)

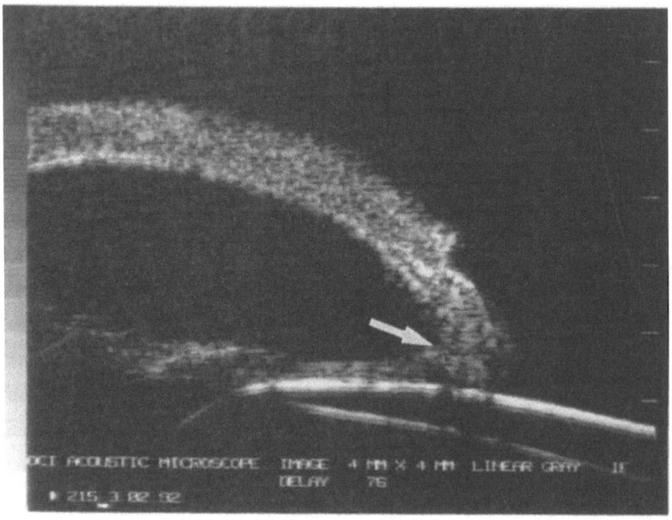

(b)

FIGURE 10.14. (**a**) Iris bombé in a case of pseudophakic pupil block. (**b**) The iris is adherent to a membrane on the surface of the lens (arrow).

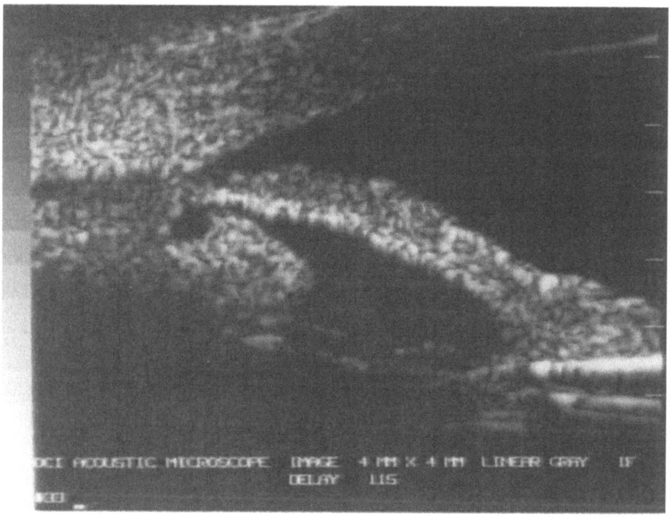

FIGURE 10.15. Pupil block with a wide iris adhesion to the lens margin.

Lens Dislocation

Lens dislocation was a relatively common problem with iris-fixated lenses. Figure 10.16a shows an eye with corneal edema. The anterior chamber could not be visualized. Ultrasound biomicroscopy shows the dislocated intraocular lens margin superiorly, lodged in the inner corneal surface (Figure 10.16b). This lens haptic was most likely the cause of the corneal decompensation. Lens dislocation is less common with posterior chamber lenses, but can occur if adequate capsular fixation is not present. Ultrasound biomicroscopy can aid in the analysis of these complications if the lens remains in the anterior part of the eye.

Wound Leak

Wound leak is less common with smaller incisions, but still occasionally occurs. Figure 10.17 shows the wound margin of an eye that had low pressure and a small filtering bleb. The gap in the wound is clearly imaged.

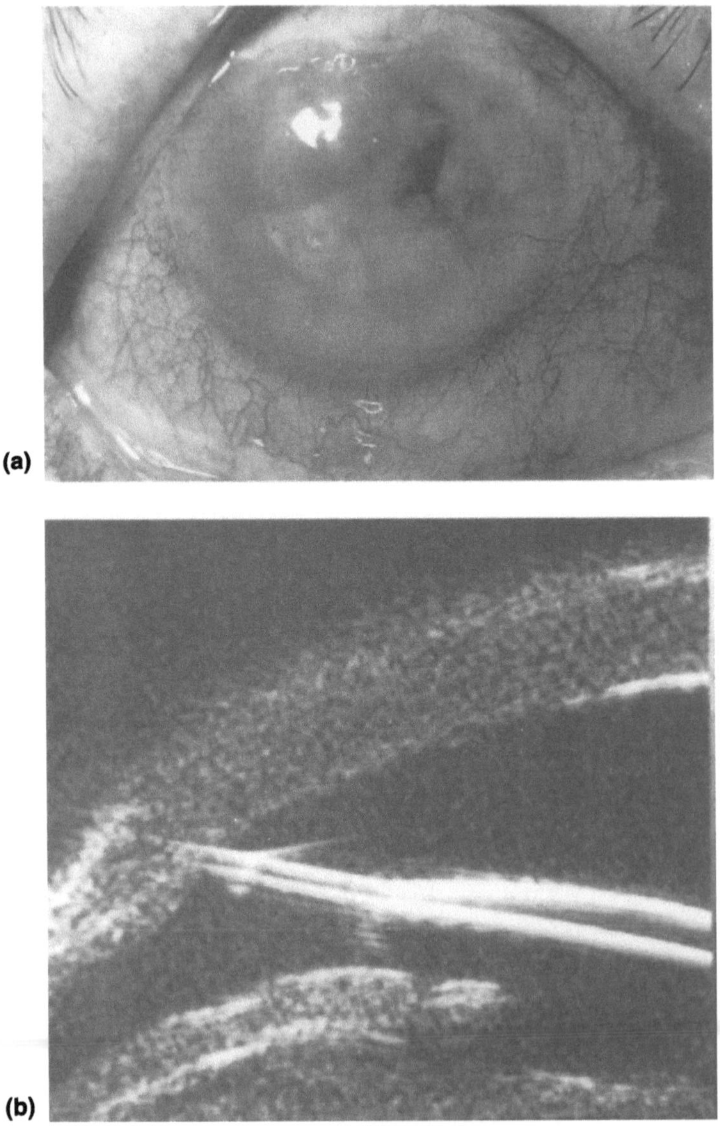

FIGURE 10.16. **(a)** Clinical photograph of a pseudophakic eye with corneal edema. **(b)** Ultrasound biomicroscopy shows the haptic of the iris-fixated lens is dislocated and lodged in the internal corneal surface (arrow).

FIGURE 10.17. Wound leak after cataract surgery. Ultrasound biomicroscopy shows the gap in the surgical incision at the site of leakage (arrow).

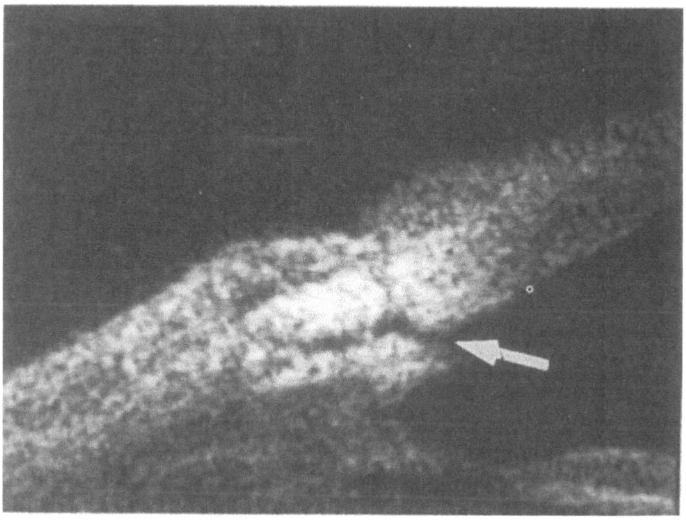

Summary

Intraocular lenses are easily outlined with ultrasound biomicroscopy because of the high reflectivity of the IOL material. Ultrasound biomicroscopy presents the unique ability to image and locate the position of haptics below the iris without the need for a pathological specimen. The relationships of haptics to surrounding structures can be determined. The surgeon can use this knowledge to monitor and refine surgical techniques. Ultrasound biomicroscopy also allows analysis of surgical complications and provides new insight into their etiology.

References

1. Pavlin CJ, Rootman D, Arshinoff S, Harasiewicz K, Foster FS. Determination of haptic position of transsclerally fixated posterior chamber intraocular lenses by ultrasound biomicroscopy. *J Cataract Refract Surg* 1993;19:573–577.
2. Stark WJ, Gottsch JD, Goodman DF, Goodman GL, et al. Posterior chamber intraocular lens implantation in the absence of capsular support. *Arch Ophthalmol* 1989;107:1078–1083.
3. Spigelman AV, Lindstrom RL, Nichols BD, Lindquist TD, et al. Implantation of a posterior chamber lens without capsular support during penetrating keratoplasty or as a secondary lens implant. *Ophthalmic Surg* 1988;19:396–398.
4. Cowden JW, Hu BV. A new surgical technique for posterior chamber lens fixation during penetrating keratoplasty in the absence of capsular or zonular support. *Cornea* 1988;7:231–235.
5. Hu BV, Shin DH, Gibbs KA, Hong YJ. Implantation of posterior chamber lens in the absence of capsular and zonular support. *Arch Ophthalmol* 1988;106:416–420.
6. Duffey RJ, Holland EJ, Agapitos PJ, Lindstrom RL. Anatomic study of transsclerally sutured intraocular lens implantation. *Am J Ophthalmol* 1989;108:300–309.
7. Swan KC. Hyphema due to wound neovascularization after cataract extraction. *Arch Ophthalmol* 1973;89:87–90.
8. Johnson SH, Kratz RP, Olson PF. Iris transillumination defect and microhyphema syndrome. *J Am Intraocul Implant Soc* 1984;10:425–428.
9. Khaw PT, Chisholm IH, Elkington AR, McGill JI. Iris pigment loss and hyphema secondary to anteriorly tucked posterior chamber intraocular lens loops [Letter]. *J Cataract Refract Surg* 1987;13:453–454.
10. Hakin K, Batterbury M, Hawksworth N, Khaw P, McGill J. Anterior tucking of the iris caused by posterior chamber lenses with polypropylene loops. *J Cataract Refract Surg* 1989;15:640–643.
11. Pavlin CJ, Harasiewicz K, Foster FS. Ultrasound biomicroscopic analysis of haptic position in late onset recurrent hyphema following posterior chamber lens implantation. *J Cataract Refract Surg* 1994;20:182–185.

11
Conjunctival and Adnexal Disease

Many adnexal structures are accessible to examination by ultrasound biomicroscopy. In general, any structure that can be approached over the surface can be examined. An eye cup of the same design used for examination of the globe can often be used. For example, an eyelid lesion can usually be examined by placing the eye cup on the surface of the lid, applying light pressure, and filling with 2.5% methyl cellulose. Viscous solutions such as 2.5% methyl cellulose are required during this type of examination to minimize fluid loss during examination. Occasionally a water bath constructed with a surgical drape may be required because of the irregularity of the surfaces being examined. A small amount of pressure from a cotton swab may be necessary to bring pathology into a position in which it can be examined. This is often true of lid margin tumors and lateral fornix tumors, where some lid eversion may be required. The keratinized epithelium of the skin causes significantly more attenuation than conjunctiva or cornea and limits the penetration over skin surfaces. The lower frequency range (50 MHz) is usually preferable for these conditions.

Conjunctival and Limbal Disease

Ultrasound biomicroscopy can be performed on all limbal disease, and at least part of most conjunctival disease. Conjunctival lesions involving the fornices are difficult to image for technical reasons. Ultrasound biomicroscopy can provide information on internal acoustic characteristics and depth of pathology.

Conjunctival Melanoma

Conjunctival melanoma can occur as a nodular mass or in a more diffuse form. Thickness of lesions can have a bearing on prognosis [1,2]. Figure 11.1a shows the clinical appearance of a localized conjunctival melanoma. Ultrasound biomicroscopy images the lesion as having a very uniform low-level reflectivity (Figure 11.1b). These lesions are generally composed of small cells in a very regular arrangement accounting for the relatively low reflectivity and lack of internal features. The depth of the lesion can be ascertained, and the relationship of the lesion to underlying sclera determined. Ultrasound biomicroscopy is important in differentiating this type of lesion from other causes of a pigmented lesion on the scleral surface, such as a scleral staphyloma or extrascleral extension of a choroidal or ciliary body tumor.

Conjunctival Lymphoma

Conjunctival lymphomas can occur as primary lesions, or can be associated with disease elsewhere in the body [3]. Conjunctival lymphoma is imaged as a low-reflective lesion, generally not involving the underlying sclera (Figure 11.2). Most lesions that are composed of a uniform distribution of small cells have a similar ultrasound appearance of low internal reflectivity, and a very regular structure. This is because of the uniform low backscatter from the small cells and the lack of internal structure that would vary the appearance.

FIGURE 11.1. (**a**) Clinical photograph of a conjunctival melanoma. (**b**) Ultrasound biomicroscopy shows a nodular, uniformly low-reflective lesion near the limbus.

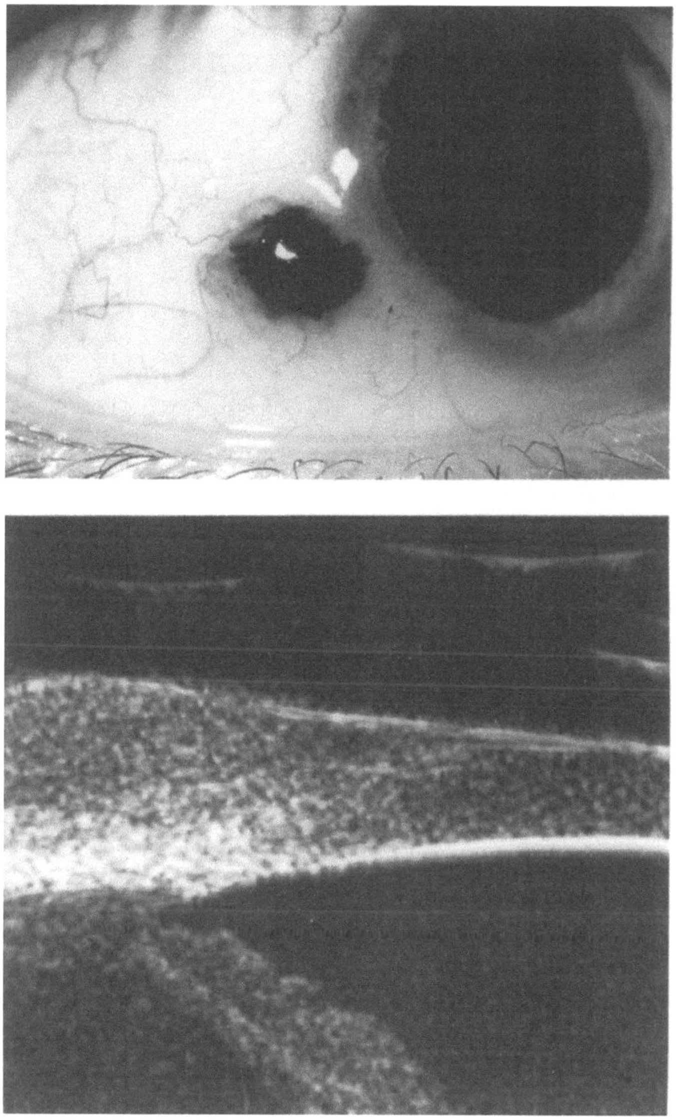

(a)

(b)

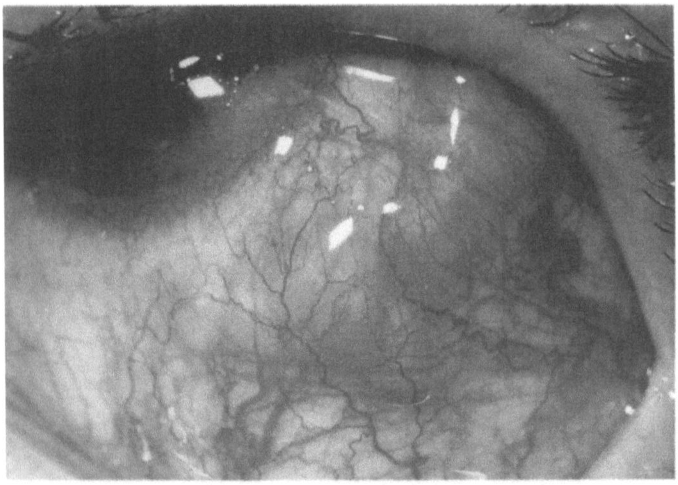

(a)

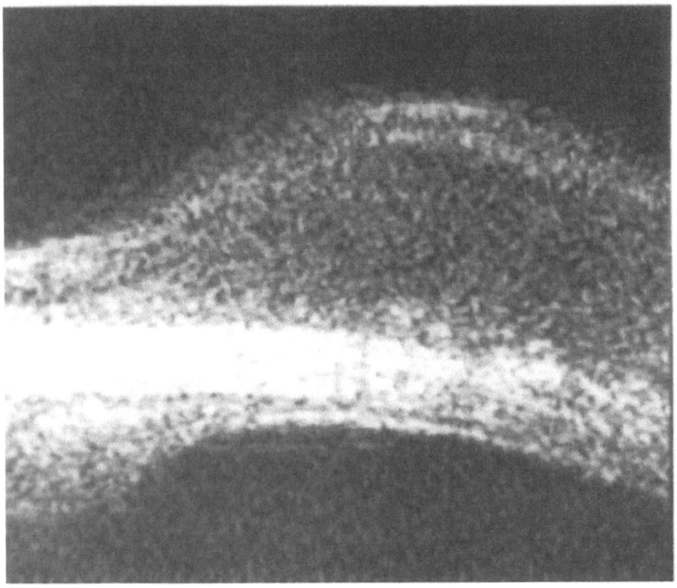

(b)

FIGURE 11.2. **(a)** Clinical photograph of a conjunctival lymphoma. **(b)** Ultrasound biomicroscopy shows a solid, elevated subconjunctival mass with low, uniform internal reflectivity. It does not involve the sclera.

Kaposi's Sarcoma

Kaposi's sarcoma can involve the conjunctiva, especially in people with AIDS [4]. Figure 11.3a shows the clinical appearance of a conjunctival lesion. The ultrasound biomicroscopic appearance is that of a discrete elevated lesion extending to the sclera, with a medium internal reflectivity with slight irregularity (Figure 11.3b).

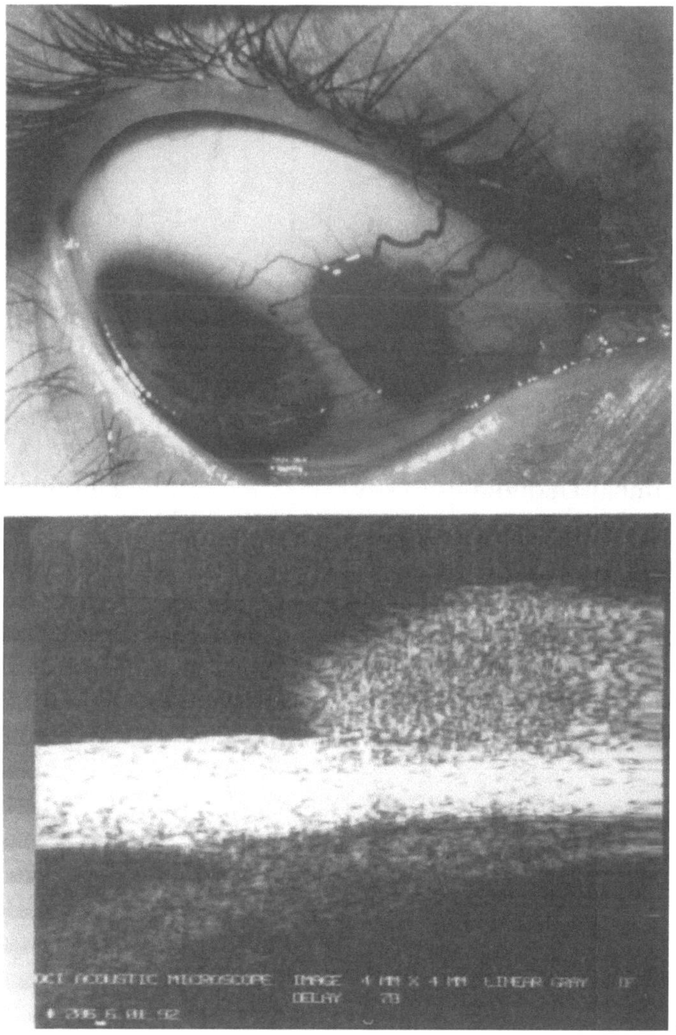

(a)

(b)

FIGURE 11.3. **(a)** Clinical photograph of a conjunctival Kaposi's sarcoma. **(b)** Ultrasound biomicroscopy shows a discrete, medium reflective, elevated lesion with slight internal irregularity.

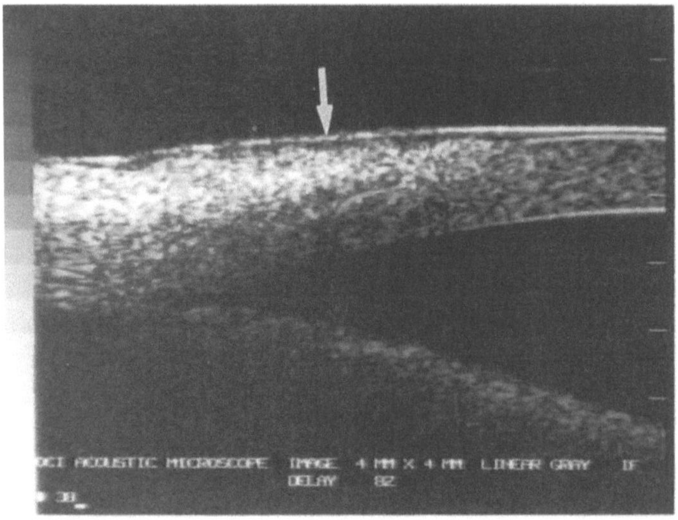

FIGURE 11.4. Ultrasound biomicroscopic image of a limbal dermoid (arrow) shows diffuse thickening and increased reflectivity involving the peripheral cornea and adjacent sclera.

Limbal Dermoid

Limbal dermoids are congenital lesions that produce opacification of the involved cornea [5]. A limbal dermoid is imaged by ultrasound biomicroscopy as a smooth diffuse thickening of the limbal region with a high reflectivity and involvement of the superficial layers of the cornea and sclera (Figure 11.4).

Pterygium

Pterygia are imaged as superficial limbal lesions extending over the cornea (Figure 11.5). The penetration level is usually just below Bowman's membrane. Internal reflectivity is relatively high.

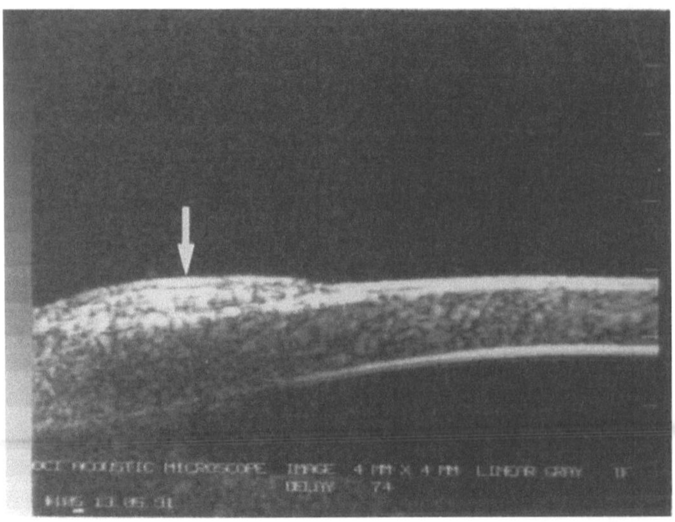

FIGURE 11.5. Ultrasound biomicroscopic image of a pterygium (arrow) shows high reflectivity and penetration to just below Bowman's membrane.

Chemosis

Chemosis can be a manifestation of local pathology or generalized edema. Ultrasound biomicroscopy shows elevated and thickened subconjunctival tissue. A fluid space is seen only occasionally (Figure 11.6). The appearance is similar to that of a filtering bleb.

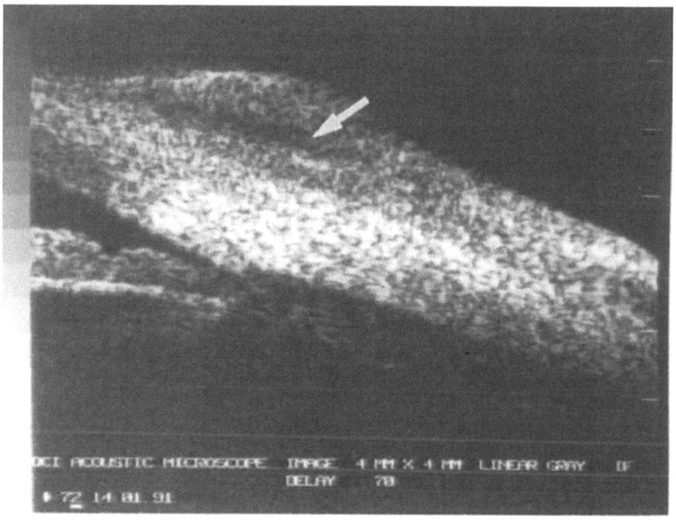

FIGURE 11.6. Chemosis of the conjunctiva shows thickened episcleral tissue with some evidence of low-reflective fluid accumulation (arrow).

Tumors in the Superotemporal Quadrant

Space-occupying lesions of the superotemporal conjunctival fornix can have similar clinical appearance. High-frequency ultrasound penetration of tumors of this size is limited, varying with the histological makeup and the resulting sound attenuation. Ultrasound biomicroscopy can image the superficial aspect of these lesions in depth and provide some diagnostic information that can be useful in differentiating them [6].

Fat Prolapse

Fat prolapse generally presents clinically as a mobile, yellow, smooth-surfaced mass that can create cosmetic problems [7]. Figure 11.7a shows the clinical appearance of a region of prolapsed orbital fat. Ultrasound biomicroscopic features include a smooth surface without a distinct capsule, and a regular, high internal reflectivity (Figure 11.7b). Penetration is usually good. The ultrasound biomicroscopic appearance is compatible with the histological findings of uniform fat cells.

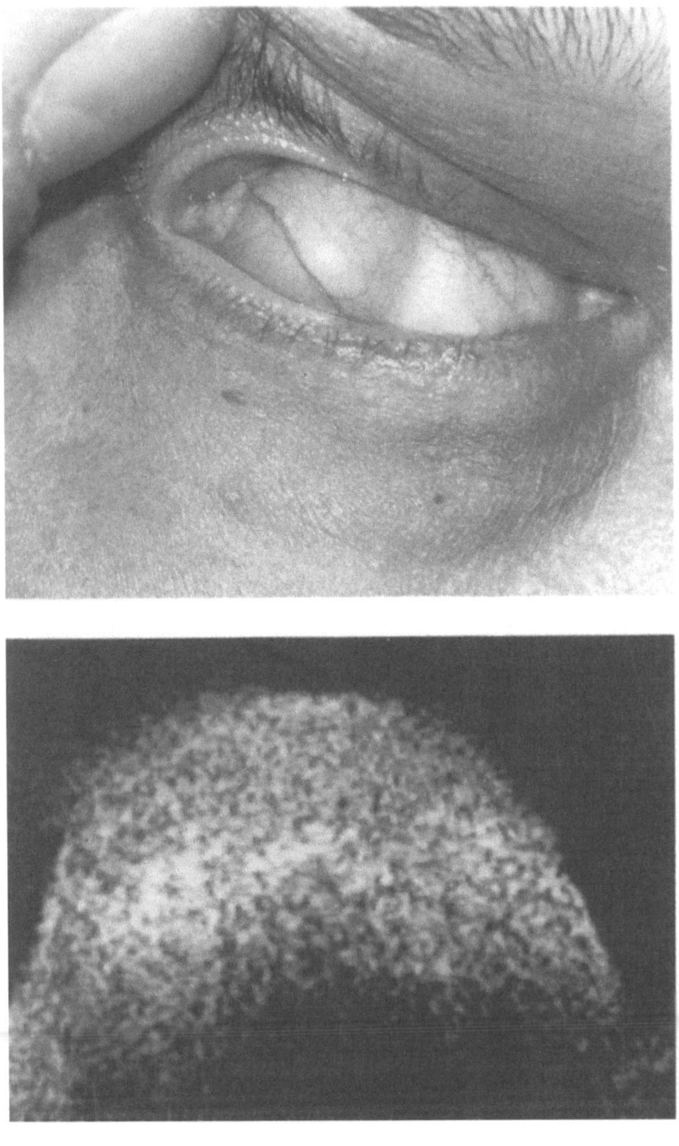

(a)

(b)

FIGURE 11.7. **(a)** Clinical photograph of orbital fat prolapsing into the palpebral aperture superiorly. **(b)** Ultrasound biomicroscopy shows absence of a distinct capsule and uniform high internal reflectivity. Published with permission from the journal *Orbit* [6].

Lipodermoid

Lipodermoids are congenital lesions usually presenting as nonmobile yellow-white lesions, occasionally bearing fine surface hairs [8,9]. Figure 11.8a shows a clinical photograph of such a lesion. Ultrasound biomicroscopic features include a dense, highly reflective capsule, variable internal reflectivity, and shallow penetration (Figure 11.8b). Ultrasound biomicroscopic appearance is compatible with the histological findings of keratinized squamous epithelium covering these lesions and their dense content of fat admixed with collagen bundles.

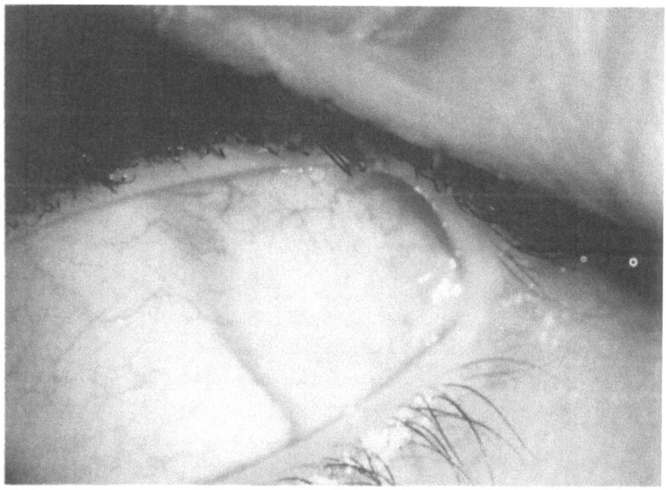
(a)

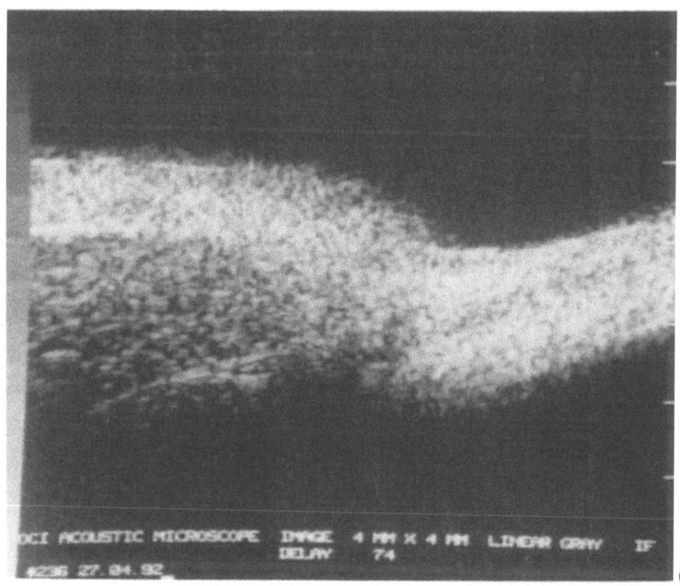

(b)

FIGURE 11.8. (**a**) Clinical photograph of a subconjunctival lipodermoid. (**b**) Ultrasound biomicroscopy shows a dense capsule and variable internal reflectivity. Published with permission from the journal *Orbit* [6].

Prolapsed Lacrimal Gland

Prolapsed lacrimal glands usually present as bluish lesions that do not transilluminate (Figure 11.9a). Ultrasound biomicroscopic features include absence of a distinct capsule, and multiple small cystic spaces (Figure 11.9b). Ultrasound biomicroscopic appearance is compatible with the histological findings of normal or mildly ectatic lacrimal gland ductules present in these lesions.

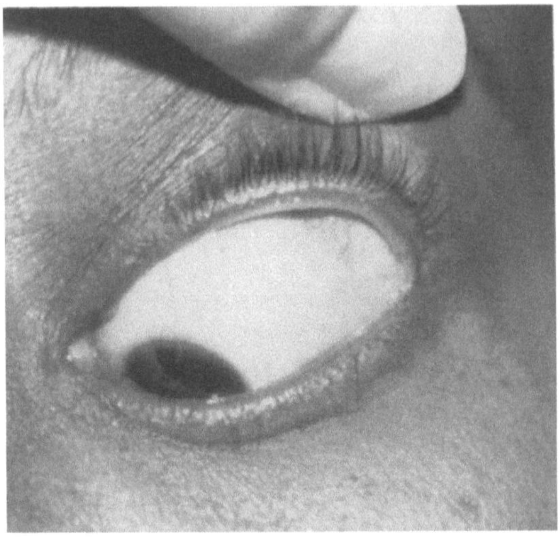

(a)

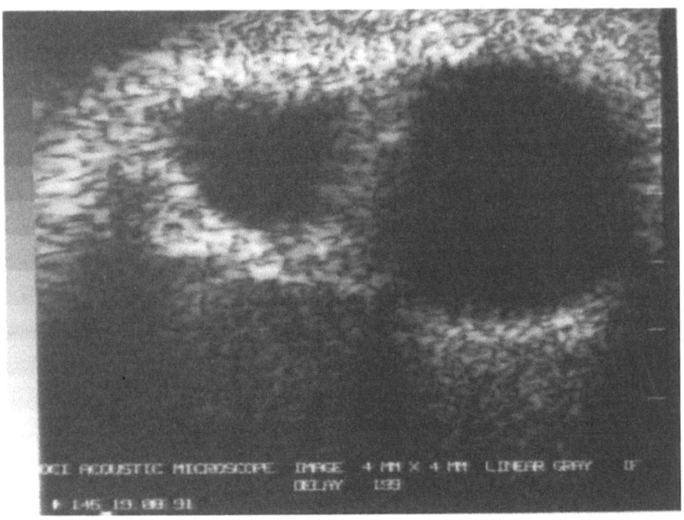

(b)

FIGURE 11.9. **(a)** Clinical photograph of a prolapsed lacrimal gland. **(b)** Ultrasound biomicroscopy shows no distinct capsule and multiple small cystic spaces. Published with permission from the journal *Orbit* [6].

Lacrimal Cysts

Lacrimal ductal cysts usually present as large bluish masses that transilluminate readily [10]. Figure 11.10a shows the clinical appearance of a lacrimal cyst. Ultrasound biomicroscopic features include a thin outer wall, and a single cystic mass acoustically hollow except for the presence of flecks floating in the cystic space (Figure 11.10b). Ultrasound biomicroscopic appearance is compatible with the histological findings of a single cyst with the floating secretory globoid bodies described by Stern et al. as pathognomonic of dacryops [11].

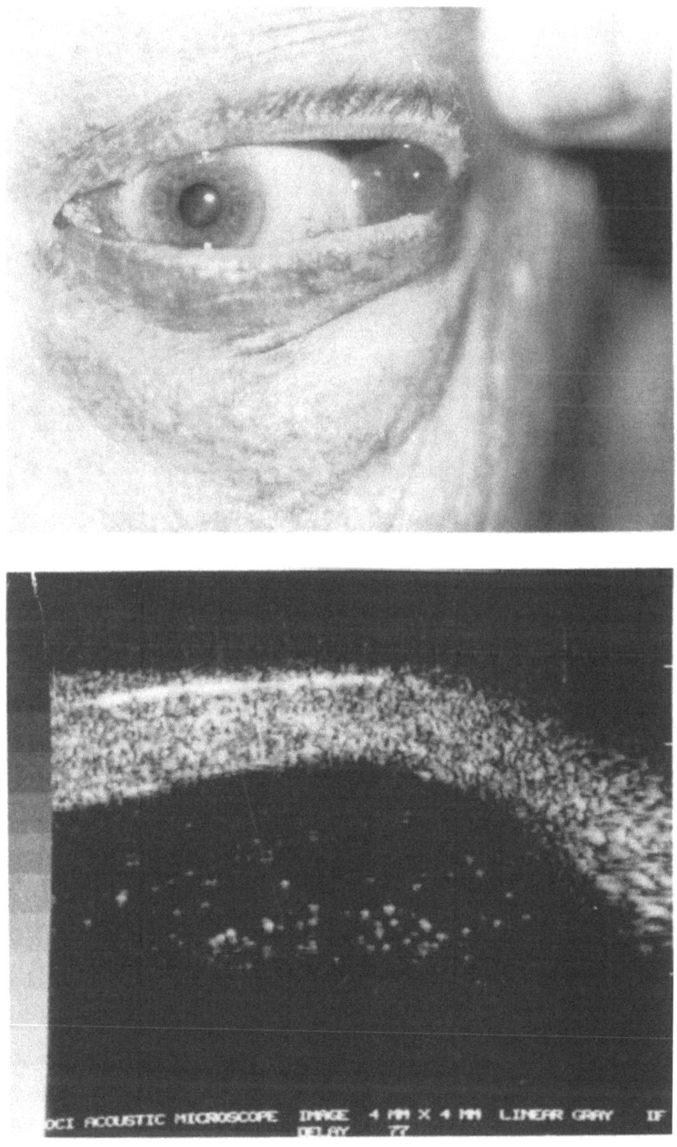

(a)

(b)

FIGURE 11.10. **(a)** Clinical photograph of a lacrimal gland duct cyst. **(b)** Ultrasound biomicroscopy shows a single, large, thin-walled cyst containing numerous particles. Published with permission from the journal *Orbit* [6].

Eyelid Disease

Eyelid Tumors

Lesions of the skin of the eyelid as well as lesions of skin elsewhere can be assessed by ultrasound biomicroscopy. If the lesion is too large, such as in larger melanocytic lesions, penetration may not be adequate to measure the lesion at higher frequencies. Figure 11.11a shows a melanocytic lesion of the lid margin. Ultrasound biomicroscopy shows a low-reflective lesion extending into the lid margin (Figure 11.11b). The depth of this lesion can be ascertained.

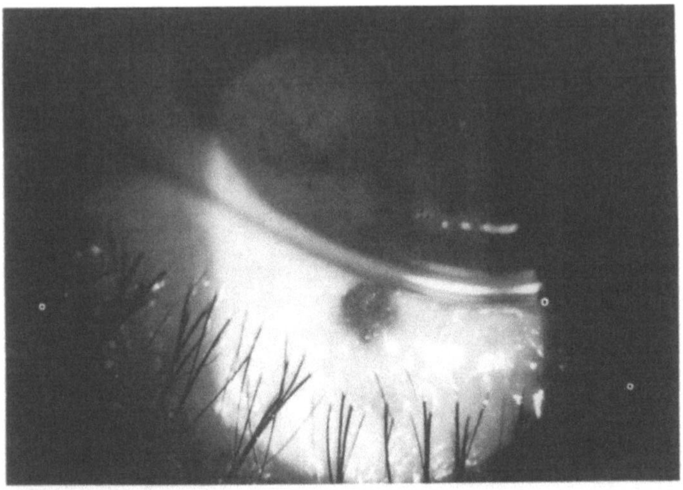

(a)

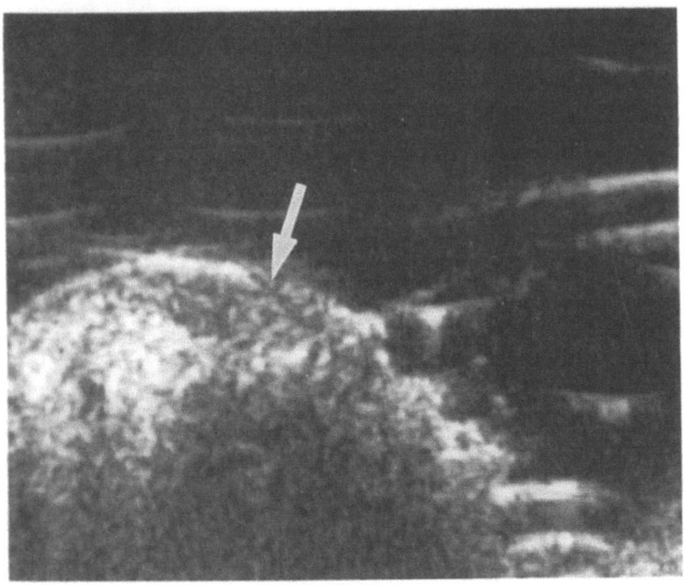

(b)

FIGURE 11.11. **(a)** Clinical photograph of a melanocytic lesion of the lid margin. **(b)** Ultrasound biomicroscopic image of this lesion shows a low-reflective lesion involving the lid margin (arrow).

Ptosis

The levator tendon can be consistently imaged by ultrasound biomicroscopy. In cross-sectional images of the upper lid it appears as a linear area of low reflectivity inserting into the anterior tarsal border. Figure 11.12a shows an ultrasound biomicroscopic image of a normal levator tendon. Certain types of ptosis have a defect or dehiscence of the levator tendon. Ultrasound biomicroscopy provides a method of determining the levator tendon status prior to surgery. Figure 11.12b shows the appearance of a cross section of an upper lid in the same orientation as Figure 11.12a in a patient with ptosis. The levator tendon is completely absent in this image. Lesser degrees of levator abnormality can also be imaged as irregularity of the tendon. The tendon can also have variable configuration as one scans through the lid.

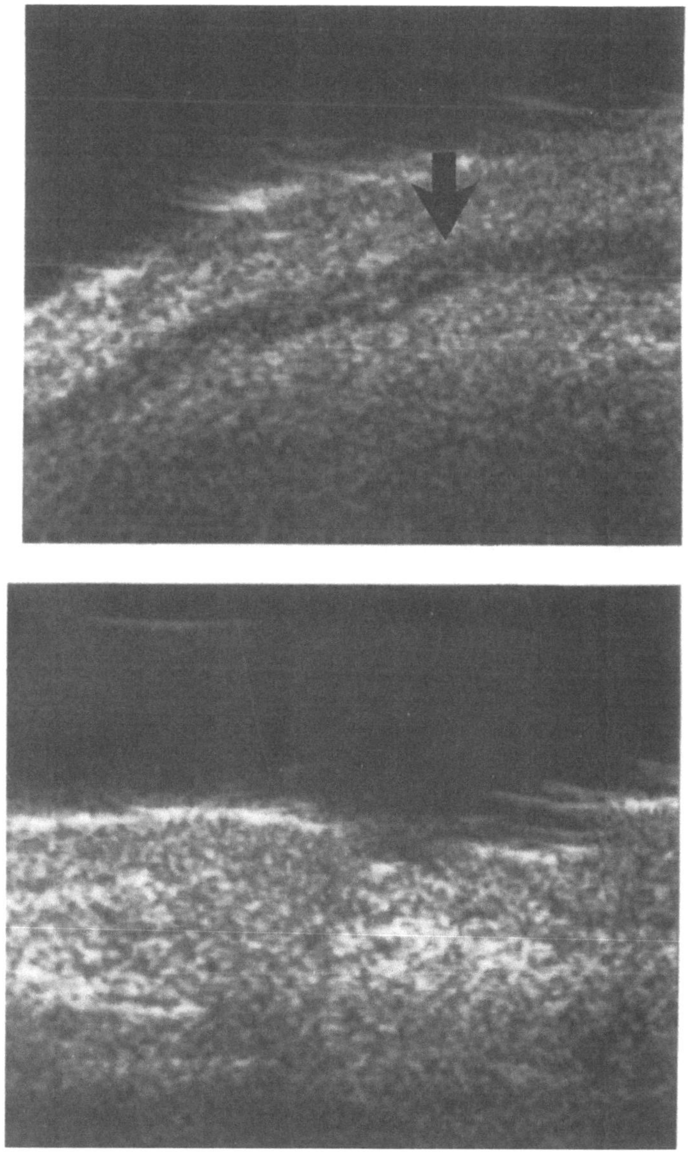

(a)

(b)

FIGURE 11.12. **(a)** Ultrasound biomicroscopic image of a cross section of a lid shows the levator tendon clearly outlined as a low-reflective line. **(b)** Ultrasound biomicroscopic image of a lid with levator disinsertion and ptosis does not image the levator tendon.

Summary

Conjunctival and limbal pathology is well imaged by ultrasound biomicroscopy. Information on internal structure and degree of involvement of underlying tissue can aid in the clinical assessment of these lesions. Examination of other adnexal structures by ultrasound biomicroscopy is somewhat limited by problems with penetration. Frequently, only the superficial region of adnexal masses can be examined. Keratinized epithelium is also a barrier to good sound penetration. Nevertheless, the high resolution of ultrasound biomicroscopy provides improved imaging of subsurface structures and can aid in differential diagnoses even if the entire tumor cannot be imaged.

References

1. Jeffery IJ, Lucas DR, McEwan C, Lee WR. Malignant melanoma of the conjunctiva. *Histopathology* 1986;10:363–378.
2. Jakobiec FA, Folberg R, Iwamota T. Clinicopathological features of premalignant and malignant lesions of the conjunctiva. *Ophthalmology* 1989; 96:147–166.
3. Knowles DM, Jakobiec FA, McNally L, Burke JS. Lymphoid hyperplasia and malignant lymphoma occurring in the ocular adnexa (orbit, conjunctiva, and eyelids): A prospective multiparametric analysis of 108 cases during 1977 to 1987. *Hum Pathol* 1990;21:959–973.
4. Panton RW, Sugar J. Excision of limbal dermoids. *Ophthalmic Surg* 1991;22:85–89.
5. Shuler JD, Holland GN, Miles SA, Miller BJ, Grossman I. Kaposi sarcoma of the conjunctiva and eyelids associated with the acquired immune deficiency syndrome. *Arch Ophthalmol* 1989;107:858–862.
6. Molgat YM, Pavlin CJ, Hurwitz JJ. Ultrasound biomicroscopy as a diagnostic tool in space-occupying lesions of the supero-temporal conjunctival fornix. *Orbit* 1993;12:121–126.
7. Glover AT, Grove AS. Subconjunctival orbital fat prolapse. *Ophthalmic Plast Reconstr Surg* 1987; 3:83–86.
8. Spencer WH. Congenital and developmental abnormalities. In: Spencer WH, ed. *Ophthalmic Pathology*. 1986; p. 123. WB Saunders, Philadelphia.
9. McNab AA, Wright JE, Caswell AG. Clinical features and surgical management of dermolipomas. *Aust NZ J Ophthalmol* 1990;18:159–162.
10. Smith S, Rootman J. Lacrimal duct cysts. Presentation and management. *Surv Ophthalmol* 1986;30: 245–250.
11. Stern K, Jakobiec FA, Harrison WG. Caruncular dacryops with extruded secretory globoid bodies. *Ophthalmology* 1983;90:1447–1451.

Index

A
Absorption
of acoustic wave energy, 6–7
and thermal damage, 25
defined, 7
Accuracy of measurements, 23–25
optimizing, 44–46
Acoustical impedance Z, 10
Acoustic streaming, and tissue damage, 25
Acoustic waves, fundamental properties of, 5–6
Age, and pigmentary glaucoma, 88
AIDS, conjunctival involvement in Kaposi's sarcoma, 199
Amplification, gain and, 44
Amplitude scan, 13
Anatomy, of the eye and adnexa, 47–60
Angle closure
cystic, 86–87
in inflammatory disease, 76
traumatic, 159
Angle closure glaucoma, 63–87
cysts causing, 127
Angle opening distance (AOD), 51
Angle region
open angle glaucoma, 88–93
recession in, due to trauma, 140, 141
ultrasound biomicroscopic anatomy of, 51–52
Anterior chamber
in plateau iris syndrome, 70
ultrasound biomicroscopic anatomy of, 50–51
Anterior segment
abnormalities due to trauma, 140
three-dimensional image of, 27–28
tumors of the, 98–139
Aphakic pupil block, 66–67
Art, ultrasound examination as, 40–41
A-scan signal, 17
historic development of, 20–21
Attenuation
of acoustic waves, 7–9
due to protective contact lens, 34–35
Attenuation coefficient, α´, 8
and penetration, 14
Axial resolution, 14–15, 18–19
versus measurement precision, 24–25
ultrasound biomicroscopy versus conventional ultrasound, 44

B
Backscatter coefficient μ_b
defined, 11
variation with frequency, 11–12
Backscattered radiofrequency spectra, for differentiating ocular masses, 7
Backscattering, effect on image, 11, 12–13
Bleb, filtering, 94–95, 201
Blood
scattering by red cells, 148
vitreous hemorrhage, 148–149
Blood vessels, ultrasound imaging of, 4
B-mode imaging
components of, 17
historic development of, 19, 21
Boundaries
of ciliary body tumors, 119, 120–121
of iris tumors, 106–108
Bowman's membrane
image of, 47, 155
loss of, in keratectomy, 163–165, 166
in pterygium, 200
Bruch's membrane, 60, 106
B-scan imaging systems, 5
orientation of, 38–39
Bullae, epithelial, 157

C
Calcification, corneal, 156, 157
Calipers, 46
Cataract surgery, and aphakic pupil block, 66
Cavitational streaming, and tissue damage, 25
Chemosis, 201
Choroid, 173
anterior, detachment of, in lymphoma, 139
ciliochoroidal effusion, 78–82
images of, 19–20
peripheral, ultrasound biomicroscopic anatomy of, 60
Choroidal tumors
anterior, defining the anterior margin, 128–132
differentiating from conjunctival melanoma, 196
peripheral, 127–135

Ciliary body, 52–53
  anterior rotation of, in angle closure glaucoma, 78
  attenuation coefficients for, as a function of frequency, 8
  backscatter coefficients for, as a function of frequency, 11–12
  in cyclodialysis due to trauma, 143–144
  defect in, with scleral thinning, 171
  disinsertion of, due to trauma, 143–144
  images of, historic development, 19
  speed of sound in, 9
  tear into, due to trauma, 140
  tumors of, 119–123
  ultrasound biomicroscopic anatomy of, 55–58
Ciliary processes, 55–56
  anterior rotation of, in phakic malignant glaucoma, 83–85
  and etiology of glaucoma, 63
  in plateau iris syndrome, 68–70
Ciliary sulcus
  depth of, 54
  location for placement of haptics, 186, 188
  in pupillary block, 68
  ultrasound biomicroscopic anatomy of, 52–53
Ciliochoroidal effusion, 78-82
Collagen, role of, in attenuating ultrasound energy, 8
Coloboma, ciliary, 170, 171
Complications
  in excimer laser keratectomy, 167–168
  of intraocular lenses, 186–188
Computers, imaging programs, 46
Congenital disorders
  limbal dermoid, 200
  lipodermoid, 203
  See also Hereditary disorders
Conjunctival disease, 196–199
Conjunctival flaps, and assessment of the cornea, 160
Contact lens, protective, in examination, 34–35
Control system, commercial scanner, 41–42
Conventions, for ultrasound biomicroscopy, 39–40
Cornea
  attenuation coefficients for, as a function of frequency, 8
  backscatter coefficients for, as a function of frequency, 11–12
  blood staining in, due to trauma, 150–151
  diseases of, 155–169
  edema of, 194
  images of, historic development, 19–20
  mapping of, after refractive surgery, 28
  precision of measurement of, 25
  reflection in, 10
  speed of sound in, 7, 9
  ultrasound biomicroscopic anatomy of, 47–49
Corneoscleral junction
  image plane through, 19–20
  ultrasound biomicroscopic anatomy of, 47–48, 51
Coupling medium, fluid, 31, 33
Crypts, iris, 53
Cyclodialysis, due to trauma, 142–44
Cycloplegia
  cyclodialysis after treatment with, 147
  supraciliary effusion in, 78, 80–81
  zonule and lens after, 58–59
Cysts
  anterior segment, 123–127
  clinical image of, historic development, 22
  at the iridociliary junction, 123–124
  iris, 86–87, 126, 153
  lacrimal, 205

D

Decibel, defined, 8
Delay, setting for, instruments, 43
Density, and acoustical impedance, 10
Depth of field (DOF), of a transducer, 14
Dermoid, limbal, 200
Descement's membrane, 47, 161
Development, future, of instrumentation, 28
Differential diagnosis
  in aphakic pupil block, 66
  choroidal tumors versus ciliary body tumors, 127–128
  ciliary body tumors versus anterior choroidal tumors, 132
  of conjunctival melanoma, 196
  hypotony versus cyclodialysis, 189
  iris tumor versus foreign bodies, 152
  iris versus ciliary body tumors, 119, 122
  iris versus iridociliary tumors, 106–107
  melanomas versus nevi, 112
  of scleral staphylomas, 170
Dilator muscle, 53
Doppler ultrasound, for mapping blood flow in ocular tissues, 28
Dystrophy
  corneal, 163–165
  granular, 164–165

E

Ectropion uvea, 53
Edema, corneal, 155, 156, 194
Effusion
  ciliochoroidal, 78–82
  supraciliary, 78–85
Elastic properties, and reflectivity, 9
Episcleritis, 170, 173
Epithelium, downgrowth of, due to trauma, 153
Examination, techniques for, 30–46
Extrascleral extension, of tumors, 170
Eye cups, for ultrasound examination, 31, 32
Eyelids
  diseases of, 206–207
  tumors of, 206

F

Fat, prolapse of, 202
Fixation device, 30
Fluid standoff, creation of, 31–34
f-number
  defined, 14
  and image quality, 23
  of a transducer, 18–19
Focal zone, setting, 43
Food and Drug Administration, standards for exposure to

high-frequency ultrasound, 25
Foot switch, 42
Foreign bodies, trauma due to, 152
Frequency
for clinical ultrasound imaging, 4
and scanner design, 17
for corneal assessment, 169
defined, 6
and image quality, 23
relationship to resolution, 47
relationship to resolution and penetration, 14
resonant, of a transducer, 18
Frequency domain techniques, 25
Frictional loss, component of attenuation, 7
Full width at half maximum amplitude (FWHM), 13–14
Fusiform lesion, iris, 110

G

Gain, 44
Gastrointestinal trace, ultrasound imaging of, 4
Glaucoma, 63–97
cyclodialysis as surgical procedure for, 140
from an iris melanoma, 113
late onset, with angle recession due to trauma, 140
pigmentary, posterior bowing in, 53
pupil block, 192–193
Globe
radial sections of, image, 40
transverse sections of, image, 40
Gonioscopy, for estimating an angle of opening, 51
phakic pupil block, 63–66
Graft, corneal, 161–162
Graft-host junction, corneal grafts, 161–162
Granulomatosis, Wegener's, 180

H

Haptics
position of, 182–183
reflectivity of, 182
Heat conduction loss, component of attenuation, 7
Hemorrhage, vitreous, 148–149
Hereditary disorders, cysts of the iris, 86–87.
See also Congenital disorders
Hyphema
corneal blood staining with, 150–151
due to posterior lens placement, 190–191
due to trauma, 148
Hypotony, in intraocular lens implantation, 189

I

Image (computer program), 46
Images
clinical, historic information, 21–22
historic information, 19–22
optimizing, 37–38
probe orientation versus screen appearance, 38–39
quality of, 23
Imaging
A-mode and B-mode, 12–13
applications to the body, 4
physics of, 3–15
pulse echo, 12–13, 15
real time systems, 5
transmission, 5
Impedance, discontinuities of, and imaging, 12–13
Infantile glaucoma, 63
Inflammatory disease, angle closure as a complication of, 76
Information, from sound, 3
Instrumentation, 17–28
Interference, constructive and destructive, from backscattering, 11
Intraocular lenses, 182–195
transcleral fixation, 55
Iridociliary junction, cysts at, 123–124
Iridocyclectomy
amelanotic iris lesion, 114
monitoring of, 123
Iridodialysis
after cycloplegia, 147
due to trauma, 140, 142
Iridoplasty, laser, 96
Iridotomy
change in curvature following, 64–65
and chronic angle closure, 72–75
concavity following, 88
laser, in cystic angle closure, 86–87
and hyphema, with intraocular lenses, 190–191
peripheral, in pigmentary dispersion syndrome, 90–91
in reverse pupil block, 88
and supraciliary effusion, 80
ultrasound biomicroscopic image of, 93
Iris
attenuation coefficients for, as a function of frequency, 8
backscatter coefficients for, as a function of frequency, 11–12
convex profile, in phakic pupil block, 63–66
in a corneal graft, 162
curvature of, defined, 64–65
cysts of, 126, 153
familial, 86–87
dilation of, and measurements of angle opening, 52
elevated, with lymphoma, 136–137
images of, historic development, 19
pinning to the trabecular meshwork, 186
in recurrent hyphema, 190–191
transillumination defects in, 88
tumors of, 98–119
ultrasound biomicroscopic anatomy of, 52–55
See also Plateau iris syndrome
Iris bombe, 192
Iris-lens contact (ILCD), zone of, 55
in angle closure glaucoma, 66
Iris-zonule distance (IZD), 59–60
in plateau iris syndrome, 70

K

Kaposi's sarcoma, conjunctival lesions in, 199
Keratectomy, excimer laser photokeratectomy, 163–164, 166–168
Keratopathy
bullous, 155
lipid, 158, 159
Kerato-precipitates, 136–137

L

Lacrimal cysts, 205
Lacrimal gland, prolapsed, 204
Laser, for keratectomy, 166
Lenses
  anterior chamber, 182, 183–184
    and pseudophakic pupil block, 68
  after cycloplegia, 58–59
  dislocated, 194
    and aphakic pupil block, 66
  intraocular, 182–195
  posterior chamber, 182–185
  removal of, in aphakic pupil block, 66
  See also Intraocular lenses
Lens extraction, plateau iris syndrome following, 72
Leukemia, hypopyon, anterior chamber, 138
Leukoma, adherent, 158
Levator tendon, 207
  imaging of, 60
Light pen, 42
Limbal dermoid, 200
Limbal disease, 196–199
Lipodermoid, 203
Lymphoma, 136–139
  conjunctival, 196, 198

M

Machine controls, positioning of, 30
Macintosh computer, 44
Malignant glaucoma, 83–85
  aphakic, 66
  phakic, following filtering surgery, 83
Measurement
  accuracy of, 23–25
  techniques for, 44–46
Mechanical damage, from high-frequency ultrasound measurement, 25
Mechanical motion, and measurement accuracy, 23
Melanomas
  anterior, 128–132
  ciliary body, 123
  conjunctival, 170, 196, 197
  iris, 110, 112
  mixed cell, 112–113
  posterior uveal, 98–139
  spindle cell, 114–115, 116–117
Methyl cellulose, for fluid coupling, 33, 196
Mice, 102–103
Modeling, thermal, 26
Moguls, 100–101
Molecular exchange of energy, component of attenuation, 7
Molteno implants, ultrasound biomicroscopic analysis of, 94–95
Monitoring
  of changes in iris tumors, 108–112
  of iridocyclectomy sites, 123
Monitor, positioning of, 30
Morphology, of iris nevi, 99–106

N

National Institutes of Health, Image program, 46
Nephropathy, IgA, supraciliary effusion in, 78–80
Nevi, iris, 98–111
Nuclear layers, imaging of, historic, 19, 21

O

Ocular adnexa, attenuation by, 60
Ocular tissues, acoustical properties of, at high frequencies, 6–12
Onscreen labeling, of estimate thermal and mechanical indices, 25
Opacification, corneal, 155–159
Open angle glaucoma, 88–93
Optical drive, for image storage, 44
Orientation, in anterior chamber examination, 50–51

P

Pars plana, ultrasound biomicroscopic anatomy of, 60
Patients
  positioning of, for examination, 35
  preparation of, for examination, 30–35
Penetration, and resolution, 13-15
Period, of a wave, 6
Phakic pupil block, 63–66
Phantom, for evaluating measurement accuracy, 23–25
Piezoelectric material, for a transducer, 17–18
Pigmentary dispersion syndrome, 88–93
Pigment epithelium, 60
Plaque therapy, radioactive, for peripheral choroidal tumors, 128
Plateau iris syndrome, 68–75
  laser iridoplasty in, 96
  and postmortem distortion, 63
Poly(methyl methacrylate) (PMMA), reflectivity of, 182
Polyvinylidene difluoride (PVDF), transducers of, 4–5, 17–18
Positioning, of the patient, 30
Posterior chamber, ultrasound biomicroscopic anatomy of, 59–60
Pressure wave, 6
  exponential loss of amplitude, 8
Probe, positioning of, 38
  and landmarks locating tumors, 121
Procedure, eye examination, 35–37
Proline lenses, reflectivity of, 182
Pseudophakic malignant glaucoma, anterior ciliary process rotation in, 85
Pseudophakic pupil block, 68, 192
Pterygium, 200
Ptosis, 207
Pulse duration, and image quality, 23
Pulse echo imaging, 12–13
  length of pulse, and axial resolution, 15
Pupil
  occlusion of, 151
  size of, 54
Pupil block
  anterior bowing in, 53
  in cyclodialysis due to trauma, 143, 145, 147
  in intraocular lens placement, 192
  reverse, posterior bowing in, 88, 92–93

R

Real time, image frame rates in, 13

Red blood cells, scattering by, 148
Reflection, of acoustic wave
energy, 6
Reflectivity
of choroidal melanomas, 132
of ciliary body tumors, 120
of haptics, 182
of the sclera, 49–50
of tissue, 9
Refraction, corrective surgery,
166–168
Resolution
axial, 18–19
and penetration, 13–15
Retina
changes in, in episcleritis, 173
detachment of, 60
images of, 19–20
peripheral, ultrasound
biomicroscopic anatomy of,
60
reflection in, 10
Rubeosis iridis, and angle closure,
76–77

S

Safety, of high-frequency
ultrasound, 25–28
Scan converter, 17
Scanners
commercial, 41–44
design of, 17
Scanning acoustic microscopy
(SAM), 5
Scarring, in excimer laser
keratectomy, 167–168
Scatter, of reflected waves, 6
Scattering, 7–8
from tissue, 10-12
Scatter number density, of tissues, 7
Scatter size, of tissues, 7
Scheimpflug technique, 64–65
Schlemm's canal, 88
Schwalbe's line, 47–48
Sclera
attenuation coefficients for, as a
function of frequency, 8
backscatter coefficients for, as a
function of frequency,
11–12
corneoscleral junction, 19–20
diseases of, 170–181
images of, historic development,
19
speed of sound in, 9
ultrasound biomicroscopic
anatomy of, 49–50
Scleral nodule, with an extrascleral
extension, 134–135
Scleral spur
as a landmark, 49–50, 51, 54
ultrasound biomicroscopic
anatomy of, 51
Scleritis
diffuse, 175
necrotizing, 178–180
nodular, 176–177
Screen, operating, 42–43
Settings, standardized, commercial
scanner, 43–44
Size, in pixels, of an image, 23
Skin, ultrasound imaging of, 4
Snell's law, 10
Soft tissues, speed of sound in, 9
SONAR (sound navigation and
ranging), 3
Spatial peak intensity, averaged
(SPA), 26
Spectrum, acoustic, 3–5
Specular component of reflected
waves, 6–7
defined, 9
geometry, 10
Speed of sound
in tissues, 7, 9
and accuracy of measurement,
23, 45
in water, 9
Sphincter muscle, iris, imaging
after pilocarpine
administration, 53
Staphyloma, scleral, 170, 171, 172,
196
Storage and retrieval, of images, 44
Superotemporal quadrant, 202–205
tumors of, 202–205
Suprachoroidal space, lymphoma
cells in, 139
Surface acoustic wave devices
(SAW), 5
Surface plaques, in iris nevi, 99,
109
Surgery
cyclodialysis following, 140
defining boundaries of ciliary
body tumors before,
120–121
for glaucoma, 93–96
refractive, 166–168
Synechiae
anterior, 76–77, 159
differentiating from traumatic
injury, 152

T

Techniques
measurement, 44–46
removing air bubbles, 33
Temporal width, of an ultrasound
pulse, 18–19
Three-dimensional studies, 27–28
Time-gain compensation (TGC), 17
Time gain control, 43
Tools, for measurement, 45–46
Toxicity, of ultrasound, estimates,
26–28
Trabecular-ciliary process distance
(TCPD), 54
average measurement, 56
in plateau iris syndrome, 70
Trabecular-iris angle, 52
Trabecular meshwork
as a landmark, 54
pigment in, 88
Trabeculectomy, ultrasound
biomicroscopy following,
94
Transducers, 17–22
higher frequency, for corneal
assessment, 169
polyvinylidene difluoride, 4–5
role in backscatter imaging,
12–13
Transfer functions (TF), 43
Transmission imaging, 5
Transmission scanning acoustic
microscopes, 5
Transscleral intraocular lens
fixation, 55
Trauma, 140–154
Tumors
anterior segment, 98–139
ciliary body, 119–123, 126, 196
extrascleral extension of, 170
eyelid, 206
iris
from a testicular primary
tumor, 136–137
differentiating from foreign-
body trauma, 152
local spread of, 118–19
peripheral choroidal, 127–35
small, following with ultrasound

Tumors (*cont.*)
superotemporal quadrant, 202–205

U

Ulceration, in episcleritis, 170, 173–174
Ultrasound biomicroscopy (UBM), defined, 5
Ultrasound interferometer, 7
Units, nepers/mm, for the attenuation coefficient, 8
Uvea, ectropion, 53

V

Video monitor, 17
Viscoelastic tissues, attenuation characteristics of, 8–9
Vitrectomy, in aphakic pupil block, 66, 85
Vitreous face, posterior bowing of, 66–67
Vitreous fibrils, in necrotizing scleritis, 180–181
Vitreous humor, reflection in, 10

W

Water bath approach, 21–22, 34
Water, speed of sound in, 9
Wave number, defined, 6
Wegener's granulomatosis, 180
Wound leak, in intraocular lens placement, 194–195

Y

Yag laser iridotomy, 63–65, 93

Z

Zonule
in pigmentary dispersion syndrome, 88
ultrasound biomicroscopic anatomy of, 58–59

MIX
Papier aus verantwortungsvollen Quellen
Paper from responsible sources
FSC® C105338

If you have any concerns about our products,
you can contact us on
ProductSafety@springernature.com

In case Publisher is established outside the EU,
the EU authorized representative is:
Springer Nature Customer Service Center GmbH
Europaplatz 3, 69115 Heidelberg, Germany

Printed by Libri Plureos GmbH
in Hamburg, Germany